EORTC Genitourinary Group
aph 2, Fritz H. Schroeder, Brian
, *Editors*. Published in two volumes:
'herapeutic Principles in Metastatic
Cancer. Part B: *Superficial Bladder*

Carcinoma of the Large Bowel and
rsors, John R.F. Ingall, Anthony J.
arino, *Editors*

Normal and Abnormal Bone Growth:
d Clinical Research, Andrew D.
ernard G. Sarnat, *Editors*

Detection and Treatment of Lipid
protein Disorders of Childhood, Kurt
, Herbert K. Naito, *Editors*

Bacterial Endotoxins: Structure,
cal Significance, and Detection With
lus Amebocyte Lysate Test, Jan W.
Harry R. Büller, Augueste Sturk, Jack
litors

The Interphotoreceptor Matrix in
nd Disease, C. David Bridges, *Editor*,
Adler, *Associate Editor*

Vol 191: **Experimental Approaches for the Study of Hemoglobin Switching,** George Stamatoyannopoulos, Arthur W. Nienhuis, *Editors*

Vol 192: **Endocoids,** Harbans Lal, Frank LaBella, John Lane, *Editors*

Vol 193: **Fetal Liver Transplantation,** Robe
Peter Gale, Jean-Louis Touraine, Guido Lucarelli, *Editors*

Vol 194: **Diseases of Complex Etiology in Small Populations: Ethnic Differences and Research Approaches,** Ranajit Chakraborty
Emőke J.E. Szathmary, *Editors*

Vol 195: **Cellular and Molecular Aspects o**
Aging: The Red Cell as a Model, John W. Eaton, Diane K. Konzen, James G. White, *Editors*

Vol 196: **Advances in Microscopy,** Ronald F
Cowden, Fredrick W. Harrison, *Editors*

Vol 197: **Cooperative Approaches to Resea**
and Development of Orphan Drugs, Melvi
Van Woert, Eunyong Chung, *Editors*

contact the publisher for information about previous titles in this series.

S McGarvey

PROGRESS IN CLINICAL AND BIOLOGICAL R

RECENT TITLES

Vol 163: **Prevention of Physical and Mental Congenital Defects**, Maurice Marois, *Editor*. Published in 3 volumes: Part A: *The Scope of the Problem.* Part B: *Epidemiology, Early Detection and Therapy, and Environmental Factors.* Part C: *Basic and Medical Science, Education, and Future Strategies*

Vol 164: **Information and Energy Transduction in Biological Membranes,** C. Liana Bolis, Ernst J.M. Helmreich, Hermann Passow, *Editors*

Vol 165: **The Red Cell: Sixth Ann Arbor Conference**, George J. Brewer, *Editor*

Vol 166: **Human Alkaline Phosphatases,** Torgny Stigbrand, William H. Fishman, *Editors*

Vol 167: **Ethopharmacological Aggression Research**, Klaus A. Miczek, Menno R. Kruk, Berend Olivier, *Editors*

Vol 168: **Epithelial Calcium and Phosphate Transport: Molecular and Cellular Aspects,** Felix Bronner, Meinrad Peterlik, *Editors*

Vol 169: **Biological Perspectives on Aggression,** Kevin J. Flannelly, Robert J. Blanchard, D. Caroline Blanchard, *Editors*

Vol 170: **Porphyrin Localization and Treatment of Tumors,** Daniel R. Doiron, Charles J. Gomer, *Editors*

Vol 171: **Developmental Mechanisms: Normal and Abnormal,** James W. Lash, Lauri Saxén, *Editors*

Vol 172: **Molecular Basis of Cancer,** Robert Rein, *Editor*. Published in 2 volumes: Part A: *Macromolecular Structure, Carcinogens, and Oncogenes.* Part B: *Macromolecular Recognition, Chemotherapy, and Immunology*

Vol 173: **Pepsinogens in Man: Clinical and Genetic Advances,** Johanna Kreuning, I. Michael Samloff, Jerome I. Rotter, Aldur Eriksson, *Editors*

Vol 174: **Enzy 2: Aldehyde Reductase, a** Geoffrey Flyr

Vol 175: **Adv Research,** A Robert C. Se

Vol 176: **Con** Manning J. C *Editors*

Vol 177: **Me Future,** Kå r

Vol 178: **Blu** T. Lynwood *Editors*

Vol 179: **Ta Clinical Per** Ahtee, Pirjo

Vol 180: **Int** Edward A. W.C. Bird,

Vol 181: **Ge Control an Sciences,** B R. Pleasant Morris Wag

Vol 182: **In Transfusio** Barker, *Edi*

Vol 183: **Al** Michael A.

Vol 184: **H** Eugene P. P. McCaffr *Editors*

Vc **M** Ri Pa *Pr Tu*

Vo **Its** Ma

Vo **Ba** Di

Vol **and** Wi

Vol **Bio the** ten Lev

Vol **Hea** Alic

Pleas

DISEASES OF COMPLEX ETIOLOGY IN SMALL POPULATIONS

ETHNIC DIFFERENCES AND RESEARCH APPROACHES

DISEASES OF COMPLEX ETIOLOGY IN SMALL POPULATIONS

ETHNIC DIFFERENCES AND RESEARCH APPROACHES

Proceedings of a Symposium on Genetic Epidemiology in an Anthropological Context
Held in Victoria, British Columbia, Canada
August 18 and 19, 1983

Editors

RANAJIT CHAKRABORTY
Center for Demographic and Population Genetics
University of Texas Graduate School
of Biomedical Sciences
Houston, Texas

EMŐKE J.E. SZATHMARY
Department of Anthropology
McMaster University
Hamilton, Ontario, Canada

ALAN R. LISS, INC • NEW YORK

Address all Inquiries to the Publisher
Alan R. Liss, Inc., 41 East 11th Street, New York, NY 10003

Printed in the United States of America

Library of Congress Cataloging in Publication Data

Symposium on Genetic Epidemiology in an Anthropological
Context (1983 : Victoria, B.C.)
Diseases of complex etiology in small populations.

Includes bibliographies and index.
1. Medical genetics—Congresses. 2. Genetic epidemiology—Congresses. 3. Ethnic groups—Diseases—Congresses. I. Chakraborty, Ranajit, 1946–
II. Szathmary, Emöke J. E. III. Title. [DNLM:
1. Anthropology—congresses. 2. Epidemiologic Methods—congresses. 3. Ethnic Groups—congresses. 4.Genetics, Population—congresses. W1 PR668E v. 194 /
QH 455 S9885d 1983]
RB155.s9376 1983 616′.042 85-15986
ISBN 0-8451-5044-8

Contents

Contributors

J. Adams, Division of Biological Sciences, University of Michigan, Ann Arbor, MI 48109 **[283]**

A. Basu, Human Adaptability Programme, Biological Sciences Division, Indian Statistical Institute, Calcutta 700 035, India **[345]**

J. Benoist, Laboratoire d'écologie humaine de l'Université de Droit, d'Economie et des Sciences d'Aix-Marseille, 13100 Aix-en-Provence, France **[227]**

P. Bharati, Human Adaptability Programme, Biological Sciences Division, Indian Statistical Institute, Calcutta 700 035, India **[345]**

E. Boerwinkle, Department of Human Genetics, University of Michigan, Ann Arbor, MI 48109 **[39]**

C. Bonaïti, Groupe de recherches de génétique épidémiologique, Institut national de la santé et de la recherche médicale, 75016 Paris, France **[227]**

D.G. Bonett, Department of Psychology, The University of Southern California, Los Angeles, CA 90089 **[67]**

S. Castillo, Departamento de Medicina, Facultad de Medicina, Universidad de Chile, Santiago 7, Chile **[325]**

R. Chakraborty, Center for Demographic and Population Genetics, University of Texas Graduate School of Biomedical Sciences, Houston, TX 77225 **[xi,3,21,105,247]**

L.P. Greksa, Department of Anthropology, Case Western Reserve University, Cleveland, OH 44106 **[255]**

R. Gupta, Human Adaptability Programme, Biological Sciences Division, Indian Statistical Institute, Calcutta 700 035, India **[345]**

J.D. Haas, Division of Nutritional Sciences, Cornell University, Ithaca, NY 14853 **[255]**

H. King, Royal Southern Memorial Hospital, Melbourne, Victoria 3162, Australia **[119]**

R.L. Kirk, Human Biology Department, John Curtin School of Medical Research, Canberra, A.C.T. 2601, Australia **[119]**

J.M. Lalouel, Laboratoire d'Anthropologie, Université de Paris VII, 75221 Paris, France **[97]**

G.M. Lathrop, Laboratoire d'Anthropologie, Université de Paris VII, 75221 Paris, France **[97]**

Ph. Lefèvre-Witier, C.N.R.S., Centre d'Hémotypologie, 31300 Toulouse, France **[367]**

F.M. Mayer, Centre de recherches caraïbes, Université de Montréal, Montréal, Québec H3C 3J7, Canada **[227]**

P.P. Moll, Department of Human Genetics, University of Michigan, Ann Arbor, MI 48109 **[39]**

The number in brackets is the opening page number of the contributor's article.

B. Mukhopadhyay, Human Adaptability Programme, Biological Sciences Division, Indian Statistical Institute, Calcutta 700 035, India **[345]**

C. Ritenbaugh, Department of Family and Community Medicine, School of Medicine, University of Arizona, Tucson, AZ 85721 **[67]**

D.F. Roberts, Department of Human Genetics, The University of Newcastle Upon Tyne, Newcastle Upon Tyne NE2 4AA, England **[9]**

F. Rothhammer, Departamento Biología Celular y Genética, Facultad de Medicina, Universidad de Chile, Santiago 7, Chile **[325]**

S.K. Roy, Human Adaptability Programme, Biological Sciences Division, Indian Statistical Institute, Calcutta 700 035, India **[345]**

F.M. Salzano, Departamento de Genética, Instituto de Biociências, UFRGS, 90000 Porto Alegre, Brazil **[301]**

W.J. Schull, Center for Demographic and Population Genetics, University of Texas Graduate School of Biomedical Sciences, Houston, TX 77225 **[325]**

S.W. Serjeantson, Human Biology Department, John Curtin School of Medical Research, Canberra, A.C.T. 2601, Australia **[119]**

C.F. Sing, Department of Human Genetics, University of Michigan, Ann Arbor, MI 48109 **[39]**

S.L. Smalley, Department of Anthropology, University of California, Los Angeles, CA 90024 **[67]**

P.E. Smouse, Department of Human Genetics, University of Michigan, Ann Arbor, MI 48109 **[283]**

E.J.E. Szathmary, Department of Anthropology, McMaster University, Hamilton, Ontario L8S 4L9, Canada **[xi,3,105,199,247]**

F. Vogel, Institut für Anthropologie und Humangenetik, University of Heidelberg, D-6900 Heidelberg, Federal Republic of Germany **[401]**

R.H. Ward, Department of Medical Genetics, University of British Columbia, Vancouver, British Columbia V6T 1W5, Canada **[147]**

K.M. Weiss, Center for Demographic and Population Genetics, University of Texas Graduate School of Biomedical Sciences, Houston, TX 77225 **[179]**

B.J. Williams, Department of Anthropology, University of California, Los Angeles, CA 90024 **[67]**

J.A. Woodward, Department of Psychology, University of California, Los Angeles, CA 90024 **[67]**

P. Zimmet, Royal Southern Memorial Hospital, Melbourne, Victoria 3162, Australia **[119]**

Preface

The papers in this volume were written for a symposium entitled "Genetic Epidemiology in an Anthropological Context." The symposium, held on August 18–19, 1983 in Victoria, British Columbia, Canada preceded the XI Congress of the International Union of Anthropological and Ethnological Sciences held in Vancouver.

The purpose of the symposium was to bring together two groups of scientists whose academic training and orientation differ, but who have common interests that focus on health and disease, including chronic diseases. One of these groups was field workers who have experience conducting biomedical research in population isolates, in migrant groups, and in small, rural, traditional communities in non-Western societies. The other group, smaller in number than the first, was theoreticians who have developed research strategies and methods of data analysis that have been widely used in genetic epidemiological investigations carried out in large, technologically sophisticated, and primarily "Western" societies. In our opinion, both groups of scientists have much to offer each other and much to learn from each other. The small sizes and complex interrelationships that characterize most population isolates, for example, require the development of research approaches that extract the maximum amount of information from small amounts of data. Statistical methods that require samples as "small" as 500, for example, to show significant differences may be useless applied to data gathered in a group whose total population size approximates 1600. Complex segregation analysis, an increasingly more common and very high profile research approach, is rarely employed by anthropologists, again because of the limitation imposed by the nature of the populations in which they work. On the other hand, statistically able geneticists may be more interested in turning their attention to the special problems of statistical resolution in small population research, if they learn that some of these groups possess attributes that make them uniquely suitable to test various etiological models that have been proposed for the onset of chronic diseases. Because research results obtained from analysis of data obtained in small societies sometimes question the conventional widsom concerning a particular causal model of disease, small populations can also serve to generate new and more appropriate hypotheses of causation.

The papers in this volume illustrate the range of research that is being done in different parts of the world on a variety of biomedical problems. We think they are interesting in their own right and serve as a good introduction to the kinds of issues that engage the attention of anthropologists and some genetic epidemiologists.

As is always the case we would not have been able to hold either the symposium or produce this volume without the assistance of individuals and institutions. For financial support to hold the symposium we are grateful to the Faculty of Social Sciences, McMaster University, Hamilton, Ontario, Canada. The XI Congress of IUAES organizing committeee was kind enough to provide logistic support for this symposium. For assistance with the production of this book we thank the Graduate School of Biomedical Sciences of the University of Texas at Houston and our publisher, Alan R. Liss, Inc. Ms. Sara A. Barton has earned our gratitude for her painstaking editorial assistance. The printing format and special symbols were produced by software developed by Robert J. Schwartz for which we owe him appreciation. Lastly, we thank our participants for their contributions.

Ranajit Chakraborty
Houston, Texas

Emőke J.E. Szathmary
Hamilton, Ontario

SECTION I

COMMON DISEASES, THEIR RESEARCH DESIGNS, AND ANALYTICAL STRATEGIES

Diseases of Complex Etiology in Small Populations:
Ethnic Differences and Research Approaches, pages 3–8

SECTION I. INTRODUCTORY REMARKS

R. Chakraborty and E.J.E. Szathmary

Intervention in and prevention of chronic diseases depends heavily on detection of the underlying risk factors for such maladies. Past experience indicates that the methods used to delineate the etiology of chronic illnesses cannot rest solely on either epidemiologic or genetic principles. A hybrid discipline, 'genetic epidemiology', is most likely to produce tools for the study of the causal risk factors for common diseases of complex etiology. This section presents some ideas on research designs for this hybrid field. By highlighting these presentations, we do not mean to imply that we have covered the entire spectrum of underlying risk factors for all possible common, chronic illnesses. That is clearly not the case. The papers here focus primarily on research designs that are important and interesting from the perspectives of public health and the clinical sciences.

Roberts begins with a definition of "genetic epidemiology". Many think that the later rubric is just another name for 'statistical genetics', but Roberts shows that the field contains new concepts that are true hybrids between those of genetics and those of epidemiology. Roberts draws our attention to the distinctions among epidemiologic, clinical genetic, and formal population genetic approaches to understand the etiology of variation in the prevalences of anencephaly and multiple sclerosis in different parts of Newcastle Upon Tyne. Roberts' insights concerning the nature of genetic epidemiology can be best appreciated by comparing them with other judgments. Certainly the need for a merger of these two disciplines was first expressed and elaborated in a chapter called 'Genetics and Epidemiology' by Neel and Schull (1954). Many treatments of this subject have since been presented. Contrasting opinions on the scope of the field are evident from the descriptions in Neel et al. (1965), Morton and Chung (1978), Schull and Weiss (1980), Morton (1982), Neel (1984), King et al. (1983) and Motulsky (1984).

The familiality of some chronic illnesses suggests that genetic and/or common environmental factors are causally involved in the onset of these conditions. Chakraborty discusses some analytical methods used to discern whether the aggregation of a disease is truly familial or whether it is due to a random co-incidence of the condition in different members of a single family. Epidemiologists often use measures that are 'aggregate' in nature, contrasting observations on a group of individuals with expectations on this same set of individuals (e.g., Schlesselman, 1982). Geneticists, on the other hand, test the pattern of occurrence in families by contrasting the 'chance' hypothesis with a 'genetic' hypothesis (e.g., Elandt-Johnson, 1971) when segregation of disease traits in families is predicted under well-defined rules. In contrast, Chakraborty discusses the use of 'model-free' methods that relate the observation on each individual to its random (or genetic) expectation. The methods discussed depend heavily on a proper definition of expected risk for each individual, a definition that depends critically on how the age of each individual is reported. This problem, we might add, is not unique to model free methods; it affects any treatment that employs age-dependent penetrance probabilities. Competing tests of familiality for complex diseases that take into account the variable size and age structure among families and variable disease predisposition rates have also been presented by Swift et al. (1974) and Lynch et al. (1981).

Sing et al. open the discussion of a complex issue: the role that genetic heterogeneity plays in the identification of a discrete endpoint, the presence (or absence) of a chronic disease. They surmise that heterogeneity may be the etiologic consequence of a wide spectrum of genotype-environment interactions that are expressed as intervening phenotypes between genotypes and the ultimate disease endpoint. Sing et al. note that we use statistical methods to recognize genetic heterogeneity because we are unaware of the nature of the genes responsible for chronic diseases. The scope of these statistical studies has been limited in the past, for one major reason: While the 'genetic control of sensitivity to the environment' (Mather and Jinks, 1982), can be experimentally resolved in fungi, plants, insects, and mammals, similar studies are impossible in humans. With the increasing resolution provided by the molecular delineation of chronic diseases, the intervening gene-actions that make individuals disease-prone have begun to clarify. This allows the development of more realistic statistical models for the study of genetic heterogeneity and its underlying cause -- genotype-environment interaction (e.g., Maciejko et al., 1983).

Smalley at al. discuss an important analytical procedure for dealing with the quantitative genetics of correlated traits. The theory of co-inheritance of associated traits has a lengthy history in biometrical genetics (e.g., Hazel, 1943; Robinson et al., 1951; Nei, 1960), although its usage in the study of the genetics of chronic diseases is quite recent (e.g., Eaves and Gale, 1974; Martin and Eaves, 1977; Moll et al., 1978; Lange and Boehnke, 1983; Hanis et al., 1983). A preliminary analysis by Smalley et al. indicates that the association of glucose tolerance impairment and obesity in Pima Indians is not due to a set of common genes, but is rather due to non-familial environmental factors. It must be remembered, that such inferences may well be model-dependent when genetic, environmental, and regression sources of co-aggregation of traits are all simultaneously employed in family data analysis (Hanis et al., 1983). Nevertheless, a covariance structure analysis of associated traits should prove valuable (1) in establishing the utility of multivariate models that explicitly parameterize the sources of correlation among variables, (2) in identifing the sources of co-aggregation, (3) in tracking phenotypic changes in individuals during a lifetime, and (4) in establishing directions for a more thorough understanding of the risk factors of common diseases of complex etiology.

Lathrop and Lalouel describe the efficiency of multi-point linkage analysis, relative to that of traditional two-point linkage studies. Linkage analysis enriches our understanding of the structural organization of disease-susceptibility genes along the chromosome, and has utility in predicting recurrence risks for genetic counseling purposes. More and more DNA polymorphisms that are associated with diseases of complex etiology are being reported. It is natural to enquire whether there is any gain in the efficiency of detecting gene carriers by employing the multi-point linkage techniques. The authors indicate that there are situations where multi-point linkage analysis provides more efficient estimates of recombination rates than available from pairwise linkage studies. A full description of the strategies of multi-point linkage analysis is also available in another recent paper by these authors (Lathrop et al., 1984).

In summary, these presentations cover a wide array of theoretical issues, ranging from a general over-view of some concepts of genetic epidemiology, to multi-point linkage analysis. Model-free methods of detecting familiality of complex diseases, genotype-environment interaction and heterogeneity of disease end-points, and co-aggregation of associated risk factors are matters of current debate and concern. While previous publications (e.g., Sing and Skolnick, 1979; Rao et al., 1984) cover some of these issues in oblique fashion, the presentations here are more direct. Hopefully, they will facilitate understanding of the scope and limitations of some current, large scale epidemiologic studies on chronic disease and should provide useful tools for the development of new ones.

LITERATURE CITED

Eaves LJ, Gale JS (1974). A method for analyzing the genetic basis of correlation. Behav Genet 4:253.

Elandt-Johnson RC (1971). "Probability Models and Statistical Methods in Genetics." New York: Wiley.

Hanis CL, Sing CF, Clarke WR, Schrott HG (1983). Multivariate models for human genetic analysis: Aggregation, coaggregation, and tracking of systolic blood pressure and weight. Amer J Hum Genet 35:1196.
Hazel LN (1943). The genetic basis for constructing selection indexes. Genetics 28:476.
King MC, Lee GM, Spinner NB, Thomson G, Wrensch MR (1984). Genetic epidemiolgy. Ann Rev Publ Hlth 5:1.
Lange K, Boehnke M (1983). Extensions to pedigree analysis. IV. Covariance component models for multivariate traits. Amer J Med Genet 14:513.
Lathrop GM, Lalouel JM, Julier C, Ott J (1984). Strategies for multilocus linkage analysis in humans. Proc Natl Acad Sci USA 81:3443.
Lynch HT, Fain PR, Golgar D, Albano WA, Mailliard JA, McKenna P (1981). Familial breast cancer and its recognition in an oncology clinic. Cancer 47:2730.
Maciejko JJ, Holmes DR, Kottke BA, Zinsmeister AR, Dinh DM, Mao SJT (1983). Apolipoprotein A-1 as a marker of angiographically assessed coronary-artery disease. New Eng J Med 309(7):385.
Martin NG, Eaves LJ (1977). The genetic analysis of covariance structure. Heredity 38:79.
Mather K, Jinks JL (1982). "Biometrical Genetics: The Study of Continuous Variation." London: Chapman and Hall.
Moll PP, Sing CF, Brewer GJ, Gilroy TE (1978). Multivariate analysis of the genetic effects on red blood cell glycolysis. In Brewer GJ (ed): "The Red Cell," New York: Alan R. Liss, p 385.
Morton NE (1982). "Outline of Genetic Epidemiology." Basel: Karger.
Morton NE, Chung CS (1978). "Genetic Epidemiology." New York: Academic Press.
Motulsky AG (1984). Genetic epidemiology. Genet Epidemiol 1:143.
Neel JV (1984). Editorial. Genet Epidemiol 1:5.
Neel JV, Shaw MW, Schull WJ (1965). "Genetics and the Epidemiology of Chronic Diseases." Washington DC: US Dept Hlth Education and Welfare.
Neel JV, Schull WJ (1954). "Human Heredity." Chicago: University of Chicago Press, p 283.
Nei M (1960). Studies on the application of biometrical genetics to plant breeding. Memoirs of the College of Agriculture. Kyoto University, No. 82.
Rao DC, Elston RC, Kuller LH, Feinleib M, Carter C,

Havlik R (1984). "Genetic Epidemiology of Coronary Heart Disease: Past, Present, and Future." New York: Alan R Liss.

Robinson HF, Comstock RE, Harvey PH (1951). Genotypic and phenotypic correlations in corn and their implications in selection. Agron Jour 43:283.

Schlesselman JJ (1982). "Case Control Studies." New York: Oxford University Press, p 171.

Schull WJ, Weiss KM (1980). Genetic epidemiology: Four strategies. Epidemiol Rev 2:1.

Sing CF, Skolnick M (1979). "Genetic Analysis of Common Diseases: Applications to Predictive Factors in Coronary Disease." New York: Alan R Liss.

Swift M, Cohen J, Pinkham R (1974). A maximum-likelihood method for estimating the disease predisposition of heterozygotes. Amer J Hum Genet 26:304.

Diseases of Complex Etiology in Small Populations:
Ethnic Differences and Research Approaches, pages 9–20

Chapter 1

A DEFINITION OF GENETIC EPIDEMIOLOGY

D.F. Roberts

Department of Human Genetics, University of Newcastle Upon Tyne, Newcastle Upon Tyne, England

INTRODUCTION

That the whole is different from the sum of its parts is well illustrated by genetic epidemiology. Genetics, of course, refers to what is inherited, what is transmitted biologically from parent to child, from generation to generation, and the mechanisms by which transmitted biological information is acted on. Epidemiology may be defined as the study of the distribution of disease in space and time, its object being to elucidate etiological factors. Space and time refer not only to locality but also to population, and subdivisions of populations. It is in its emphasis on population variations in incidence and occurrence that epidemiology is distinguished from clinical study. Epidemiological incidences and occurrences, frequencies, probabilities and similarly, are conceptual entities. Clinical investigation draws inferences from the facts that are observed in examination of individual patients or groups of patients by sight, touch, smell, sound and similarly. In epidemiology there is no attempt at experimental alteration of environmental factors to test hypotheses. In clinical studies, advances in management and treatment may be based on controlled trials in which there is experimental alteration of the internal environment of the body.

An integral element in epidemiology is the calculation of risk factors, referred to elsewhere in this discussion, which barely enter into clinical study though their application is increasingly important in patient management. They provide one illustration of the way in which an epidemiological approach is complemented by the genetic. Risk factors themselves are twofold. First, there are those deriving from background and environment, elucidated epidemiologically, that are relevant in the disease prognosis and treatment of a patient, and secondly there are those relating to the individual - his clinical history and his own inheritance, which one applies for example in the genetic counselling situation. They may be quite different. Epidemiologically, one can produce risk factors for Huntington's chorea, say, according to particular localities where the families with the disease may concentrate, where therefore the epidemiological risk, the chance for an individual taken at random from the population, will be greater than from an area where the disease does not occur. From the point of view of genetic risk, one may start with two members of a family, say two sibs, who have an affected parent. For each of them, the *a priori* risk is 50% that he will develop the disease some time in his life. But those risks otherwise may differ, particularly as the years pass. First they vary according to the presence or absence of particular restriction enzyme polymorphisms and other chromosome markers in the two subjects, established possibly presymptomatically, possibly prenatally. Secondly, the risks vary according to the age of onset in other members of the family, and also with the age of the individual himself. Such variation is taken into account in the genetic calculation of risk by Bayesian probabilities, and by observation of what is actually happening in each individual.

Epidemiology may be said to have been born with the work of Dr. William Farr who in 1839 was assigned responsibility for medical statistics in the office of the Registrar-General for England and Wales. As a result of his influence, the annual reports of that office over the following 40 years contained a remarkable series of essays on topics such as mortality in the metal mines of Cornwall, the distribution of cholera, the consequences of emigration, the effect of imprisonment on mortality, and these laid the foundations for later work in their establishment of fundamental ideas - the concept of the population at risk, the need to consider features other than disease in the groups concerned, the biases that may operate on the selection of subjects, ways of measuring excess risk, the concept of attributable risk.

In the early days of epidemiology, almost all the diseases known were essentially infectious, and it was in these and especially those that were associated with poor hygiene, that epidemiology had its main impact. One of the earliest and best-known examples was the work of Dr. John Snow, who identified the Broad Street pump as the source of an epidemic of cholera in the city of London in 1854. He did this simply by plotting the distribution of cases of cholera in the houses and factories in that neighborhood. He was able to show that it was only among the women or workers who went to this particular pump to get their water that cases of cholera developed, while among those who used other sources of water (wells in their gardens, for instance) there were no such cases. He went so far as to put a lock on the handle of the pump, and that was the end of that particular outbreak of cholera.

WHAT IS GENETIC EPIDEMIOLOGY?

What then is genetic epidemiology? One possible definition is the application of classic epidemiological methods to genetic disease, the quantitation of its incidence in a particular population or in segments of it. This of course is not of great help in a disorder that is totally inherited with negligible variation in penetrance or expressivity, but it may be of help in those disorders in which there is interaction between genotype and the developmental milieu. One example was the identification of environmental influence on neural tube defects by establishing their concentrations in the disadvantaged sections of the population, for example in lower socioeconomic classes (Carter and Evans, 1973), an effect recently elucidated as being mediated by a specific dietary deficiency. Figure 1 shows the concentration of anencephalics in the poorer

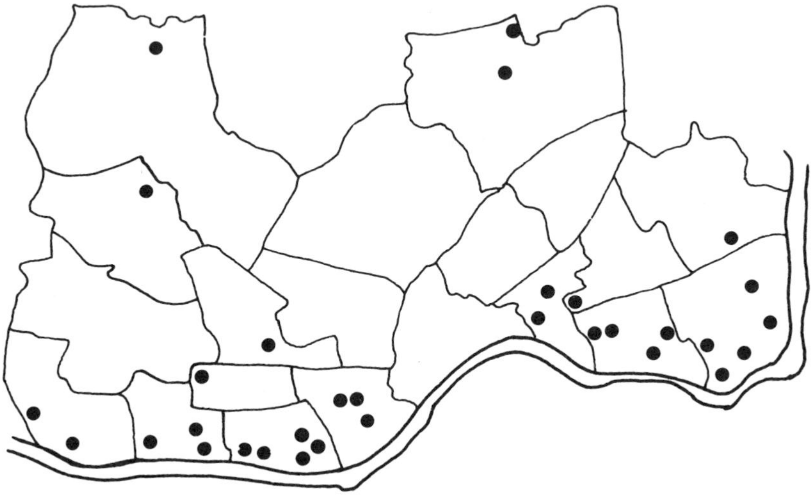

Figure 1. Anencephalus in Newcastle Upon Tyne, 1960-62.

quarters of Newcastle upon Tyne. As defined by Morton and Chung (1978) and Morton (1982), genetic epidemiology is concerned with etiology, distribution, and control of disease in relatives and with inherited disease in populations; but this definition is somewhat unspecific, for it would apply to clinical genetics generally, or indeed much of clinical work. MacMahon (1978) sees the key characteristic distinguishing genetics and epidemiology as the time at which the relevant species/environmental interaction took place. When investigating a particular feature of an individual, the geneticist seeks determinants which are now largely intrinsic to the species, the results of all the diverse environments that have existed since its origin, and transmitted to that individual by the mechanism of inheritance. The epidemiologist, on the other hand, seeks causes in events that have occurred and circumstances that have existed during the lifetime of the individual. Much of the literature that has appeared in the last few years in genetic epidemiology is concerned mainly with methods of analysis, and again here many of these are fundamental to work in clinical genetics.

In genetic epidemiology there is something more. To the equation of space/time/disease of classical epidemiology, a further group of variables is added, the concepts of genetic constitution and genetic structure of the population. Not only is one interested in comparison of disease incidence amongst genetically identifiable subdivisions of a population, but also in its distribution within the subpopulations in relation to the other genes and genotypes that occur there, that is to say, the genetic structure itself. The question to be asked is not "How does a particular disease vary in occurrence in space and time?" and so point to factors relevant to etiology. Instead, one asks "How do the differing frequencies of the disease between populations relate to their differences in genetic constitution? How does a particular disease vary in relation to the distribution of genes and genotypes within the population, that is to say with the genetic structure of that population?" The specific object is to elucidate the role of genetic factors in the etiology.

Its utility depends on the disease itself that is being investigated. Diseases may be envisaged as occurring in a spectrum. At one end of the spectrum are those disorders that are totally genetic, which occur no matter what environment an individual grows up in; that is to say, the role of genetic factors is absolute. At the other end of the spectrum, there are those disorders that are totally independent of the genetic constitution of the individual. There is little point in carrying out an epidemiological analysis of those disorders at the totally genetic end of the spectrum, for that would principally tell us where the individuals with the disorder live, where the families cluster, and so would really be an index of past migration and settlement, though examination of age distributions has delineated prognosis and helped with the attendant family, social and emotional problems for those that are progressive, e.g. Duchenne muscular dystrophy. The classical epidemiological approach has been particularly useful at the infectious end, the non-genetic end, of the spectrum. But the real contribution of genetic epidemiology comes in those disorders from the middle of the spectrum where it is not known how extensive is the genetic contribution to the etiology of the disorder.

GENETIC EPIDEMIOLOGY OF MULTIPLE SCLEROSIS

A series of studies of multiple sclerosis illustrates the utility of genetic epidemiology as here defined (Roberts, 1980; Roberts and Bates, 1982; Roberts et al., 1979, 1983). They were undertaken partly because there was no satisfactory explanation of its etiology, partly because one of the established methods of genetic epidemiology (examination of the association of a disease with a particular Mendelian polymorphic variant) had shown that one of the HLA antigens, HLA-B7, was present at increased frequency in patients with the disorder, and led to its inclusion amongst the group of disorders conceptualized as autoimmune diseases. Whereas such an association was reported in several populations, in multiple sclerosis patients in Newcastle there was no such excess of B7. We therefore decided to go to the localities with the world's highest incidence of multiple sclerosis, the islands north of Scotland - Orkney and Shetland. They are particularly useful for the type of investigation envisaged. First, each is a geographically well-defined area, vital records are accurate, there is a strong sense of identity of the population. There is, moreover, relative constancy of the population for although there has been a steady flow of emigrants from the islands, there has been very little in the way of immigration except in the last few years with the discovery of North Sea oil. The incidence figures from the four surveys of 1954, 1962, 1970 and 1974 show a rapid rise (Figure 2). Rises of this degree of steepness do not occur with simple genetic disorders, unless there has been an influx of an immigrant group bringing the genes for a disease into an established population (such as has occurred with thalassemia in England), and this clearly is not the case in Orkney and Shetland. Instead, it appears to be due to differential survival; that, as a result of modern chemotherapy, people with multiple sclerosis do not succumb to lethal infections and so survive longer, while new cases are developing at the same rate as in the past.

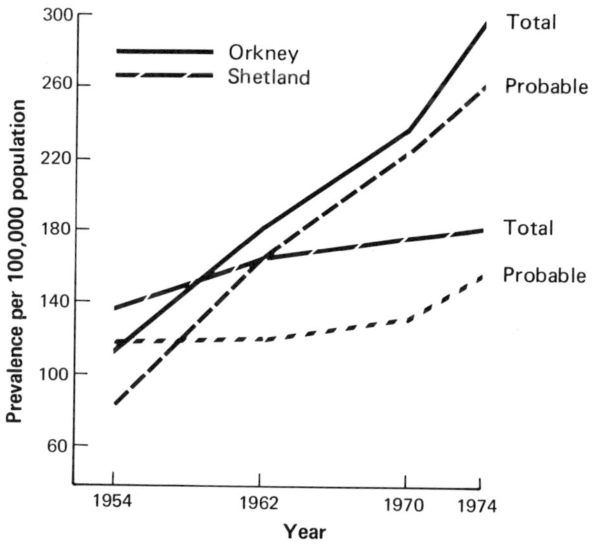

Figure 2. Change in prevalence of multiple sclerosis in Orkney and Shetland.

For every case of multiple sclerosis alive in Orkney on December 1, 1974, a contiguous control of the same sex was obtained who was born in the same parish in the same year and who had lived in that parish for the first 15 years of his life, and also a discontiguous control of the same sex, born in a discontiguous parish. By examining these two sets of controls it was possible to take into account the effect of local environment. From each patient and contiguous control a detailed family history was obtained. With multiple sclerosis there are reports in the literature of the disorder occurring in several members of the family. Some of these reports are unfortunately written by people inexperienced in clinical genetics, who regard as irrelevant (and therefore ignore), or are unaware of, the many unaffected members in the family. The patients' pedigrees in the islands proved to be remarkably empty of cases, no matter what mode of inheritance one envisaged as involving any major gene. The cases were then examined in relation to the genetic structure of the population. The Orkney measures of genetic structure were calculated on the basis of record searching of each case tracing the antecedents over a period of at least 200 years; that is to say to before 1776 for all cases, and indeed for many even before 1750. For each case and for each control, the inbreeding coefficient was calculated, because if a disorder has a recessive component then the distribution of the inbreeding coefficients will be displaced towards the right. Similarly, the kinship coefficients were calculated between all possible pairs of patients, between all possible pairs of controls, and between all patients and all controls, because if a disorder has an appreciable dominant or codominant or polygenic element in its etiology, the distribution of kinship coefficients among the affecteds would be expected to shift towards the right. Incidentally, Jorde et al. (1983) showed such a shift in the kinship coefficients among the patients with neural tube defects.

The results came as something of a surprise. First, 12% of the Orkney patients were inbred to some extent. There are no directly similar data with which this finding could be compared, but indirect evidence indicated that it was considerably higher than that expected for a population elsewhere in the British Isles. In the Republic of Ireland the first-cousin marriage rate amongst Catholics was 0.16%, and in Northern Ireland it was 0.06%. Parental consanguinity for inpatients in general hospitals in London was 0.84%, and in the provinces 0.79% (Bell, 1940; Masterson, 1973). However, the Orkney contiguous controls showed a very similar rate, 10.4%. Clearly the consanguinity of the patients' parents was a function of the population, not the disease. The mean inbreeding coefficients of patients and controls also were very similar. Kinship, too, was high amongst the patients, but it was no higher than in controls or between patients and controls.

A similar analysis was carried out in Shetland. Again, consanguinity was high, 16% in patients and 21%

in controls. Mean inbreeding coefficients were high, mean kinship was high, but there was very little difference between patients and controls. In neither population did any association with HLA-B7 appear.

These findings give information on several genetic hypotheses. In the consanguinity analysis the inbreeding is a phenomenon of the population as a whole, rather than of the patients. The lack of elevation of the number of inbred patients by comparison with the controls, or of any pronounced displacement of the distribution of the inbreeding coefficients, appears to argue against, though not eliminate conclusively, recessive involvement of rare genes. In the kinship analysis the similarity of the mean kinship coefficients and their distribution within patients, within contiguous and within discontiguous controls, and their similarity moreover to those between patients and controls, appears to eliminate involvement of genes of dominant or co-dominant effect recently introduced in the population. The kinship analysis does not eliminate involvement of such genes widely distributed, long established in the population, but of very low penetrance.

The family histories and inspection of pedigrees suggest that single locus inheritance of multiple sclerosis is unlikely. There is little evidence for dominance or codominance, such as is implied in recent discussions of a "gene" for multiple sclerosis linked to the histocompatibility complex. If such a gene exists its effects are grossly outweighed by environmental factors, and the kinship analysis indicates that it must have been introduced very early in the history of the population. While the consanguinity analysis does not totally exclude a hypothesis of recessive involvement of rare genes, the family analysis gives no support to this hypothesis, for if it were correct one would expect many more of the siblings of patients to be affected than appears to be the case. Again, however, if such genes recessive in effect exist they must be heavily obscured by environmental factors. Sex linkage also may be eliminated from the sex distribution of the disorder that is in the opposite direction to that required on this hypothesis. The pedigrees themselves appear much more compatible with the alternative, polygenic hypothesis.

On this hypothesis, heritabilities were calculated, by comparing the incidence of the disorder in relatives of the patients with the incidence in the controls and in the population at large. For Orkney these estimates range from 31 to 47%, depending on which comparisons are made, but slightly lower it seems than the remarkably consistent figures from other series (Roberts et al., 1979). For Shetland, pooling estimates from first, second and third-degree relatives gives a weighted heritability of 23%, rather lower than the Orkney estimates and considerably lower than those calculated from other studies. Particularly interesting was the comparison with the heritability of multiple sclerosis in the Newcastle region, about 52% (Roberts and Bates, 1982), for the studies leading to the estimates were carried out in the same way. These parallel studies in different localities indicate what genetic theory has always emphasized, that estimates of heritability only relate to a particular population in a particular environment at a particular time, so that heritability calculated in one population cannot be applied for the same disorder in some other population elsewhere. But the demonstration of these differences between populations is extremely important, for one practical application of any heritability estimate is in calculating the risk to relatives. From the theoretical point of view, however, the apparent gradient in heritabilities - to be interpreted with caution for the standard errors attaching to each estimate are high - may suggest a concentration of some exogenous factors in the etiology of multiple sclerosis at its northern end. The findings, moreover, do not preclude environmental components in the etiology, such as possible viral infection or diet. They explain the variability in the HLA association from one population to another, for on the multifactorial hypothesis, the association with each allele is merely one in the polygenic system, and so essentially contributes to the loading for susceptibility, rather than determines it. The reason why so many patients do not have HLA-B7 is that they have a sufficient loading of other contributing polygenes in the system, and the varying strength of the association with the histocompatibility loci in different surveys is explicable in terms of the differing importance of the polygenes at other loci.

There remains now to take the particular model proposed, a multifactorial model, and to examine the likelihood of its occurrence. Unfortunately, this cannot yet be done with the Orkney and Shetland data, because in the families there is an insufficient number of affected individuals for the models to be tested. But with the passage of time, one expects that further cases would occur, and the necessary additional data accumulate. Nevertheless, the studies as a whole, analyses of multiple sclerosis in total, relatively compact populations, applying modern methods of population genetics to etiological problems, show how much there is to be gained from defining genetic epidemiology, as here, for they have produced valuable results. They indicate that any genetic component that there may be in multiple sclerosis is not simple. Monogenic inheritance in any form appears unlikely, unless there is greatly reduced penetrance and gross environmental interference. The results are more compatible with a more complex etiology, in which the genetic contribution is polygenic. The heritability estimates, however, suggest that this is moderate to slight, particularly in the northernmost populations, by comparison with non-genetic elements in the etiology. The findings point to the possible existence of a gradient in relevant exogenous factors.

CONCLUSION

This study argues the distinction of genetic epidemiology from epidemiology in general. It is not merely the application of the central concept of epidemiology, the study of the distribution of disease in space and time, to genetic disease. Instead in genetic epidemiology the concept is extended to include the additional variables of the genetic structure of a population, with the object of elucidating the etiology of a disease in which there may be a genetic component. The studies carried out on multiple sclerosis show how useful that approach can be in indicating whereabouts in the genetic to environmental spectrum is located the disorder under investigation.

LITERATURE CITED

Bell J (1940). A determination of the consanguinity rate in the general hospital population of England and Wales. Ann Eugen, London 10:370.

Carter CO, Evans K (1973). Spina bifida and anencephalus in Greater London. J Med Genet 10: 209.

Jorde LB, Fineman RM, Martin RA (1983). Epidemiology and genetics of neural tube defects: an application of the Utah genealogical data base. Amer J Phys Anthrop 62:23.

MacMahon B (1978). Epidemiologic approaches to family resemblance. In Morton NE, Chung CS (eds): "Genetic Epidemiology," New York: Academic Press, p 3.

Masterson JC (1973). Cousin marriage in Ireland. In Roberts DF, Sunderland E (eds): "Genetic Variation in Britain," London: Taylor & Francis, p 59.

Morton NE (1982). "Outline of Genetic Epidemiology." Basel: Karger.

Morton NE, Chung CS (1978). "Genetic Epidemiology." New York: Academic Press.

Roberts DF (1980). Multiple sclerosis in the Orkney and Shetland Isles. In Clifford Rose F (ed): "Clinical Neuroepidemiology," Tunbridge Wells: Pitman, p 208.

Roberts DF, Bates D (1982). The genetic contribution to multiple sclerosis: evidence from North-East England. J Neurol Sci 54:287.

Roberts DF, Roberts MJ, Poskanzer DC (1979). Genetic analysis of multiple sclerosis in Orkney. J Epidemiol Commun Hlth 33:229.

Roberts DF, Roberts MJ, Poskanzer DC (1983). Genetic analysis of multiple sclerosis in Shetland. J Epidemiol Commun Hlth 37:281.

Diseases of Complex Etiology in Small Populations:
Ethnic Differences and Research Approaches, pages 21–37

Chapter 2

SOME ANALYTICAL EXPLORATIONS FOR DETECTING FAMILIAL AGGREGATION OF DISEASE TRAITS

R. Chakraborty

Center for Demographic and Population Genetics, University of Texas Graduate School of Biomedical Sciences, Houston, Texas

INTRODUCTION

A primary step in studying the etiology of a chronic disease is to detect excess risk of it in a sampled group of individuals. In genetic epidemiology, because the sampling unit is often a group of biologically related individuals, the object is to measure familial risk and to determine if it is in excess of the expected risk given the age, sex, and birth cohorts of the individuals. Since the early 1950's several statistical procedures have been described with the above objective in mind (e.g., Penrose, 1953; Williams et al., 1979; Chakraborty et al., 1980a; Hill, 1980; Thompson, 1980; Chakraborty et al., 1984). In these approaches the excess risks have been defined in various ways. For example, when excess risk is measured in terms of excess number of cases, detection of excess familial risk is done in most epidemiological studies by a chi-square statistic or various relative risk measures (e.g., Kleinbaum et al., 1982). Alternatives to this procedure involve definition of biological distances between affected members of a pedigree and to determine excess familial risk by showing that the affected individuals are biologically closer than the control normals (e.g., Williams et al., 1979; Chakraborty et al., 1980a; Hill, 1980; Thompson, 1980).

When excess risk of disease is manifested only by an unusual value of a risk variable, such as a lower age of onset, excess risk may not be detected by comparing the numbers of affecteds alone. With this possibility in mind, recently Chakraborty et al. (1984) suggested an alternative method to detect excess risk by relating the individual observations (e.g., disease status) with their own expectations (expected risk given the age, sex, birth-cohort, etc).

The purpose of this presentation is to examine various statistical properties relating to these alternative methods of detecting familial risks. In describing these properties, the main issue is to determine if any of these approaches adequately answer the following questions: (1) Is there evidence of increased risk of disease in members of a given sampled pedigree? (2) In a collection of sampled pedigrees, what is the minimum proportion of pedigrees at increased risk? (3) Among these pedigrees, which are most likely to reflect unusually high susceptibility?

In this context, the test based on the Genealogical Index (Williams et al., 1979; Hill, 1980) is also modified in this paper to make it applicable in situations where the study does not emerge from genealogy based data.

FAMILIAL RISKS OF GENETIC DISEASES AND ITS VARIABILITY IN DIFFERENT POPULATIONS

Before a comparison of the different methods of familial risks is made, it is important to establish that the extent of familial risk of a disease may vary widely in different populations. Hence, a comparison of the relative efficiency of one method over another by comparing their applications in two different populations may not be valid.

To illustrate this point, we may note that genetic as well as environmental factors play a complex role in the etiology of most common chronic diseases. Since environmental factors as well as gene frequencies at disease susceptibility loci vary within a population as well as between populations, estimation of the relative importance of genetic versus environmental factors should take into account variability among individuals at both intra- and inter-population levels. Simple familial risk ratios, relative risk (RR) or odds ratio (OR), the tools employed in epidemiological research, can thus be very different in different ethnic groups even if the disease is simply inherited in Mendelian fashion.

Following Penrose (1953), Chakraborty et al. (1980b) demonstrated this analytically by plotting PRR (P, the probability of a relative being affected given the proband is affected) and RR (R, relative risk defined as PRR as a ratio of the risk of the disease in the population at large) as functions of gene frequency of the disease for a few common pairs of relatives. The summary of their findings may be shown in the form of Figure 1 where the PRR and RR values are computed for the parent-offspring (o/p) and sib-sib (s/s) pairs for an autosomal dominant (d) and an autosomal recessive (r) disease. It is interesting to note that for an autosomal dominant disease, the conditional probability of an offspring or a sib being affected given that the proband is affected ($P_{o/p}{}^{d}$, or $P_{s/s}{}^{d}$) hardly changes over a wide range of disease frequency and this is also the case of a sib-sib contrast for an autosomal recessive disease $P_{s/s}{}^{r}$). The relative risk measures for both of these two contrasts (parent-offspring and sib-sib), on the other hand, are sensitive functions of the disease frequency for both dominant and recessive diseases. Thus a low relative risk value for a disease may in fact be due to high population-at-large risk of the disease, and may not be a reflection of non-genetic factors responsible for the disease. This phenomenon was noted by Penrose in 1953 although in the epidemiologic literature this fact is not commonly recognized (Lilienfeld, 1965).

We must note that the simple calculations above may not immediately apply to common diseases since they often involve sporadics and incomplete penetrance of genes even if the environmental factors are totally neglected. Majumder et al. (1983) showed that rejection of genetic involvement for a disease on the basis of low values of a single relative risk measure may be quite erroneous, particularly when sporadics and incomplete penetrance of genes are involved.

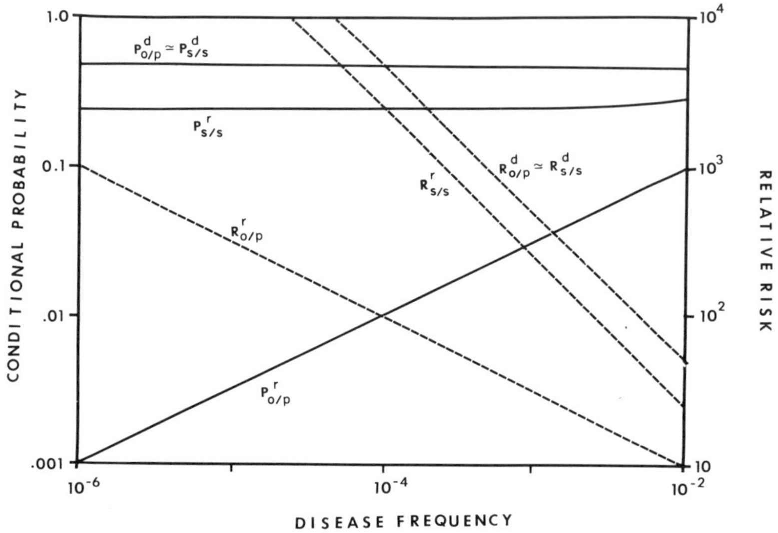

Figure 1. Conditional probabilities of a first degree relative (sib or offspring) to be affected given the disease status of the proband and relative risks (R) for simple Mendelian disorders as functions of the disease frequency in the population.

It is possible to conceive examples of genetic diseases for which familial aggregation may be rather weak, and often not detectable by a single summary measure which pools data from different families. To illustrate this let us consider the case of rheumatoid arthritis (RA) which has been reviewed recently by del Junco et al. (1984). They found that the frequency distribution of 17 relative risk values from the HLA-DR 4 versus RA studies conducted during 1977 - 1982 range from 2.5 to 12.2, with a weighted average of 4.5 with no significant heterogeneity. In contrast, there is considerable variability of 17 earlier reports of familial aggregation of RA for which the relative risk in first degree relatives ranges between 0.8 to 15.2 with significant heterogeneity. The significant heterogeneity of familial RR values, and their often insignificant (not different from 1.0) values cast doubt regarding genetic involvement in RA. However, these two sets of findings are not contradictory to each other.

Del Junco et al. (1984) reported data on 496 first degree relatives of 78 RA patients from which the familial RR is obtained as 1.7 (95% confidence limit 1.0 to 2.9). They concluded that this low and insignificant RR does not contradict with the high HLA DR-4 versus RA association (RR = 4.5). This may be shown by computing the distribution of familial RR of RA as a function of HLA-DR 4 antigen prevalence, as

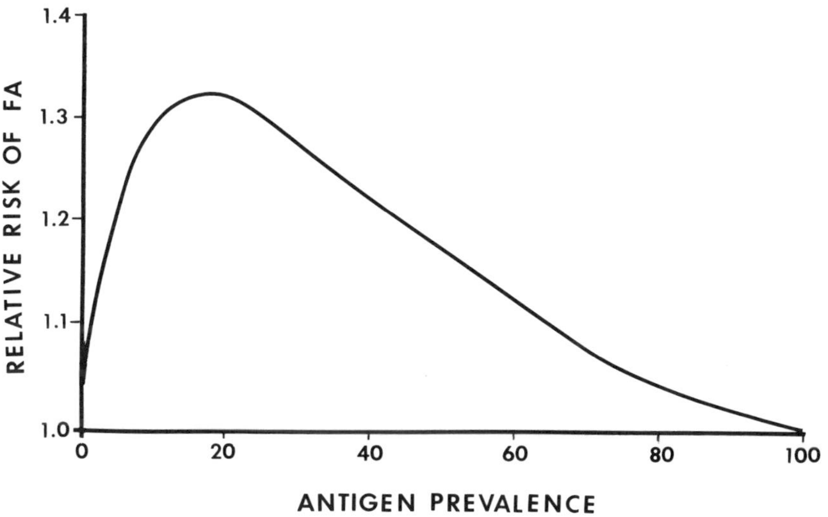

Figure 2. Relative risk (RR) of familial aggregation in the first degree relatives as function of antigen prevalence in the population for antigen relative risk equal to 4.5.

done in Chakraborty et al. (1980b). For example, let us consider the prevalence of HLA-DR 4 antigen among the RA patients (63% in the present example). With the association of HLA DR-4 and RA of 4.5 the expected relationship between the familial RR of RA in first degree relatives and the DR-4 antigen prevalence in the population is shown in Figure 2. Note that for the observed antigen prevalence of 28% the expected RR in first degree relatives is 1.32 which is not statistically different from 1.7 suggesting that the low familial aggregation of RA is in almost perfect agreement with the high HLA DR-4 and RA association. Of course, in this computation we make the assumption that the sole factor influencing the familial aggregation of RA is due to the Mendelian inheritance of the HLA DR-4 factor.

MODEL-FREE TEST PROCEDURES TO DETECT EXCESS RISK IN PEDIGREES

Geneticists, customarily, spend very little time in demonstrating familial aggregation before proceeding to identify the mode of causation of disease traits. Most commonly the involvement of non-genetic factors are ruled out in the process of segregation analysis by rejecting a sub-hypothesis of only sporadic occurrences of the disease. Since this is conducted by a likelihood ratio criterion, what is really inferred in this process is that the likelihood of observing the pattern of distribution of disease in the families examined under a specific genetic model is more in comparison with that under random occurrences of the disease. In this approach, thus, one does not answer the question: How often can we expect to find the observed distribution of the disease in a family of the given structure and size under a random occurrence hypothesis?

Two possible alternative test criteria may be considered to address this question in a model-free manner.

1. T-test Procedure:

Suppose that we have a family where the age, sex, and disease states of each individual are known.

Examples of kindreds are available in the study of cancer occurrences in a family collected through a unilaterally affected retinoblastoma patient (Strong et al., 1984). Let us assume that we have data on this pedigree and some others, each of different structure and size, from an underlying population for which we know the age, sex, and cohort specific incidence rates for the disease of interest. On each individual we record the sex, disease status and age at which the disease is contracted (age of onset) or if the individual is normal, the age at last observation. To each individual we can assign a value of an indicator variable X that takes value 0 if the individual is normal, and 1 if affected. We can then transform the observation on this family by a string of 0's and 1's counting all non-proband individuals of the family.

Let p_i be the probability that the i-th individual is affected (i.e., $X_i = 1$) given that he/she is a random member of the population. Each p_i is assumed to be known for a person in the population, specific for age, sex, and other relevant risk categories. Under the null hypothesis that the risk for an individual in uncorrelated with his/her relationship with the proband or any other individual in the data, is the vector $p = (p_1, p_2, \ldots, p_N)$, and its variance-covariance matrix is diagonal matrix with elements $p_i(1 - p_i)$, $i = 1, \ldots, N$. To test if the observed vector X differs significantly from its expectation, Chakraborty et al (1984) constructed the statistic T(X) where

$$T(X) = \sum_{i=1}^{N} \frac{(X_i - p_i)^2}{p_i(1 - p_i)} \qquad (1)$$

This test statistic takes value $T(x) = \sum_{i=1}^{N} (x_i - p_i)^2 / [p_i(1 - p_i)]$ with probability

$$\text{Pr. } (X = x) = \prod_{i=1}^{N} \text{Pr. } (X_i = x_i) \qquad (2)$$

from which the significance of the observed pattern of distribution of disease in the family may be judged (see Chakraborty et al., 1984 for details).

We have applied this test procedure to data on 80 families where our concern was to detect aggregation of cancers (of all sites) in family members related to 80 retinoblastoma patients (probands, one per family). The families were subdivided into 47 families with bilateral and familial and 33 with unilateral sporadic retinoblastoma affected probands. Of these families, 18 bilateral and 15 unilateral showed no other cancer cases by the time of observation. Since these are clearly uninformative as far as familial aggregation is concerned, they were excluded from evaluation of T(x) and its distribution. Of the remaining, 11 of 18 families obtained through a single unilateral retinoblastoma patient and 15 of 29 families gathered through a single bilateral retinoblastoma patient demonstrated significant T(x) values when the 5% level of significance was used. These figures clearly show that excess risk of cancers of all sites are exhibited in families ascertained through both unilateral and bilateral retinoblastoma families. While this analysis is consistent with the earlier findings of Strong et al. (1984), application of the T-statistic also enabled us to identify the specific families who are at high risk which did not always result in larger number of affecteds as compared to that expected by chance alone. The significant T values also emerged in families where the ages of onset were younger than those in nonsignificant families. Such findings would not have been seen in any aggregate test based on relative risk computations based on person-year at risk.

The advantage of the T statistic over the standard relative risk measures are also elaborated in Chakraborty et al. (1984). Briefly, when the expected risks, p_i's, differ from person to person, T may be regarded as more exact than the aggregate test. This occurs because T uses each specific p_i for the computation of the mean and variance of the indicator variables X_i's, whereas the aggregate test the variance of the number of cases (affecteds) is computed with average p for all individuals.

One caution should, however, be mentioned in the

application of T test procedure. This relates to the computation of expected probability of a disease in a given set of data. While in our previous application (Chakraborty et al., 1984) we computed the expected probability of cancer by cumulative incidence, this may not be the best measure of p_i for a single individual at his/her age of observation. This is so because retrospectively gathered family data involve competing causes of death and non-uniform distributions of individuals are withdrawn from observation. The effects of these sources of decrements on the expected cumulative incidence of disease are often not known. When risk must be assigned to individuals specifically at their observed ages, a precise measure of their expected risk may be the age-specific hazard rate rather than the cumulative incidence by that age. This does not essentially depend on other decrements, in particular on the age at which an individual was last observed. In the applications of the T statistic in cancer aggregation, this modification did not change our qualitative conclusions. However, in other applications this should be checked before applying the test procedure described above.

The construction of T suggests that deviation from the expected risk is detected in either direction. When p_i's are small (say, less than 0.5, which will be the case when hazard rates are used), existence of excess risk only elevates the value of T; a deviation in the other direction (deficiency of risk) makes T values smaller. On the contrary, if all p_i's are equal, for $p > 1/2$, the more excess the risk, the smaller the value of T becomes, because in this case for a given value of n and p ($>1/2$), T is a decreasing function of r, the total number of affecteds. So, if all individual risk probabilities, p_i's are larger than 0.5, instead of computing the upper tail area of the distribution of T, we need to evaluate the lower tail [Pr. $(T < T_*)$] probability of the T - distribution to construct the critical region of T. Of course, for almost all rare chronic diseases, we will be interested in the upper tail region of T. Should one wish to construct an analogous test criterion for a disease with moderately high p_i values, one possible alternative of T of equation (1) can be

$$t(X) = \sum_{i=1}^{N} \frac{(X_i - p_i)}{\sqrt{p_i(1 - p_i)}} \qquad (3)$$

whose distribution may be computed by the method as outlined in Chakraborty et al. (1984).

2. Genealogical Index Approach:

Williams et al. (1979) and Hill (1980), in connection with a study of cancer epidemiology in Utah Mormon genealogies, proposed a test for familial

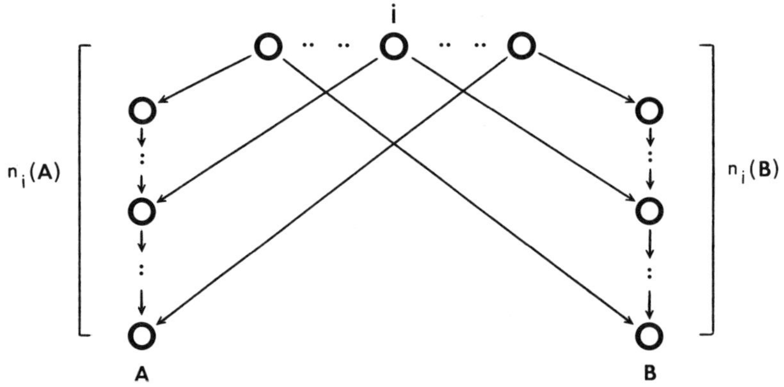

Figure 3. Genealogical index (GI) between two individuals A and B.

aggregation that compares the genetic relationships between affected members of a population with the expected relationships between two randomly chosen matched controls from the same population. In this approach, the Genealogical Index between two individuals is defined by Malecot's coefficient of kinship (Malecot, 1969). Specifically, if A and B are two individuals whose ancestral lines of descent can be represented as shown in Figure 3, the genealogical index of A and B can be written as

$$GI(A,B) = \sum_i (1/2)^{n_i(A) + n_i(B) + 1} \qquad (4)$$

The steps involved in GI computation in a population-based genealogical study constitute: (1) definition of cases individuals with the disease trait) and their matched controls (often multiples of them matched according to pre-selected criteria to remove sources of epidemiological bias), (2) listing of all known ancestors for each case and control, (3) searching for common ancestors of all pairs of cases and controls, (4) tabulation of the number of related pairs by specific degree of kinship (with the same GI values), and (5) comparison of the case-pairs and control-pairs with multiple selection of controls to attain stability of the distribution) with regard to the mean GI as well as with regard to its distribution wherever possible.

Current applications of the Genealogical Index (GI) suffer from a number of short-comings, some of which limit the potential use of this approach only to population-based genealogical studies. Some of these limitations are: (1) the scope of repeated sampling for selecting multiple controls may be limited where the disease is rare, or suitable controls are not available in the sample drawn from the same population, (2) the test procedure as described above depends critically on the choice of controls, (3) test of aggregation is done at the population level and no genealogy-specific test procedure is available with the above approach, (4) the dependence of the GI between two members of a genealogy on the total number of individuals in the genealogy is not taken into account explicitly, and (5) when more than one pair of cases occur in a pedigree, the GI values for each pair are not statistically independent, and no adjustment for such statistical dependence has been proposed.

To circumvent these limitations, let us imagine a situation where our object is to answer the following questions: (1) Given that a pedigree is sampled from a population of known age-sex specific risk schedule, is the GI between an affected pair (or the average GI of all pairs of affected individuals) larger than the GI of two randomly picked individuals from the same pedigree matched for all other characteristics of the affected pair? and (2) Is the extent of aggregation more in some pedigrees than in others?

We may avoid control selections by computing the expected distribution of GI values between pairs of individuals under the hypothesis that the affection status of individuals is independent of their biological relationship with any other individual in the pedigree. Consider a pedigree consisting of N individuals of k relationship categories. Let n_i be the number of individuals in the i-th category, and

t_{ij} = Age of the j-th individual in the i-th relationship category,

$P_{i\ell}$ = Probability that a random individual of the same sex and birth-cohort as that of the ℓ-th individual of the i-th relationship catgory will develop the disease at age $t_{i\ell}$,

Φ_{ii} = GI between two individuals belonging to the i-th relationship category,

Φ_{ij} = GI between two individuals one of whom belongs to the i-th relationship category and the other to the j-th.

Under the hypothesis of no familial aggregation of disease, the probability that two randomly chosen affected individuals will have GI equal to Φ_{ii} or Φ_{ij}, is given by Q_{ii} or Q_{ij} respectively, where

$$Q_{ii} = \sum_{\ell \neq} \sum_{m=1}^{n_i} P_{i\ell} P_{im} \Big/ \{ (\sum_{i\ell}\sum P_{i\ell})^2 - \sum_{i\ell}\sum P_{i\ell}^2 \}$$

and (5)

$$Q_{ij} = \Big(\sum_{\ell=1}^{n_i} P_{i\ell} \Big) \Big(\sum_{m=1}^{n_j} P_{jm} \Big) \Big/ \{ (\sum_{i\ell}\sum P_{i\ell})^2 - \sum_{i\ell}\sum P_{i\ell}^2 \} .$$

From these probabilities we may compute the

expectation and variance of the distribution of GI between two randomly chosen affected individuals as

$$E(\Phi_{obs}) = \sum_{i=1}^{k} \Phi_{ii}Q_{ii} + \sum\sum_{i<j} \Phi_{ij}Q_{ij} ,$$

and (6)

$$Var(\Phi_{obs}) = \sum_{i=1}^{k} \Phi_{ii}^2 Q_{ii} + \sum\sum_{i<j} \Phi_{ij}^2 Q_{ij} - [E(\Phi_{obs})]^2,$$

respectively.

Note that since the n_i's, k and P_{ij} values are specific to each pedigree, the observed GI can be contrasted with $E(\Phi_{ij})$ to see if the observed GI is significantly higher (suggesting familial aggregation) than its expectation. Unfortunately, unless the pedigree size is large, the distribution of GI cannot be approximated by any standard distribution. As we have done for T(X) discussed earlier, we can enumerate the distribution of GI between pairs, or the distribution of average GI's of all pairs of affected individuals by considering all possible combinations of individuals in the pedigree. Table 1 demonstrates the nature of the necessary calculations to be done for triplets of affected individuals in a pedigree.

Suppose that we have K different pedigrees in each of which we can compute the distribution of the average GI between all pairs of affected individuals. Denoting the averages by $X_1, X_2, \ldots, X_K$ we have the average GI in the entire data set as

$$\overline{X} = \sum_{i=1}^{K} X_i / K . \tag{7}$$

Since the pedigrees may be regarded as independent (otherwise, they may be lumped together into larger pedigrees), the distribution of X can be computed by convolution of the distributions of $X_1, X_2, \ldots, X_K$; namely,

$$Pr.\ (\overline{X} = \overline{x}) = Pr.\ (X_1 = x_1,\ X_2 = x_2, \ldots,\ X_K = x_K)$$

$$= \prod_{i=1}^{K} Pr.\ (X_i = x_i)\ , \quad (8)$$

where $\overline{x} = \sum_{i=1}^{K} x_i\ /\ K$.

From these exact distributions, suitable test criteria for testing familial aggregation or extent of excess aggregation in some subsets of pedigrees in comparison with others can be computed by usual normal deviate type of statistics.

Table 1. Example for constructing expected distribution of genealogical index (GI) between all possible pairs of affected cases in pedigrees consisting of three affected cases.

Affected cases	Average GI	Probability
1,2,3	$(\Phi_{12}+\Phi_{23}+\Phi_{13})/3$	$P_1P_2P_3/T$
1,2,4	$(\Phi_{12}+\Phi_{24}+\Phi_{14})/3$	$P_1P_2P_4/T$
..	..	..
i,j,k	$(\Phi_{ij}+\Phi_{jk}+\Phi_{ik})/3$	$P_iP_jP_k/T$
..	..	..
N-2,N-1,N	$(\Phi_{N-2,N-1}+\Phi_{N-2,N}+\Phi_{N-1,N})/3$	$P_{N-2}P_{N-1}P_N/T$

where $T = \sum_{i<j<k}\sum\sum P_iP_jP_k = \{(\Sigma P_i)^3 - 3(\Sigma P_i)(\Sigma P_i^2) + 2\,(\Sigma P_i^3)\}\ /\ 6.$

Note that in this approach there is no need of

control selection since the distribution of GI is computed for each pedigree under the null hypothesis of no familial aggregation. Furthermore, the size and structure of the pedigrees are explicitly taken into account in constructing such null distributions. This method has an added advantage over the T statistic described earlier. While the T approach reveals the pedigrees where aggregation occurs, it does not provide any scope to examine if the extent of aggregation is stronger in any subgroup of pedigrees as compared with others. The GI approach resolves this issue since we may compare the average GI values over any subclasses of pedigrees by methods outlined above. If we make sure that the sampled pedigrees are representatives of the population from which sampling has occurred, with reference of the used P_{ij} values, the above approach will enhance the applications of the Genealogical Index beyond its current applicability (Skolnick et al., 1981).

DISCUSSION

The approaches of testing excess risk described in this paper are essentially non-parametric, and are not dependent on any model of causation of familial aggregation. In this sense, these are "model-free" approaches and can be regarded as more general than the usual approach of rejection of the null hypothesis of no familial aggregation practiced in conjunction with a complex segregation analysis. As demonstrated in two recent applications (Chakraborty et al., 1984; Bale et al., 1984), these are more powerful than other procedures involving relative risk or odds ratio where an entire pedigree structure is not utilized in drawing inferences from the relative risk types of statistics.

When familial aggregation is detected by either of the two methods described above, the nature of clustering of a disease can be examined by studying the joint occurrences of the affected individuals in different branches of a pedigree. This is achieved in the use of the T statistic where we may compute the T values for different categories of relatives in the pedigrees (Chakraborty et al., 1984). The covariance matrix of these components computed over all pedigrees available for analysis may provide clues as to the cause of aggregation since its expectation is easy to derive under any specific genetic model. This may then be contrasted with the observed covariance matrix to identify possible etiology of genetic causation of the disease under study.

We argue that the approaches discussed here are by no means alternatives of segregation analyses. We only set up grounds to establish that the observed pattern of occurrences of affecteds in a family cannot be explained by chance alone and hence some specific models must be examined to understand the etiology of the disease in question.

ACKNOWLEDGEMENTS

This research is supported by US Public Health Service research grant CA 19311 from the National Institutes of Health. Some of the findings reported here are from collaborative works done with Dr. L. C. Strong, K. M. Weiss, and P. P. Majumder. Their help is greatly appreciated.

LITERATURE CITED

Bale SJ, Chakravarti A, Strong LC (1984). Aggregation of colon cancer in family data. Genet Epidemiol 1:53.

Chakraborty R, Weiss KM, Schull WJ (1980a). A test for the randomness of occurrence of a disease trait in familial or other epidemiological data. Proc Natl Acad Sci USA 77:2974.

Chakraborty R, Weiss KM, Ward RH (1980b). Evaluation of relative risks from the correlation between relatives: A theoretical approach. Med Anthrop 4: 397.

Chakraborty R, Weiss KM, Majumder PP, Strong LC, Herson J (1984). A method to detect excess risk of disease in structured data: Cancer in relatives of retinoblastoma patients. Genet Epidemiol 3:229.

del Junco DJ, H. S. Luthra HS, Annegers JF, Worthington JW, Kurland LT (1984). The familial aggregation of rheumatoid arthritis and its relationship to the HLA-DR4 association. Amer J Epidemiol 119:813.

Hill JR (1980). A survey of cancer sites by kinship in the Utah Mormon population. In Cairns J, Lyons J, Skolnick M (eds): "Banbury Report 4: Cancer Incidence in Defined Populations", New York: Cold Spring Harbor Laboratory, p 299.

Kleinbaum DG, Kupper LL, Morgenstern H (1982). "Epidemiological Research." London: Lifetime Learning Publications, p 140.

Lilienfeld AM (1965). Epidemiological concepts applied to studies of chronic diseases. In Neel JV, Shaw M, Schull WJ (eds): "Genetics and Epidemiology of Chronic Diseases," Washington DC: National Institutes of Health, p 87.

Majumder PP, Chakraborty R, Weiss KM (1983). Relative risks of diseases in the presence of incomplete penetrance and sporadics. Statistics in Med 2:13.

Malecot G (1969). "The mathematics of heredity" (translated by Yermanos DM). San Francisco: Freeman.

Penrose LS (1953). The genetic background of common diseases. Acta Genet Stat Med 4:257.

Skolnick M, Bishop DT, Carmelli D (1981). A population based assessment of familial cancer risk in Utah Mormon genealogies. In Arrighi F, Rao PN, Stubblefeild E (eds): "Genes, Chromosomes, and Neoplasia," New Yok: Raven Press, p 477.

Strong LC, Herson J, Elder K, Chakraborty R, Weiss KM, Majumder PP (1984). Cancer mortality in relatives of retinoblastoma patients. J Natl Cancer Inst 73:303.

Thompson EA (1980). Genetic etiology and clusters in a pedigree. Heredity 45:323.

Williams RR, Skolnick M, Carmelli D, Maness AT, Hunt SC, Hasstedt S, Reiber GE (1979). Utah pedigree studies: Design and preliminary data for premature male CHD deaths. In Sing CF, Skolnick (eds): "Genetic Analysis of Common Diseases: Applications to Predictive Factors in Coronary Disease," New York: Alan R. Liss, p 711.

Diseases of Complex Etiology in Small Populations:
Ethnic Differences and Research Approaches, pages 39–66

Chapter 3

STRATEGIES FOR ELUCIDATING THE PHENOTYPIC AND GENETIC HETEROGENEITY OF A CHRONIC DISEASE WITH A COMPLEX ETIOLOGY

C.F. Sing, E. Boerwinkle, and P.P. Moll

Department of Human Genetics, University of Michigan, Ann Arbor, Michigan

INTRODUCTION

Definitions of Diseases with Complex Etiologies

It is generally accepted that the genetic mechanisms for the chronic diseases, whether they are common or rare in frequency, have a complex etiology. Few of the chronic diseases are directly inherited according to simple Mendelian principles even though most aggregate in families. As a class of diseases, the chronic illnesses that are not inherited according to simple Mendelian patterns have a greater impact on the health of the adult population than the simply inherited inborn errors of metabolism or chromosomal abnormalities (Trimble and Doughty, 1974; Trimble et al., 1977). The complexity of the etiological links between genetic and environmental variations and the endpoints for diseases such as anemia, diabetes, coronary heart disease, arthritis, epilepsy and the psychiatric disorders is characterized by 1) continuous variation in clinical, biochemical and molecular phenotypes that are measures of health, 2) environmental modification of the biological predisposition of an individual to disease and 3) multiple genotypes giving rise to the same disease endpoint.

Although genetic variation may determine a large fraction of human disability, human geneticists have been less successful in understanding the links between genes, environments and endpoints for most of the chronic diseases. In contrast to the successes with the inborn errors of metabolism, only rarely has research revealed a simple relationship between the genotype and the endpoint for a chronic disease. Familial hypercholesterolemia (Goldstein and Brown, 1983) is one disease where a single gene mutation is directly responsible for a discrete class of individuals who have extreme levels of the LDL cholesterol and are predisposed to early coronary heart morbidity and mortality (Gagne et al., 1979).

At least two very different biological models have been used to describe chronic diseases. We present them in Figure 1 as being the typical points of departure for research into the genetic basis of diseases having complex etiologies and not representative of any one disease in particular. The first model (Figure 1A) relates the discrete disease endpoint to a mutation at any one of many genetic loci. The disease and the healthy state are made up of subgroups of genotypes. Each subgroup is distinguishable from other subgroups by a combination of clinical, biochemical and molecular phenotypes that are involved in the hierarchical network that connects a specific genetic locus with the endpoint. This approach has been successful in the study of diseases with discretely defined endpoints. Cystic fibrosis, PKU and diabetes are examples. Separate dominant or recessive mutations at multiple loci (A, B, or C in Figure 1A) are hypothesized to lead to disease. Adherents to this model have focused on identifying traits that discriminate among subgroups and on the gene loci that cause variation in those traits. Continuous variation in the liability to disease in the population is considered to be a consequence of environmental modifications of the combinations of molecular, biochemical, and clinical phenotypes associated with genotypic variation. Considerations of the interactions between genetic and environmental factors has, for most studies that are based on this model definition, been limited to the discrete phenomenon of phenocopy (Rimoin and Rotter, 1982). Phenocopy is defined as the occurrence of the disease as a consequence of an environmental insult to individuals who have the genotypes that are involved with the nondisease state.

An alternative to this multiple unilocus conceptualization of the etiology of the chronic diseases is given in Figure 1B. This multifactorial model emphasizes the interaction between multiple environmental and multiple genetic factors in the determination of the phenotypic variation for traits in the hierarchy between genotype and endpoint. Here the continuously distributed liability phenotype is a direct consequence of interaction between many genetic and many environmental factors. Genetic analysis may proceed without direct measurement of the liability phenotype by considering one or more of the biological risk factors that predict liability to disease. Hyperglycemia and diabetes, hypercholesterolemia and cardiovascular disease, and elevated levels of serum uric acid and arthritis are examples of diseases modeled this way.

In this model many gene loci are hypothesized to determine the alternative phenotypes within and across the levels of the hierarchy. Allelic differences at these loci, each with a small impact on liability, determine a polygenotype that interacts as a unit with environmental inputs at all levels. A disease with such a multifactorial etiology may result from many different combinations of genetic and environmental inputs. Genetic effects are modified by the environment at all levels and the expression of their interaction is age dependent in most cases.

One complicating feature of many chronic diseases is the continuous nature of the phenotypes that define health and disease. The separation of individuals into classes that do and do not have the genetic predisposition for disease becomes arbitrary. The use of a threshold to define disease is both a weakness and a strength of both of the models given in Figure 1. On one hand, clinically defined disease is a discrete endpoint that is, operationally, the medical problem. However, an arbitrary, fixed classification of the endpoint cannot reflect the multiple patterns of preclinical phenotypes and multiple etiological causations that underlie the endpoint. Since genotypes are revealed to us only as phenotypes, the exploration of the nature of action of a genotype becomes a search for the informative phenotypes that discriminate among genotypes.

Recent reviews of the genetics and epidemiology of common chronic diseases (Morton and Chung, 1978; Sing and Skolnick, 1979) summarize the following six characteristics that should be considered in studies of the etiology of chronic diseases. 1) Multiple genetic and environmental causative factors are correlated. Hence the study of chronic disease is a multivariate problem, rather than a series of multiple univariate problems. 2) There is a hierarchical relationship among the phenotypes that link genotype and disease endpoint. The study of the chronic disease is a level crossing problem that involves cell, tissue and organ systems as they change through development and are modified by aging and changes in the environment. 3) The vector of phenotypes that link genotype with endpoint is a consequence of the interactions between the effects of the genotype and the nongenetic environment. The chronic diseases are a result of an interplay between the effects of nature and nurture. 4) Information at the genotype level is often discrete, but combines to yield intervening phenotypes that are continuous. These continuous intervening phenotypes are often the basis for diagnosis into discrete classes of health and disease. The genetic analysis of the discrete endpoint can obfuscate the true nature of gene action across the hierarchy of biological organization. 5) The definition of the endpoint may change as a result of studies of the clinical, biochemical and molecular phenotypes that link genotype to endpoint. Studies of the etiology of a chronic disease very often lead to a redefinition of the disease. 6) When many loci are involved in determining the diseased class, no single individual or nuclear family is likely to represent all of the genetic mechanisms that may give rise to the endpoint.

The failure of the two widely used models for the chronic diseases (Figure 1) to encompass all of the above complicating features has led Murphy (1981) to question the meaningfulness of inferences that can be drawn from their application. His efforts to develop alternative models that take into account many of those characteristics listed above is one approach. We

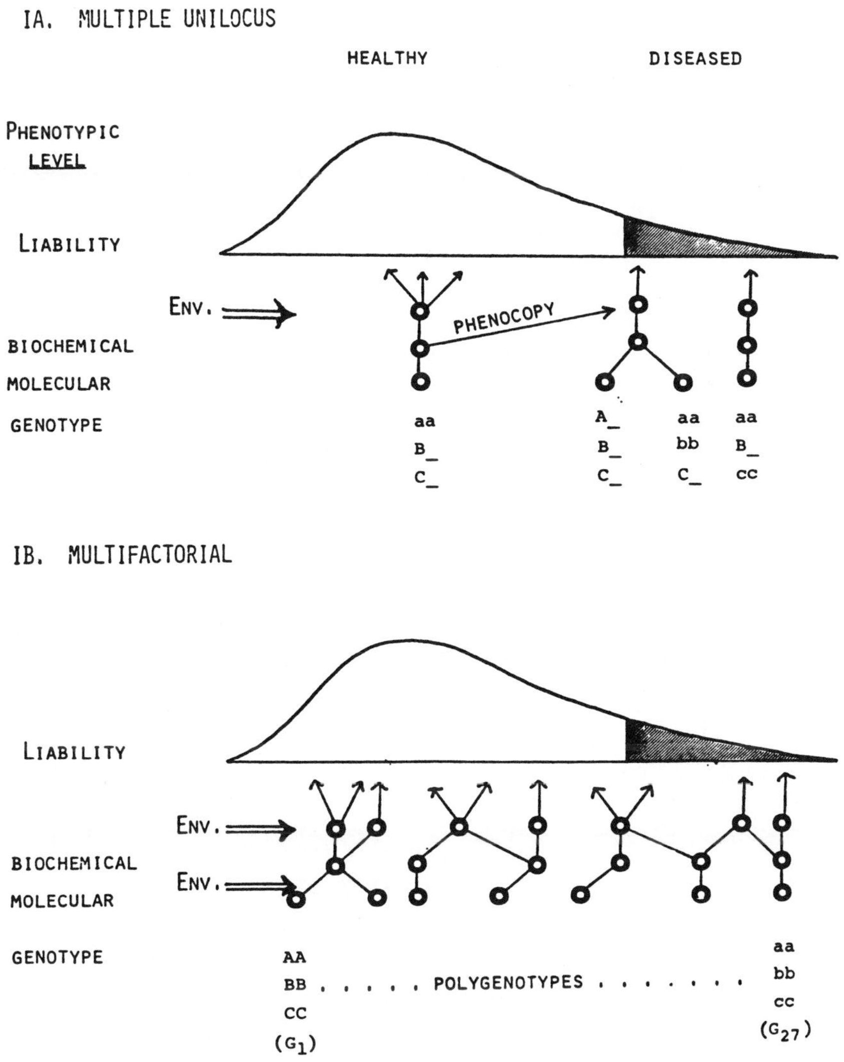

Figure 1. Models for the chronic diseases.

take the approach here that it is equally important to gather information about these features of the disease, in the belief that more realistic biological models of disease will follow from such knowledge. We specifically address the issue of determining the extent and nature of the genetic heterogeneity that underlies a single diagnostic class of disease. By investigating genetic heterogeneity, information on genetic architecture -- number of loci, frequency of alleles at each, effects on the intervening phenotypes and the impact on the endpoint -- will ultimately be understood for a chronic disease.

Definitions of Genetic Heterogeneity

There is no universal agreement on the definition of genetic heterogeneity. Vogel and Motulsky (1982) review the evidence for the presence of genetic heterogeneity: 1) children from a mating between two affected individuals for a recessive condition are phenotypically normal, 2) linkage analysis shows close linkage of the endpoint to two independent marker genes, 3) a different protein defect is responsible for the clinical defect in different individuals. Recently, Rimoin and Rotter (1982) suggest genetic heterogeneity is involved if the same clinical phenotype can be shown to be associated with the inheritance of two or more clinical, metabolic or immunological variations. They include as evidence for genetic heterogeneity the occurrence in different populations or families, different patterns of Mendelian transmission of the endpoint: recessive, dominant or X-linked. This definition is consistent with the multiple unilocal model (Figure 1A). It makes the rather restrictive assumption that chronic diseases having a complex etiological basis may be subdivided into subsets of individuals having any one of many simply inherited variations. Each subset is distinguished from all other subsets by only one genetic locus. A multivariate model (Figure 1B) where multiple loci are required to produce the clinical, biochemical or immunological variations within the diseased class of individuals is not considered.

Motulsky (1980) and Harris (1974) present a

somewhat different definition. They include the entire spectrum of mutational events at single and multiple loci and the variations in the genetic mechanisms that could lead to the same disease endpoint. Genetic heterogeneity for a disease can be a result of allelic variability at a single locus, where each allele determines a different vector of intervening phenotypes that link genotype and endpoint. Genetic heterogeneity may also be due to variability at many loci, each of which is responsible for delineating a separate vector of phenotypes that leads to the same endpoint, or to different combinations of alleles for polygenes operating in concert to determine the phenotypes that sort the subtypes of the disease. This definition encompasses the full range of types of gene action and is much broader than the multiple unilocal model. Gene action at any point in the hierarchy of biological organization may be involved in the determination of phenotypes which define the subtypes of a disease. A summary of causes is presented in Table 1.

Table 1. Causes of genetic heterogeneity.

DISEASES INHERITED IN A MENDELIAN FASHION:
- Multiple alleles at a single locus
- Multiple loci
- Phenocopy
- Genetic and/or environmental background variation

DISEASES THAT AGGREGRATE IN FAMILIES WITHOUT A SIMPLE MODE OF INHERITANCE:
- Multiple gene loci, each determining a different protein (multiple unilocus model)
- Multiple gene loci determine one phenotype (polygenes)
- Multiple gene loci, each determining a step in the pathway of phenotypes from genotype to disease endpoint

---

Most of the simply inherited chronic diseases, for example, sickle cell anemia, PKU and cystic fibrosis, display genetic heterogeneity attributable to allelism or modification of the effect of an allelic variation at a single locus by the genetic and/or environmental background. In some cases, two loci have also been implicated in the disease outcome. In PKU (McKusick, 1983), variation of phenylalanine levels among persons homozygous for the basic defect in the phenylalanine hydroxylase enzyme has been attributed to environmental and/or genetic background variability. Also, at a second locus that determines the apoprotein of phenylalanine hydroxylase, a series of mutant alleles are known to be associated with one form of hyperphenylalaninemia. In contrast to PKU, those chronic diseases that aggregate in families but do not segregate in a simple Mendelian fashion are most often genetically heterogeneous because of both multiple unilocus and polygenic causes.

Consequences of Genetic Heterogeneity

Failure to take into account genetic heterogeneity can result in errors that fall into four categories. The first category includes errors in the design of studies to understand disease. Many investigators proceed with their studies assuming there is no genetic heterogeneity because of a priori biases or misinformation about the involvement of genetic heterogeneity. The second includes errors in inferences about the etiology of disease from research on subsets of individuals or families that are not representative of the population of inference. The third includes errors in prediction of disease outcome in individuals or families attributable to the genetic heterogeneity among families in the population of interest. Finally, errors can occur in selection of the appropriate intervention strategy with the greatest chance of reducing disease.

Research on the etiological basis of the chronic diseases naturally begins with an incomplete picture of the mechanisms that are involved. It is understandable that the research design and the variables selected to understand etiology will be greatly influenced by the available knowledge and by the hypotheses and experiences of individual investigators. However, progress toward understanding the role of genetic heterogeneity cannot be made if studies are not designed to detect a multiplicity of causative factors. Molecular biologists tend to pay less attention to the influences of environmental factors and their interactions with the genotype. Clinical investigators are familiar with the patterns of variation in measures of severity and tend to pay greater attention to those environmental factors that may modify the expression of the genotype. Progress towards unraveling the nature and extent of genetic heterogeneity needs to be made from both directions; from the top (diagnosis) down (to genotype) and from bottom up. Progress is slowed because there are few opportunities to study the interaction of genotypic variability with the range of environments experienced by the population at large. The alternative has been to develop bits and pieces of the puzzle in various research laboratories with delays in bringing knowledge together that enables one to alter the paradigm that suggests the next stage of studies.

When there is genetic heterogeneity, inferences about etiology that are drawn from specific research studies are not likely to be applicable to the general population. The role of the genes in determining the prevalence of a disease in the population cannot be reconstructed from a series of separate studies of a few diseased individuals or families. Studies of the phenotype of a diseased individual having only one of the many combinations of genes that are associated with disease cannot reveal with certainty the genetic etiology of other diseased individuals. Too often conclusions about the etiology of a chronic disease in the population at large are made from studies of a few individuals or a large family. The general applicability of information about the etiology of disease from studies of an individual or a family will depend on the number of alternative genetic forms of the disease and their distribution among families. It is especially important to realize that when there is genetic heterogeneity it is very unlikely that a few large families will represent all of the etiological facets of a disease having a multifactorial etiology.

As with all diseases that have a significant

impact on health, a major goal is to identify the population subset, the family and the individual that are at increased risk. When multiple genetic and multiple environmental factors are involved a sample of individuals or families is not likely to represent a homogeneous combination of etiological causations. Accuracy of risk evaluation will depend to a large extent on knowing the mode of inheritance and the frequency distribution of phenotype(s) that define the endpoint among individuals or the groups of individuals being considered. A study of the heterogeneity of the genetic etiology of hypercholesterolemia by Moll et al. (1984) serves to illustrate the point. They partitioned 33, three generation pedigrees (each ascertained by a hypercholesterolemic index child), into a subset of three that were segregating for a single locus with a large effect on cholesterol level and a subset of 30 showing no evidence for the major gene effect. The risk for death in grandparents due to coronary heart disease (CHD) when the 33 pedigrees were pooled was increased 1.89 fold (significantly different from 1.0 at the 0.01 level probability) compared to the risk in 65 three generation pedigrees ascertained by a normocholesterolemic child. Five of the 12 grandparents in the 3 pedigrees had died of CHD. This represents a 3.26 fold increase ($p < 0.01$) in risk when compared to the estimate for the control group of 65 pedigrees ascertained by a normocholesterolemic child. Grandparents in the 30 pedigrees identified by a hypercholesterolemic child that did not show evidence for a major single gene effect had a 1.75 fold increase compared to the control group of pedigrees.

We next turn to reviewing some of the alternative strategies for investigating genetic heterogeneity. We include examples of the identification and resolution of genetic heterogeneity, pointing out how such information has contributed to understanding the complexity of the etiology of a chronic disease and has the potential to improve our ability to more accurately evaluate risk.

STRATEGIES FOR STUDYING GENETIC HETEROGENEITY, WITH SELECTED EXAMPLES

Basic Questions Being Considered

The strategies taken to identify genetic heterogeneity depend on the a priori information that is available, which in turn influences the questions that will be asked. For this reason the chronic diseases with a simple Mendelian mode of inheritance and those that aggregate in families but do not exhibit a simple mode of inheritance are often approached differently. For the diseases that have a simple mode of inheritance (e.g. cystic fibrosis and sickle cell anemia) interest has been in elucidating the genetic basis for variation in clinical severity, age of onset or interaction with environmental factors, such as therapeutic drugs, that modify the impact of the disease. Often investigators begin by defining those phenotypes that are associated with variability in the disease and then turn to the study of the causes of such variation. We refer to this as the "top down" strategy. We present examples of studies of cystic fibrosis (Sing et al., 1982) and sickle cell anemia (Odenheimer et al., 1983). Here we will review the sickle cell anemia work to illustrate how studies of the phenotypic heterogeneity among those with this single gene disorder can expose the extent of the complexity of the etiology of a chronic disease. Those chronic diseases that do not follow a Mendelian pattern of inheritance like epilepsy, psychiatric disorders, coronary heart disease, and cancer present a different challenge. Here there is less information about the role of genes in determining the disease. The end point often includes a broader range of distinguishable disease subtypes as well as clinical, biochemical and molecular variation within and among the subtypes. After distinguishing a subclass of patients that are homogeneous for the endpoint, the goal has been first to identify those phenotypic variations, at all levels between genotype and endpoint, that distinguish the subclass from all other patients (a top to bottom strategy) and second to investigate the pattern of inheritance of the vector of phenotypes that is established (a bottom to top strategy). Our studies of coronary heart disease and serum cholesterol illustrate the identification of the alternative genetic mechanisms that are involved in the etiology of hypercholesterolemia and the subsequent development of CHD.

Measurement of Genetic Heterogeneity

Genetic heterogeneity cannot be exposed unless we are capable of knowing (and measuring) the phenotypes that distinguish alternative links between genotype and endpoint. Progress is directly proportional to the development of methods for the measurement of the relevant phenotypes in the hierarchy of biological

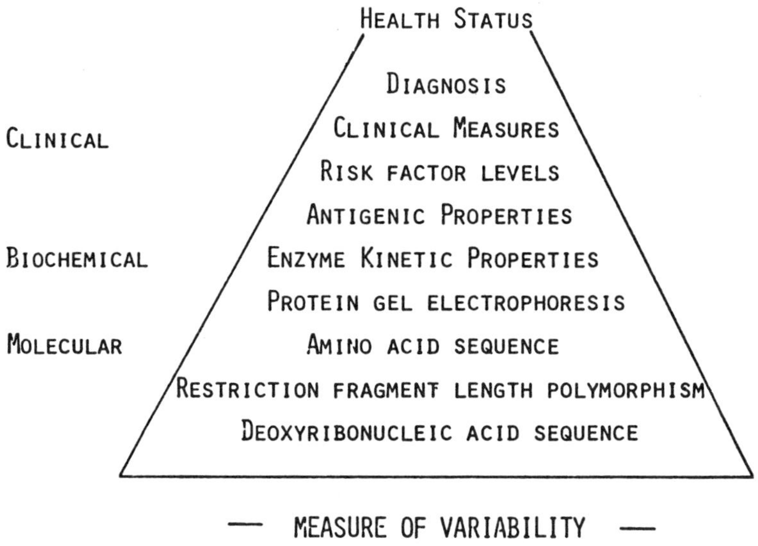

Figure 2. Intervening traits in the hierarchy of biological organization.

organization (Figure 2). Traditionally, the presence of disease heterogeneity has been established in the clinic and studies then carried out in the laboratory to identify the biological correlates of the clinically defined subtypes, a top to bottom strategy.

How much genetic variation can we expect to influence the various levels in the hierarchy of phenotypes? For many years, there has been great interest in biology in obtaining estimates of the total amount of genetic variation in a population. Biochemical and molecular analyses of the primary products of randomly selected genetic loci have established that 30 to 50% are segregating (have two or more alleles) in most plant and animal populations (Powell, 1975; Nevo, 1978). Is it reasonable to conclude that as broad a spectrum of variation exists in both the healthy and diseased subsets of the same population? How much of this genetic variation plays a role in determining disease severity in the simply inherited diseases? To what extent does this "normal" genetic variation contribute to the determination of those diseases that aggregate in families but have no simple mode of inheritance? Are the genetic polymorphisms the polygenes that are involved in the quantitative variation of intervening phenotypes?

The characterization of genetic variation is further enhanced by recent technical advances that allow more detailed molecular phenotyping of the genotype (e.g. the DNA RFLP, monoclonal antibodies to gene products and 2-D gel electrophoresis). By combining in a statistical analysis the associations between the transmission of molecular phenotypes and the transmission of clinically important phenotypes, it is becoming possible to identify the genetic variability that underlies the outcomes of health and disease. Measures of molecular markers that are correlated with specific phenotypic classes can be an important step forward in understanding the etiological progression from genotype to endpoint and also may provide more precise markers of risk to disease than are currently available in the continuously distributed risk factors.

A Top Down Strategy -- Studies of Phenotypic Heterogeneity in Sickle Cell Anemia

The factors that influence the heterogeneity of clinical severity of sickle cell anemia (SCA) are poorly understood. In a recent review, Warth and

Rucknagel (1983) have pointed out that although more is known about the physiology and pathogenesis of SCA than any other simply inherited disease, few measures have been correlated with clinical severity. The question arises as to which phenotypes are predictive of the continuous variation in severity and what combination of genetic and environmental factors causes them to vary among patients. The more we explore the phenotypic heterogeneity among those with this single gene disorder the more it becomes apparent how complex the links must be between the causes and the clinical course of SCA.

Studies in progress are designed to 1) determine if the population of children with SCA can be subdivided into distinct groups according to some combination of phenotypes hypothesized to be relevant to the etiology of the disease, 2) determine whether the subgroups identified differ in their clinical manifestations of the disease and 3) establish the genetic and environmental factors that determine the variation in the discriminating traits. To address the first issue, Odenheimer et al. (1983) studied the multivariate relationships among six hematological phenotypes: hemoglobin (HB), hematocrit (HCT), red blood cell count (RBC), percent of fetal hemoglobin (%HB F), mean cell volume (MCV), and percent of A_2 hemoglobin (%HB A_2) in a sample of 225 children with SCA. The results of a multivariate cluster analysis (Duran, 1974) are summarized for males in Figure 3A and females in Figure 3B. To aid the interpretation of the clusters, the first and second principal components are also plotted. Separate analyses of males and females gave remarkably similar clusterings. Individuals from cluster 4 are on average 7 times more similar to one another than they are similar to individuals in cluster 3 and they are 17 times more similar to one another than they are similar to any individual from cluster 1 or 2. Individuals assigned to cluster 2 are least similar to one another. The relationships among the six variables that are represented by the first principal component (PC 1) clearly separates individuals in cluster 4 from those in cluster 1 in both sexes. In cluster 4 the HB, HCT, RBC and %HB F are elevated and MCV (males) and %HB A_2 (females) are decreased compared to the mean of the

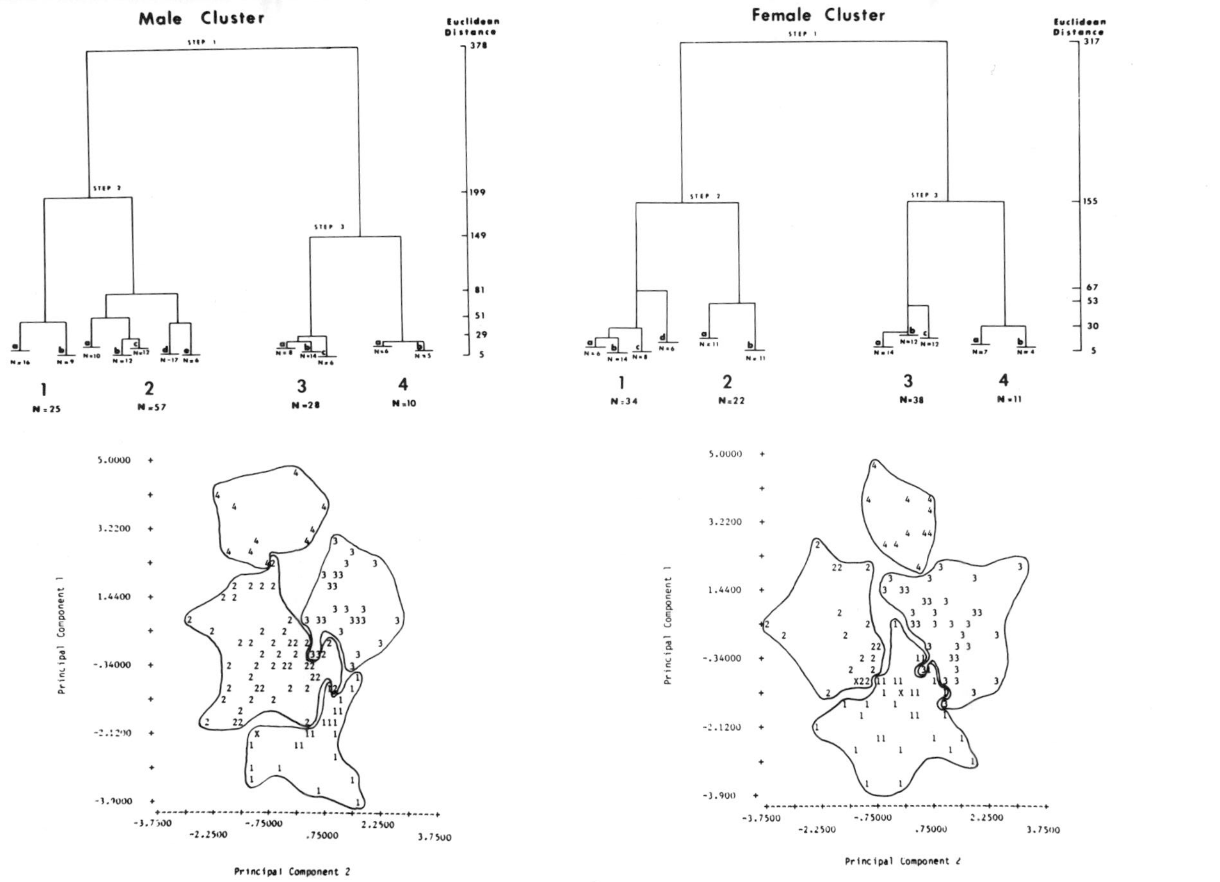

Figure 3. The identification of phenotypic heterogeneity among sickle cell anemia patients using six hematological variables.

sample (the opposite effect occurs in cluster 1). The second principal component (PC 2) separates cluster 2 from cluster 3 in each sex. Here, cluster 3 has elevated levels of %HB F and MCV and decreased levels of %HB A_2 while cluster 2 has the opposite combination of deviations from the sample mean. An inverse relationship between %HB F and %HB A_2 mean levels distinguish clusters 1 and 2 from 3 and 4. Clusters 1 and 2 have decreased %HB F levels and increased %HB A_2 levels compared to the sample mean while the means of clusters 3 and 4 have the opposite relationship between these two variables.

Table 2. Characterization of subgroups of children with sickle cell anemia.

	Clusters 1 & 2 n = 138	Clusters 3 & 4 n = 87	Significance 1 & 2 vs 3 & 4
Predictors:			
Mean %HB F (±S.D.)	8.74±3.46	15.48±3.44	< 0.001
Mean %HB A_2(±S.D.)	2.80±0.40	2.34±0.34	< 0.001
Measures of Severity:			
% Ever hospitalized	84	60	< 0.001
% Ever transfused	65	33	< 0.001
% With bone age delay greater than 1 year	35	17	< 0.01
% Ever had pneumonia	62	43	< 0.01

Sixteen measures of clinical severity were compared among the 4 subgroups of children identified by the cluster analysis. Again, the findings were similar for males and females. The results are summarized in Table 2. A retrospective evaluation of clinical records suggested that clinical findings were similar in clusters 1 and 2, and in clusters 3 and 4. A greater fraction of children in clusters 1 and 2 had been hospitalized, been transfused, had bone age delay greater than one year and had pneumonia compared to children in clusters 3 and 4. Because the inverse relationship between %HB F and %HB A_2 distinguishes clusters 1 and 2 from clusters 3 and 4, it is suggested that these hematological variables are most strongly associated with disease severity in this sample. The failure of previous studies to identify a consistent correlation of either %HB F or %HB A_2 with measures of severity is not surprising in view of the outcome reported by Odenheimer et al. (1983). This study establishes that a hematological phenotype based on a multivariate profile of variables is a useful strategy for establishing the links between underlying genetic and environmental factors and disease heterogeneity for a single gene disorder. Studies are in progress to determine whether the differences in hematological variables between clusters have a genetic basis.

Statistical and Molecular Genetic Studies of Disease: Bottom to Top Strategy

A second approach to investigating genetic heterogeneity examines the role of genes in the disease process within a class of individuals that have not been subdivided according to phenotypic properties of the disease. Using the top down strategy discussed above, it is not always possible to identify and measure the intervening phenotypes that discriminate between subgroups. A bottom to top strategy identifies genetic heterogeneity directly from genotype properties using either statistical analysis of the phenotypes in the hierarchy between genotype and disease endpoint or molecular probes that can be used to elucidate the structure of the gene itself. Differences in the properties of the genes influencing the disease status may be revealed as different modes of inheritance of the endpoint in different pedigrees or as structural DNA differences among individuals with the disease (Figure 4). Evidence for genetic heterogeneity is accepted when the population of pedigrees can be subdivided according to the mode of inheritance of the phenotype. The molecular approach reveals genetic heterogeneity by detecting those lesions (mutations) that affect the disease phenotype. The population of affected individuals can then be subdivided into those that do and those that do not carry a specific gene lesion. A

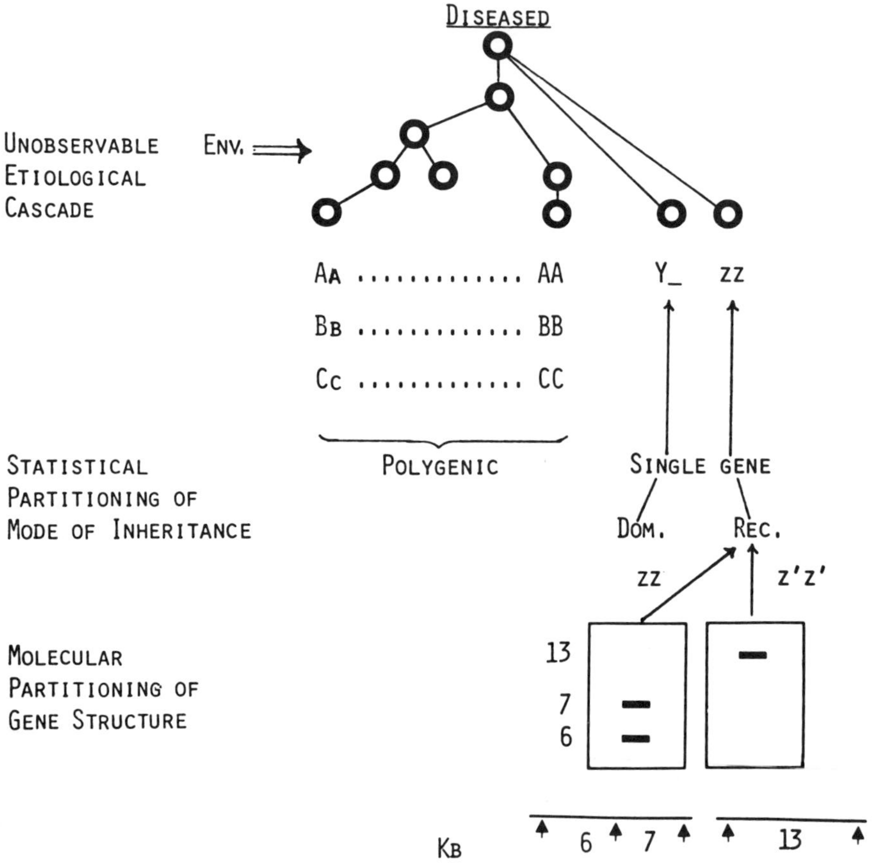

Figure 4. A schematic of the bottom to top strategy in the analysis of genetic heterogeneity.

statistical approach to sorting pedigrees among different modes of inheritance is limited by our ability to classify discretely those with the single gene effect, while the molecular approach is limited by our technical ability to probe the structure of the gene.

The statistical approach to genetic heterogeneity has a classical history and has made great contributions to understanding the diseases that have been described by the multiple univariate model (Figure 1A). The strategy is to show that an endpoint phenotype has a different mode of inheritance in different pedigrees. One typical example is provided by the early studies that established that the Hunter's and Hurler's syndromes are the result of mutations at two separate loci. Nja (1946) showed that one form on the disease (Hurler's) followed the transmission of the X chromosome and a second (Hunter's) was inherited as a autosomal recessive. Subsequent biochemical studies using fibroblast complementation tests and enzyme assays have confirmed that these two forms have very different intervening phenotypes between genotype and the clinical endpoints.

Several statistical approaches for detecting genetic heterogeneity have been applied to chronic diseases characterized by incomplete penetrance and/or multiple quantitative risk factors (see Moll et al., 1984 for a discussion). When there are no clear discrete classifications into healthy and diseased, it has been traditional to analyze the genetic basis of continuous risk factors that define the liability to disease. Complex segregation analysis, reviewed by Elston and Rao (1978), is one approach for identifying pedigrees with different genetic etiologies for variability in quantitative traits. It is based on a mixed genetic model proposed by Elston and Stewart (1971) in which one genetic locus (a major locus) is assumed to have a large effect on the trait while many loci (polygenes) each contribute small, equal and additive effects. This model is formulated under the assumption of additivity between the major locus and polygenes, and between genetic and environmental effects that are specific to each individual. Genetic heterogeneity is suggested if there are different penetrance functions for the major locus (dominance versus recessive) in different pedigrees (Williams and Lalouel, 1982) and/or there is evidence that a specific class of phenotypes is associated with the segregation at a major locus in some pedigrees while there is no evidence that a major locus explains the class in others.

Moll et al. (1983, 1984) applied complex segregation analysis to cholesterol levels to investigate the role of genetic heterogeneity in determining hypercholesterolemia (total fasting serum cholesterol levels greater than the 95th percentile expected for one's age and sex). The study involved 709 relatives of 98 healthy index cases selected from 3666 school children surveyed for lipid levels in Rochester, Minnesota. Thirty-three of the index cases and 109 relatives had hypercholesterolemia. These data suggest that both a major locus and polygenes are involved in determining cholesterol variability and that the mutant allele at the major locus is dominant rather than recessive or codominant. Using the maximum likelihood estimates of parameters obtained under the dominant mixed model, the conditional probabilities of the three possible genotypes at the hypothesized major locus were estimated for the 709 relatives. The results are summarized in Table 3. No one was judged to be homozygous for the mutant allele because the highest conditional probability for the AA genotype was 0.001. In the 28 pedigrees with no hypercholesterolemics, the highest conditional probability of an Aa individual was 0.001. In 3 of the 70 pedigrees with one or more hypercholesterolemics, all individuals with hypercholesterolemia had a conditional probability greater than 0.95 for Aa. The grandparents in the 3 pedigrees that were segregating at the major locus had the highest rates of death due to coronary heart disease as discussed earlier.

Advantages to this approach are that it does not require either _a priori_ stratification of pedigrees or dichotomization of a continuous phenotype prior to genetic analysis. There are limitations, however. If there is segregation at two or more major loci, application of the complex segregation analysis model discussed here would not differentiate between them. Specifically, we could not expect our analysis to distinguish between two subtypes of hypercholesterolemia that are both dominantly inherited. Further differentiation of the genetic etiology can only proceed by the inclusion of further phenotypic information on the nature of the genotype. However, the statistical approach provides important implications for 1) the choice of treatments for hypercholesterolemia, 2) risk assessment for coronary heart disease and 3) the directions of further studies of the molecular characterization of the inherited defects in lipid metabolism.

Table 3. Categorization of pedigrees based on the number of hypercholesterolemics and the probability of carrying the mutant allele at the major locus.

Pedigrees with	No. of Pedigrees	No. of pedigrees with individuals having P(Aa) >0.10	No. of pedigrees with individuals having P(Aa) >0.95
No hypercholesterolemics	28	0	0
One hypercholesterolemic	33	0	0
Multiple hypercholesterolemics	37	5	3
Total	98	5	3

A molecular genetic approach to the investigation of genetic heterogeneity attempts to characterize the kind and number of genetic variants that may underlie a particular phenotypic outcome. A revolution has occurred in the past decade in the tools available to probe the structure and function of the gene. These include the new research techniques provided by the recombinant DNA and monoclonal antibody techniques. Although these newer methods have been primarily applied to the study of genes involved in determining the simply inherited disorders, we feel they will soon be applied to characterize the genes and the gene products that are involved in the development of the diseases having complex etiologies. The molecular analysis of the insulin gene (Rotwein et al., 1983) to understand the complexity of the diabetes endpoint is one example. Another is the elegant work by Goldstein and Brown (1979) to define the genetic lesion that is responsible for abnormal uptake and metabolism of low density serum cholesterol.

We draw upon the work of Prochownik et al. (1983) on the genetics of antithrombin III deficiency to illustrate the power of the molecular approach to the study of genetic heterogeneity. Antithrombin III is an inhibitor of serine proteases. A deficiency of the molecule results in various thrombic disorders that are a consequence of abnormal protease levels. Antithrombin III is inherited as an autosomal dominant trait. Using the methods of recombinant DNA, a cDNA probe was isolated that could be used to identify alternative alleles for the antithrombin III gene. Two types of families were described. In one type there was evidence that segregation of the disease was explained by a gene deletion while in a second type no deletion was found. In families with the deletion, heterozygous affected individuals are missing one of the structural genes for antithrombin III. In families without the gene deletion the defect may be unlinked to the antithrombin gene itself. Other diseases, such as the hemoglobinopathies, have yielded a great deal of information about genetic heterogeneity at the molecular level (Spritz and Forget, 1983). Through the use of gene probes for specific sequences of the globin gene complex, defects have been found that include deletions of entire genes, improper messenger RNA splicing and classic point mutations. Some of this information is being used to aid in prenatal diagnosis of disease. Knowledge of the nature of specific gene defects resulting in diseases such as antithrombin III deficiency and the thalassemias also have the potential to suggest more appropriate therapeutic measures than are currently being pursued.

The contribution of molecular gene variation to resolving the problem of genetic heterogeneity depends on our ability to link such variation to the intervening phenotypes that bridge the hierarchy of biological organization from genotype to endpoint. That is, how much of the genetic variation detectable by the high resolution techniques of molecular biology is translated into a biological signal that contributes to determining health or disease? The gene region coding for alcohol dehydrogenase (ADH) was sequenced in a representative sample of _Drosophila melanogaster_ lines. Only 1 of 43 DNA sequence polymorphisms that were identified was translated into variation at the protein level (Kreitman, 1983). Many of the alterations found at the DNA sequence level may simply be natural background variation that has little or no effect on the phenotype of the organism.

INFERENCES ABOUT GENETIC ARCHITECTURE FROM STUDIES OF HETEROGENEITY

What do we know about the genetic architecture of the chronic diseases from studies of genetic heterogeneity? Few studies have considered combining the molecular information that has accumulated for the chronic diseases with the distribution in the population at large of phenotypes that link genotype with endpoint. It is reasonable to hypothesize that the gene loci involved will vary with respect to the size of their effects on each of the intervening phenotypes. At a small fraction of loci, a mutation may have a major deleterious effect at all levels and disease will be a direct consequence. These will be manifested as the single gene Mendelian disorders. At other loci mutations will have smaller effects that may act to modify, quantitatively, the effect of the major locus. In the absence of a major locus effect, the loci combine to determine a disease susceptibility phenotype. For most loci we might expect the impact of a single gene mutation on an intervening phenotype to be smaller for those phenotypes that are closer to the endpoint and larger for those near the primary gene product.

The evidence accumulated so far indicates that

the relative contribution of loci with large effects to determining the genetic heterogeneity that underlies a disease endpoint is smaller than the contribution of the loci determining small effects. The hemoglobinopathies that result in a heterogeneous class of anemias have been extensively studied using the bottom to top strategy. Most of the inherited hemoglobin variants that have a large effect on the determination of hematological status are rare in frequency. The deletion beta thalassemia variants are one example. The variants for other involved loci that are polymorphic have relatively smaller effects on the hematological status. The variants determining sickle cell anemia and alpha thalassemia are examples. Little is known about the class of variants with very small effects that contribute to normal hemoglobin variability.

Resolution of genetic heterogeneity that contributes to hypercholesterolemia has established that many genetic loci are involved in determining elevated serum cholesterol. Four polymorphic marker loci have been identified that are each associated with very small deviations from the overall mean (Sing and Orr, 1976). Polymorphic alleles (there are at least three) at the gene locus determining apolipoprotein E have intermediate effects (Bouthillier et al., 1983). On the other hand, rare mutations at the gene locus determining LDL receptors on peripheral cells are each associated with a very large effect on an individual's serum cholesterol level (Goldstein and Brown, 1983). The complexity of the biological processing of cholesterol by the body suggests that there are certainly many more loci involved in normal cholesterol metabolism that are yet to be described. Although not much data is yet available, these studies suggest that there are a small number of loci with rare alleles having large effects and a large number of loci with polymorphic alleles, each having a smaller effect on the determination of extreme values of serum cholesterol. Given the large number of loci involved and the range of effects that are present, no two individuals are likely to have the same genetic constitution for hypercholesterolemia. Whether these very incomplete data suggest an expectation for other risk factors in the chronic diseases that do not have a simple mode of inheritance remains an open question.

SUMMARY

Genetic heterogeneity is a consequence of the complexity of the biology of disease. Revealing genetic heterogeneity exposes the complexity of the genotype-environment interactions that are expressed by the intervening phenotypes that link genotype with the disease endpoint. Because we have not identified the genes involved in most common diseases, studies of genetic heterogeneity have primarily focused on a statistical analysis of either the discrete endpoint or the quantitative intervening phenotypes. Rapid progress in the development of sophisticated measures of the genotype and the intervening phenotypes will enhance our ability to characterize the etiology of the chronic disease. Both statistical and molecular methods will be required to understand the impact of each of the many genes that are expected to contribute to the chronic disease burden in the population at large.

ACKNOWLEDGEMENT

Supported in part by HL24489, HL16008 and GM07544 from NIH and DOE contract DE-AC02-82ER60089.

LITERATURE CITED

Bouthillier D, Sing CF, Davignon J (1983). Apolipoprotein E phenotyping with a single gel method: Application to the study of informative matings. J of Lipid Res 24:1060.

Duran BS (1974). "Cluster Analysis: A Survey." New York: Springer-Verlag.

Elston RC, Rao DC (1978). Statistical modeling analysis in human genetics. Ann Rev Biophys Bioeng 7:253.

Elston RC, Stewart J (1971). A general model for the

genetic analysis of pedigree data. Hum Hered 21:523.
Gagne C, Moorjani S, Brun D, Toussaint M, Lupien PJ (1979). Heterozygous familial hypercholesteremia: Relationship between plasma lipids, lipoproteins, clinical manifestations and ischaemic heart disease in men and women. Atherosclerosis 34:13.
Goldstein JL, Brown MS (1983). Familial hypercholesterolemia. In Stanbury JB, Wyngaarden JB, Goldstein JL, Brown MS (eds): "The Metabolic Basis of Inherited Diseases," New York: McGraw Hill, p 672.
Goldstein JL, Brown, MS (1979). The LDL receptor locus and the genetics of familial hypercholesterolemia. In Roman HL, Campbell A, Sandler LM (eds) Annual Review of Genet 13:259.
Harris, H (1974). Genetic heterogeneity in inherited disease. J Clin Pathol 27:32.
Kreitman M (1983). Nucleotide polymorphism at the alcohol dehydrogenase locus of Drosophila melanogaster. Nature 304:412.
McKusick VA (1983). "Mendelian Inheritance in Man. Catalogs of Autosomal Dominant, Autosomal Recessive and X-linked Phenotypes." Baltimore: Johns Hopkins University Press.
Moll PP, Sing CF, Weidman WH, Gordon H, Ellefson RD, Hodgson PA, Kottke, BA (1983). Total cholesterol and lipoproteins in school children: Prediction of coronary heart disease in adult relatives. Circulation 67:127.
Moll PP, Berry TD, Weidman WH, Ellefson R, Gordon H, Kottke BA (1984). Detection of genetic heterogeneity among pedigrees through complex segregation analysis: An application to hypercholesterolemia. Amer J Hum Genet 36:197.
Morton NE, Chung CS (1978)."Genetic Epidemiology." New York: Academic Press.
Motulsky A (1980) Approaches to the genetics of common diseases. In Rotter JI, Samloff IM, Rimoin DL (eds): "The Genetics and Heterogeneity of Common Gastrointestinal Disorders," New York: Alan R. Liss, p 3.
Murphy EA (1981). Only authorized persons admitted: The quantitative genetics of health and disease. John Hopkins Med J 148:114.
Nevo E (1978). Genetic variation in natural

populations: Patterns and theory. Theoret Pop Biol 13:121.
Nja A (1946). A sex-linked type of gargoylism. Acta paediatrica Scandinavia 33:267.
Odenheimer DJ, Whitten CF, Rucknagel DL, Sarnaik SA, Sing CF (1983). Heterogeneity of sickle-cell anemia based on a profile of hematological variables. Amer J Hum Genet 35:1224.
Powell JR (1975). Protein varition in natural populations of animals. Evol Biol 8:79.
Prowchownik EV, Antonarakis S, Bauer KA, Rosenberg RD, Fearson ER, Orkin SH (1983). Molecular heterogeneity of inherited antithrombin III deficiency. New Eng J Med 308:1549.
Rimoin DL, Rotter JI (1982). Genetic hetogeneity in common disease. In "Human Genetics, Part B: Medical Aspects," New York: Alan R. Liss, p 97.
Rotwein PS, Chirgwin J, Province M, Knowler WC, Pettitt DJ, Cordell B, Goodman HM, Permut MA (1983). Polymorphism in the 5' flanking regions of the human insulin gene: A genetic marker for non-insulin-dependent diabetes. New Eng J Med 308:65.
Sing CF, Orr JD (1976). Analysis of genetic and environmental sources of variation in serum cholesterol in Tecumseh, Michigan. III. Identification of genetic effects using twelve polymorphic blood marker systems. Amer J Hum Genet 28:453.
Sing CF, Risser DR, Howatt WF, Erickson RP (1982). Phenotypic heterogeneity in cystic fibrosis. Amer J Med Genet 13:179.
Sing CF, Skolnick M (1979)."Genetic Analysis of Common Diseases: Applications to Predictive Factors in Coronary Disease." New York: Alan R.Liss.
Spritz RA, Forget BG (1983). The thalassemias: Molecular mechanisms of human disease. Amer J Hum Genet 35:333.
Trimble BK, Doughty JH (1974). The amount of hereditary disease in human populations. Ann Hum Genet 38:199.
Trimble BK, Smith ME (1977). The incidence of genetic disease and the impact on man of an altered mutation rate. Can J Genet Cytol 19:375.
Vogel F, Motulsky AG (1982). "Human Genetics, Problems and Approaches." New York: Springer-Verlag.
Warth JA, Rucknagel DL (1983). The increasing

complexity of sickle cell anemia. In Brown EB (ed): "Progress in Hematology," Vol XIII, New York: Grune and Stratton, Inc., p 25.
Williams WR, Lalouel JM (1982). Complex segregation analysis of hyperlipoproteinemia in a Seattle sample. Hum Hered 32:24.

Diseases of Complex Etiology in Small Populations:
Ethnic Differences and Research Approaches, pages 67–96

Chapter 4

A COVARIANCE STRUCTURE MODEL FOR QUANTITATIVE GENETIC RESEARCH

S.L. Smalley[1], B.J. Williams[1],
J.A. Woodward[2], D.G. Bonett[3],
C. Ritenbaugh[4]

[1]Department of Anthropology, University of California, Los Angeles; [2]Department of Psychology, University of California; [3]Department of Psychology, University of Southern California, Los Angeles; [4]Department of Family and Community Medicine, University of Arizona, Tucson

INTRODUCTION

In recent years a number of advances have been made in the development of modeling techniques available for quantitative genetic research (Eaves et al., 1978). Many current models for the specification of genetic and environmental influences on quantitative traits arise from two traditions -- the path analysis of Wright (Wright, 1921; Morton, 1974; Rao, 1974) and the analysis of variance (Fisher, 1918; Kempthorne, 1957; Li, 1981). Each of these general approaches addresses certain unique issues in genetic research. In path analysis, causal inferences are made in correlational data through the specification and testing of simultaneous linear regression models. The analysis of variance approach, predominant in agriculture and animal breeding studies, utilizes known degrees of genetic relatedness and experimental manipulation of environment to partition quantitative traits into genetic and environmental components. In this paper we introduce a general mathematical model that merges these -- the simultaneous regression models and the analysis of variance models -- into one comprehensive formulation. The approach presented here incorporates in one model several previously separate components that are useful in genetic theory testing: specifically, a measurement model for continuous traits; a simultaneous linear regression model for studying the causal structure of a set of variables; and an analysis of variance model for representing different degrees of genetic relatedness among individuals in the sampling design.

The mathematical framework for this approach is the general class of covariance structure models that has developed in econometrics and psychometrics in the last decade (Goldberger and Duncan, 1973; Jöreskog, 1969). These general covariance structure models are just beginning to be adapted to genetic research (e.g. Eaves and Gale, 1974; Martin and Eaves, 1977). Initial applications suggest that the flexibility, generality and convenience of these models make them promising tools for quantitative genetics. Through applications to data, the power of these models for representing and testing genetic issues can be explored and the robustness of the approach when the underlying assumptions are not met can be evaluated. Furthermore, alternative approaches can be developed when existing methods prove to be inadequate. For example, an asymptotically distribution free method of estimation recently has been developed by Browne (1984) for application to data when the normality assumption (of observed variables) is not met.

This paper contains a description of our general methodological approach and of our initial applications to data on glucose tolerance and obesity in the Pima Indians of Arizona. The formulation presented is a genetic application of the general covariance structure model and estimation scheme developed by Jöreskog (1969, 1974, 1978). We have applied a specialization of the Jöreskog model that incorporates simultaneously the measurement model, components of variance model and regression model among unobserved variables (Woodward et al., 1981).

THE GENERAL MODEL

The general model may be defined by the following

set of linear equations:

$$\underset{\sim}{x} = \Lambda_x \underset{\sim}{\xi} + \underset{\sim}{\epsilon}_x \qquad (1a)$$

$$\underset{\sim}{y} = \Lambda_y \underset{\sim}{\eta} + \underset{\sim}{\epsilon}_y \qquad (1b)$$

$$\underset{\sim}{\xi} = G_x \underset{\sim}{\tau} + \underset{\sim}{e}_x \qquad (2a)$$

$$\underset{\sim}{\eta} = G_y \underset{\sim}{v} + \underset{\sim}{e}_y \qquad (2b)$$

$$\beta \underset{\sim}{v} = \Gamma \underset{\sim}{\tau} + \zeta \qquad (3)$$

The model consists of the three distinct components mentioned above: the measurement model, the components of variance model and the regression model. When multiple measures of a trait are available, an unobservable variable can be defined as the common factor contributing to the covariances among the the observed measures. The $\underset{\sim}{x}$ and $\underset{\sim}{y}$ in the equation 1(a,b) represent vectors of multiple observable variables that measure the common factors, $\underset{\sim}{\xi}$ and $\underset{\sim}{\eta}$, respectively. The matrices Λ_x and Λ_y contain factor loadings that relate observed variables to unobservable common factors. Uncommon or specific error variance is represented by $\underset{\sim}{\epsilon}_x$ and $\underset{\sim}{\epsilon}_y$. The x, y notation has developed in econometrics to differentiate exogenous from endogenous variables, respectively. An exogenous variable is one thought to be "not caused by" any other variable in the system. An endogenous variable is one that is "caused by" but may also be a causal factor among variables in the system. By convention, observed exogenous variables are denoted by $\underset{\sim}{x}$ with their common factors denoted by $\underset{\sim}{\xi}$. Observed endogenous variables are denoted by $\underset{\sim}{y}$ with their common factors represented by $\underset{\sim}{\eta}$.

Equation 2 (a,b) defines the components of variance model. Given specific sampling conditions, variance components, denoted by $\underset{\sim}{\tau}$ and $\underset{\sim}{v}$, are defined from unobserved variables ($\underset{\sim}{\xi}$ and $\underset{\sim}{\eta}$) via the design matrices G_x and G_y, respectively. The design matrices are determined by the specific sampling methodology. They reflect a parameterization of analysis of variance designs into the covariance structure model. Residual variances are represented in equation 2 (a, b) by $\underset{\sim}{e}_x$ and $\underset{\sim}{e}_y$. It is through the components of variance model that genetic applications of the present approach are realized. We will return to a more detailed development of this portion of the model in a later section.

Equation 3 defines the regression model among variance components. Structural relationships among endogenous variance components (v) are specified via the parameter matrix β. Structural relationships among endogenous and exogenous variance components (v and τ are specified via the parameter matrix Γ. Residual effects are denoted in equation 3 by ζ.

The elements of Λ_x, Λ_y, G_x, G_y, and Γ and β and the elements of the covariance matrices of τ, ζ, ϵ_y, ϵ_x, e_y, e_x are parameters of the general model. Some of the parameters must be fixed at specific values to identify the model; that is, to assure a unique estimate for each parameter. Additional parameters can be fixed at specific values or constrained to equal each other as dictated by theory or prior information. The appropriateness of overidentifying restrictions can be evaluated by a goodness-of-fit test. The remaining free parameters have unknown values and unknown variances (and covariances) all of which must be estimated from sample data. Free parameters are estimated by the method of maximum likelihood and under the assumption of multivariate normality of observed variables, the maximum likelihood estimators have been shown to be efficient, consistent and asymptotically normally distributed (Jöreskog, 1978). Estimated variances and covariances of the parameter estimates are given as the inverse of the Fisher Information matrix.

The covariance matrix predicted under the hypothesized model is found as a function of specified parameters of the system. Jöreskog and Sörbom (1981) have written a general computer program LISREL (Linear Structural Equation Relations) that can be used to obtain parameter estimates of the hypothesized model and to test the appropriateness of overidentifying restrictions by a likelihood ratio goodness-of-fit test statistic. The significance of specific parameters of the model can be tested through model comparisons. Model comparisons can be accomplished through comparisons of goodness-of-fit statistics evaluated for two alternative models where one is a restricted version of the other. The positive difference in the test statistics is known to be asymptotically distributed as a chi-square random variable with degrees of freedom equal to the difference in degrees of freedom of the alternative models (Jöreskog et al., 1981).

GENETIC APPLICATIONS

Measurement Model

We now can turn to a more detailed description of each portion of the general model as it applies to quantitative genetic research. We have seen, through equation 1 (a,b), how multiple measures of a trait can be used to define a common factor independent of measurement error. In the analysis of continuous traits, parameter estimates may be attenuated if measurement error is not taken into account. For example, heritability will be underestimated due to confounding of measurement error in the estimate of random environmental influences. Error variance may be small when due to sources such as instrument error or investigator error in measurement of physical traits such as height, weight, or blood pressure. When repeated measures are available, reliability of a measure may be assessed by the relative size of factor loadings (i.e., in the Λ matrix) and residual variances ($\underset{\sim}{\epsilon}_x$).

In contrast, error variance may be large when the phenotype of interest is more difficult to measure as in the case of behavioral traits. In this case, consistency of a measure relative to other measures becomes increasingly important. For example, a behavioral disorder such as alcoholism may be defined through a variety of measures such as degree and duration of heavy drinking, life crises related to drinking or "loss of control" while drinking (Jellinek, 1979). When multiple measures are thought to covary due to the phenotype of interest, the measures can be incorporated through equation 1 of the general model and the construct validity of the measures (relative to one another) can be assessed by goodness of fit of the model and relative size of factor loadings and residuals.

In both applications of the measurement model, a "true" phenotype (ξ or η) independent of measurement error can be defined from which genetic and environmental influences are estimated through the components of variance model. Ad hoc corrections for attenuation are available which involve taking functions of parameter estimates using the reliability coefficient of a measure (Rao et al., 1974). However, through simultaneous inclusion of a measurement model and genetic estimation, estimates are disattenuated by a statistically correct procedure (Jöreskog, 1974).

Components of Variance Model

As previously mentioned, it is through the components of variance portion of the model that genetic issues are represented. Jöreskog (1978) and Wiley et al. (1973) have shown how analysis of variance designs can be represented in structural equation models. When known degrees of genetic relatedness are introduced through specific sampling designs, variance components can be defined that have genetic interpretations as specified by theory (Kempthorne, 1957). Any familial sampling represented in an analysis of variance design can be parameterized in the components of variance portion of our general model. We have utilized the approach for full-sib, half-sib sampling and will discuss the components of variance model for this sampling condition in a later section.

Li (1981) and Kempthorne (1957) have described how full-sib, half-sib sampling can be represented in a nested random effects analysis of variance design. This design is shown schematically in Figure 1. The present depiction is that of paternal half-sibs. As can be seen in Figure 1, four offspring are measured on a trait X. Each offspring is from a sibship of size four having a common father i and within which two sets of full siblings each share a mother j or j'. The random effect model for a phenotype of the kth

child of father i and mother j is assumed to be

$$X_{ijk} = \mu + \tau_i + \tau_{ij} + e_{ijk}.$$

The population mean of the trait is the constant μ; the effect due to father i is τ_i with variance σ^2_τ; the effect due to mother ij is τ_{ij} with variance $\sigma^2_{\tau ij}$. The residual effect, e_{ijk}, has variance $\sigma^2_{e ijk}$ which represents the variation for individual k in sibship ij.

Father i			
Mother j		Mother j'	
Offspring k	Offspring k'	Offspring k''	Offspring k'''
X_{ijk}	$X_{ijk'}$	$X_{ij'k''}$	$X_{ij'k'''}$

Figure 1. Illustration of the notation of the full-sib, half-sib design for paternal half-sibs where four offspring are measured on a single trait (variable) X.

Under classic analysis of variance, parameters of the model can be estimated by ordinary least squares, and observed mean squares equated to their expections in order to solve, in a second step, for variance components (Kempthorne, 1957). This same design can be incorporated in our general formulation through the components of variance portion (equation 2 a,b). The components of variance portion can be represented schematically as in Figure 2. Boxes represent vectors of observed variables (phenotype X) measured on offsprings k through k''' in a sibship of size four sharing parent i (father, for paternal half-sibs; mother, for maternal half-sibs) with full-sibs further sharing parent j or j'. It should be noted that this is a specialized case of the measurement model where $\Lambda_x = I$ and $\underset{\sim}{\varepsilon}_x = 0$. If there are multiple measures of a trait then components of variance can be defined from unobserved common factors of the measures. The (unobserved) random effects τ_i and τ_{ij} are denoted by circles and are defined from the full-sib, half-sib sampling via the design matrix. The design matrix G_X is represented in Figure 2 by single headed arrows weighted by 1's. The residual variance is represented in $\underset{\sim}{e}$.

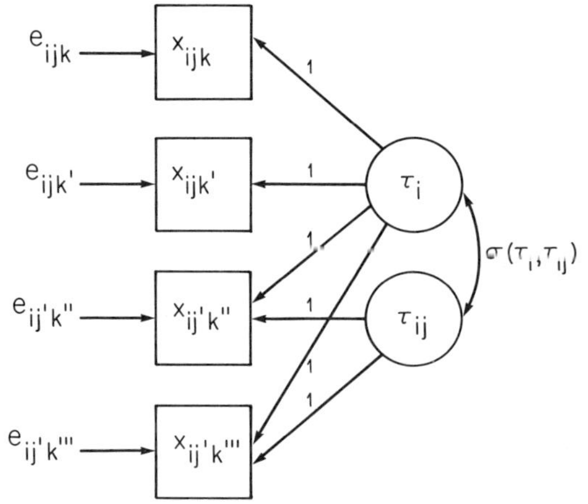

Figure 2. Illustration of full-sib, half-sib components of variance model. Variance components τ_i and τ_{ij} are defined from four offspring (X_{ijk}, $X_{ijk'}$, $X_{ij'k''}$, and $X_{ij'k'''}$) sharing parent i and parent j or j'.

The variance components have genetic interpretations as specified by theory and are shown in Table 1. The variance component estimates represent variances from sources of familial environmental effects as well as genetic effects. Heritability estimates thus can be derived as functions of variance components (Kempthorne, 1957). For example, narrow heritability, the proportion of phenotypic variance that is additive, may be found by taking $4\sigma^2_{\tau i}$ and dividing by the

Table 1. Genetic components reflected by variance components under full-sib, half-sib sampling (illustrated for paternal half-sib).

Source of Variation	Variance Component	Genetic Component
Between father	$\sigma^2_{\tau i}$	$\frac{1}{4}V_A + 1/16V_{AA} + \ldots V_{E_{t(f)}}$
Between mothers within fathers	$\sigma^2_{\tau ij}$	$\frac{1}{4}V_A + \frac{1}{4}V_D + 1/8V_{AD} + 3/16V_{AA} + \ldots + V_{E_{t(m)}} + V_{E_C}$
Between offspr. within mothers within fathers	$\sigma^2_{e ijk}$	$\frac{1}{2}V_A + 3/4V_D + 3/4V_{AA} + 7/8V_{AD} + 15/16V_{DD} + \ldots + V_{E_S}$

V_A = additive genetic variance.

V_D = non-additive genetic variance.

$V_{E_{t(f)}}$ = transmissible environmental effect (due to fathers).

$V_{E_{t(m)}}$ = transmissible environmental effect (due to mothers).

V_{E_C} = non-transmissible familial environmental effect.

V_{E_S} = specific environmental effect (non-familial).

V_{AA}, V_{AD}, V_{DD} ... represent epistatic effects.

total variance. Broad heritability, the proportion of phenotypic variance that is genetic, may be found by taking $4\sigma^2_{\tau ij}$ and dividing by the total phenotypic variance (Kempthorne, 1957). Heritability will be overestimated when familial environmental effects are present.

Through specification of variance components in the structural equation model, certain necessary restrictions in classic analysis of variance can be relaxed. As demonstrated by Wiley et al. (1973), the matrix of residuals need not be diagonal or homoscedastic. Furthermore, they have shown that the matrix of random effects need not be diagonal. These assumptions can be tested by a goodness-of-fit test using the present approach. The residuals $\underset{\sim}{e}_x$ or $\underset{\sim}{e}_y$ under full-sib, half-sib sampling represents genetic as well as environmental sources of variance (see Table 1). Unequal residual variances may reflect variations in specific (non-familial) environmental influences among siblings in a sibship. Such variation may be of interest in determining the etiology of a trait if sibling order (k through k''') corresponds to birth order or other systematic sources of variance. For the full-sib, half-sib sampling design, the covariance between the random effects τ_i and τ_{ij} reflects genetic covariance due to assortative mating when transmissible environmental effects are absent (Li, 1981). This parameter may be estimated and tested in the present context unlike the classic analysis of variance approach.

While representation of the components of variance model has been illustrated for a single trait, it can be extended to the multivariate case as shown in Figure 3. Here, the components of variance model with full-sib, half-sib sampling is defined for two traits ${}_1X$ and ${}_2X$. The genetic covariance between traits is represented by the covariance parameter $\sigma({}_1\tau_i,\ {}_2\tau_i)$ and $\sigma({}_1\tau_{ij},\ {}_2\tau_{ij})$. The former represents the covariance of linear genetic effects (under a simple model of no familial environmental effects) while the latter represents the covariance of linear and non-linear genetic effects. Genetic covariance can be tested by model comparisons of a restricted model where $\sigma({}_1\tau_i, {}_2\tau_i) = \sigma({}_1\tau_{ij}, {}_2\tau_{ij}) = 0$ against a less restricted model where these parameters are estimated. From the components of variance model, variance components that have genetic interpretations can be defined for one or more traits. Structural relationships among these variance components can be specified and tested using the third part of the general model, the simultaneous regression model among latent variables (Equation 3).

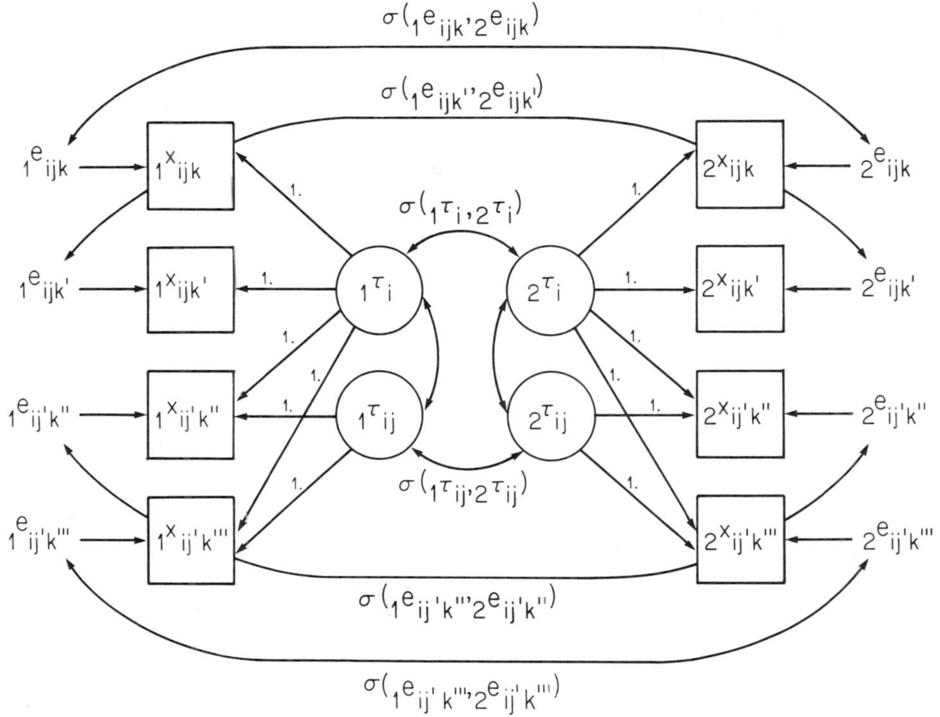

Figure 3. Illustration of full-sib, half-sib sampling and variance components defined for two traits, glucose tolerance (${}_1X$) and body mass index (${}_2X$). Variance components are denoted by τ's and residual effects by e's. Observed variables are represented by squares with unobserved variables represented by circles.

Regression Model

Through utilization of specific sampling designs random variables can be defined through the components of variance model that reflect genetic or environmental sources of variance. Hypothesized relationships among such variables can be tested using the simultaneous linear regression portion of the general model (3). The application of this part of the model may be best understood through a hypothetical example. Consider the full-sib, half-sib design previously discussed. A hypothetical depiction of this sampling design on three different traits is shown in Figure 4. The single headed arrows among the variance components (τ and v) represent the hypothesized structural relations among the three traits. In this hypothetical example, the linear genetic component (τ_i) of one trait is proposed to account for linear genetic covariance among the other two (v_i's). The same applies to the linear plus dominance component (i.e., τ_{ij} is proposed as a "cause" of covariance of ${}_1v_{ij}$ and ${}_2v_{ij}$). This representation might be appropriate when pleiotropic effects are suspected and genetic covariance of two traits is thought to be due to genetic variation underlying a third.

A second application may be in the specification of concomitant variables and their effects. For example, it may be that the random effects τ_i and τ_{ij} shown in Figure 4 do not represent linear and linear-plus-dominance genetic effects, respectively. If the independent variable was age, for example, the random effects would not have a genetic interpretation in the full-sib, half-sib design. If the age effects on a trait are linear, the random effects under the full-sib, half-sib design would reflect between sibship and between full-sibs within sibship age effects, respectively. Suppose that the closer two individuals are in age, the greater their covariance on two traits (e.g., height and weight). If full-sibs tend to be closer in age than half-sibs, this differential age effect may be removed from the covariance of two traits through regression of the genetic variance components on the age effects.

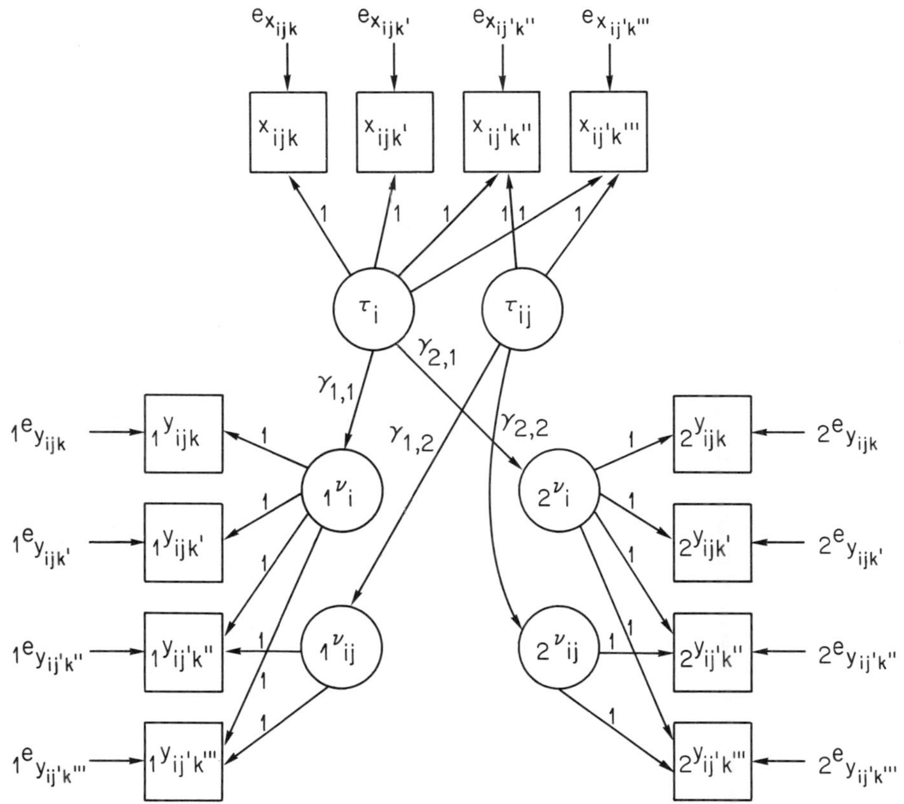

Figure 4. Schematic diagram for three traits, one exogenous (x) and two endogenous ($_1Y$, $_2Y$), measured under a full-sib, half-sib design with four offspring.

APPLICATIONS

We have applied the covariance structure model of equations (1,2,3) to data on body build and glucose tolerance in the Pima Indians. We initially applied the methodology using full-sib, half-sib sampling without parental scores. Discussion of this initial application is presented in the following section with a subsequent section containing a discussion of a preliminary application including parental scores.

FULL-SIB, HALF-SIB SAMPLING WITHOUT PARENTAL SCORES

We used a specialized case of the general model to examine genetic covariance of glucose tolerance and obesity among the Pima Indians of Arizona. Obesity and non-insulin dependent diabetes are highly prevalent among the Pima (Knowler, 1981; Bennett et al., 1971). The association of hyperglycemia (and diabetes) with obesity has been addressed using animal studies as well as research on humans (Roth et al., 1981; Stern et al., 1985). Obesity and non-insulin dependent diabetes each appear to have a genetic component as evidenced from familial studies, twin studies and animal models (Rotter et al., 1981; Smith et al., 1972; Langenbeck et al., 1976). The association of diabetes and obesity might be due to a common set of genes contributing to the two traits. We tested this hypothesis using full-sib, half-sib sampling and the components of variance model previously discussed.

Data

Subjects were selected from a larger data base collected by the National Institute of Arthritis, Diabetes, and Digestive and Kidney Diseases (NIADDK) and an Indian Health Service Sanitation Survey during 1968 and 1972 on the Gila River Indian community. Subjects were selected for this analysis that met the full-sib, half-sib criterion previously discussed. In review, the criterion is that each subject be from a sibship of at least size four sharing a common parent i within which two sets of full-siblings further share a common parent j or j'. Twenty maternal and sixteen paternal cases were identified.

We used glucose tolerance scores rather than diabetic classification for the present analysis. We were interested in examining the possible genetic covariance of degree of obesity and degree of glucose tolerance rather than diabetes per se. Glucose tolerance was measured by the NIADDK group by plasma glucose levels two hours following a 75 gram oral carbohydrate load (Ritenbaugh, 1974). Obesity was measured by the body mass index, WT/HT^2 where weight is measured in kilograms and height in meters. Glucose tolerance and body mass index scores were standardized within age and sex groupings to remove the effects of age and sex (DeFries et al., 1979; Rao et al., 1975).

The covariance matrix of standardized scores was analyzed using the structural equation model previously presented. Multiple measures of each trait (glucose tolerance and obesity) were not available; thus, the measurement model is a specialized case of the general form where $\Lambda_x = I$ and $\tilde{\epsilon}_x = 0$. The computer program LISREL V was used to compute parameter estimation and test statistics (Jöreskog and Sörbom, 1981).

Results

Univariate statistics of the standardized scores of glucose tolerance and body mass index within each sibling vector are shown in Table 2. The age groups used for standardization were 5 to 14, 15 to 24, and 25 and over. The sample ranged in age from 5 to 74 years with a mean age of 19.5 years and a median age of 15. The sample consists of 60 males and 84 females. While kurtosis values are somewhat larger than zero for two of the sibling vectors, (Xij'k'',Xij'k'''), the arithmetic average of kurtosis values for all variables is .335. This small value coupled with a visual inspection of a bivariate scatter plot of body mass index and glucose tolerance standardized scores did not provide evidence to reject the assumption of normality.

The model proposed to account for the observed

variation and covariation of glucose tolerance and obesity among the Pima is shown in Figure 3. As the goodness of fit test statistics for the model (X^2 = 30.11; d.f. = 16) is smaller than the specified cutoff criterion of 31.99 at the .01 level, the model is accepted as a plausible explanation of observed association of glucose tolerance and obesity in the Pima.

Table 2. Descriptive statistics of standarized scores (by age and sex grouping) for glucose tolerance and body mass index.

Trait	Sibling Vector	N	Mean	s.d.	Kurtosis
Glucose	$_1X_{ijk}$	36	-.288	.93	- .17
Tolerance	$_1X_{ijk'}$	36	.169	1.05	- .89
	$_1X_{ij'k''}$	36	.203	1.11	2.05
	$_1X_{ij'k'''}$	36	-.083	.74	2.05
Body	$_2X_{ijk}$	36	-.121	.91	.51
Mass	$_2X_{ijk'}$	36	.206	.90	- .60
Index	$_2X_{ij'k''}$	36	.124	1.20	-1.10
	$_2X_{ij'k'''}$	36	-.209	.87	.83

$_1X$ = observed exogenous variable for trait 1.
$_2X$ = observed exogenous variable for trait 2.

We tested the hypotheses of genetic covariance and environmental covariance through model comparisons. The goodness-of-fit statistics and results of model comparisons are shown in Table 3. The significance of non-familial environmental covariance as a parameter in the model is tested by constraining residual covariances across traits to zero and comparing the resulting chi-square value with the chi-square value of the less restricted design (i.e., where the covariance parameters are free). This model comparison (Model 1 vs. Model 2) is shown in Table 3. The chi-square difference is significant at the .01 level ($X^2 = 20.55$; d.f. = 4) and the null hypothesis of no environmental covariance is not rejected.

Table 3. Chi-square values and chi-square difference tests of alternative models.

Model	X^2	d.f.	Prob.
Model 1 (Figure 3)	30.11	16	.0174
Model 2 $\sigma({}_1e, {}_2e) = 0$	50.66	20	.0002
Model 3 $\sigma({}_1\tau_i, {}_2\tau_i) = 0$ $\sigma({}_1\tau_{ij}, {}_2\tau_{ij}) = 0$	30.97	18	.0290
Model Comparisons:			
(1) vs. (2)	20.55	4	<.0001
(1) vs. (3)	.86	2	>.5

We tested the hypothesis of no genetic covariance by constraining parameters $\sigma({}_1\tau_i, {}_2\tau_i) = \sigma({}_1\tau_{ij}, {}_2\tau_{ij}) = 0$ and comparing the chi-square value for this model with the less restricted model where parameters are free. The model comparison (Model 3 vs. Model 1), shown in Table 3 resulted in a chi-square difference value ($X^2 = .86$; d.f. = 2) that is less than the specified cutoff criterion and the genetic covariance parameters are accepted as zero. This model, designated Model 3, was used for all subsequent analyses.

Parameter estimates based on Model 3 are shown in Table 4. Heritability estimates based on these parameter estimates were found using the approach specified earlier. Narrow heritability estimates are

Table 4. Parameter estimates for model 3.

Trait	Residual variance	Components of Variance	Components of Covariance
Glucose Tolerance:			
$_1X_{ijk}$	.701±.224	.129±.150	-.182±.181
$_1X_{ijk'}$	1.018±.286		
$_1X_{ij'k''}$	.829±.277	.635±.292	
$_1X_{ij'k'''}$	.192±.131		
Body Mass Index:			
$_2X_{ijk}$	.626±.194	.195±.128	-.220±.160
$_2X_{ijk'}$	.612±.192		
$_2X_{ij'k''}$	1.149±.313	.594±.288	
$_2X_{ij'k'''}$	.383±.184		
Environmental covariances:			
$cov(_1e_{ijk}, {_2e_{ijk}})$ = .259±.141			
$cov(_1e_{ijk'}, {_2e_{ijk'}})$ = .331±.166			
$cov(_1e_{ij'k''}, {_2e_{ij'k''}})$ = .284±.201			
$cov(_1e_{ij'k'''}, {_2e_{ij'k'''}})$ = .258±.104			

$_1X$ reflects observed variable for first trait.
$_2X$ reflects observed variable for second trait.
$_1e$ reflects residual for first trait.
$_2e$ reflects residual for second trait.

0.356 and 0.526 for glucose tolerance and body mass index, respectively. Broad heritability estimates are 1.753 and 1.604 for glucose tolerance and body mass index, respectively. Environmental covariance estimates range from .258 to .331 with an average environmental correlation of .411. The covariance parameter between the variance components (τ_i and τ_{ij}) within traits are -.182 and -.220 for glucose tolerance and body mass index, respectively. This corresponds to correlations of -.6359 and -.6464, respectively.

Discussion

The association of glucose tolerance and obesity as measured by WT/HT^2 does not appear to be due to a common set of genes influencing the two traits. Our findings indicate that the covariance is primarily due to non-familial environmental effects. Familial factors appear significant in the development of both glucose tolerance and obesity as evidenced in broad heritability estimates greater than one. As familial environmental effects are indistinguishable from non-additive genetic effects in the full-sib, half-sib design, we can only deduce the presence of such effects from the broad heritability value being greater than one. To the extent that such familial environmental effects are transmissible, inclusion of parental scores may more clearly elucidate the issue. The negative covariance observed between the linear and linear plus dominance variance components for both traits may indicate the presence of assortative mating. As the covariance term reflects genetic covariation between mates under a simple genetic model, this covariance may be due to non-random mating in the population. Interpretation of this negative covariance may be clarified through inclusion of parental scores.

FULL-SIB, HALF-SIB SAMPLING WITH PARENTAL SCORES

Our second application of the covariance structure model is to data on obesity in the Pima obtained using between and within generation sampling, in this case, full-siblings, half-siblings and parents.

Data

As the data were not collected by NIADDK under this sampling design, there were only seven complete cases in the larger data base made available to us. Complete cases are ones in which at least four offspring under full-sib half-sib sampling as well as all three parents are measured. Since we were interested in illustrating the approach, we selected incomplete family sets as well as the complete family sets and estimated missing data. We selected family sets for this analysis if at least three of the four offspring under the full-sib, half-sib design (see Figure 1 for review) and all three parents (i.e. common parent i, parent j, and parent j') were measured or all four offspring and at least two of the three parents were measured. The resulting sample consists of 41 families with 25 paternal and 16 maternal cases. Obesity was measured as in the previous analysis by the body mass index (WT(kg)/HT(m)^2). Body mass index scores were standardized by age and sex groupings to remove age and sex effects. Age groupings were 5 to 14, 15 to 24, 25 to 34, 35 to 44 and 45 and older. We estimated missing data (with one score being the maximal number of values per family) using a two step regression procedure (BMD PAM, 1983).

The model proposed to explain the variation and covariation of body build among parent-offspring, full-sibs, and half-sibs is shown in Figure 5. In contrast with the earlier components of variance model on siblings without parental score (Figure 2), there are three additional vectors of observed scores (X_i, X_j, and $X_{j'}$) in the present representation. These are vectors of observed scores of common parent i and first and second mates of parent i, parent j or j'. Through specification of fixed values in the design matrix, represented by single headed arrows weighted by 1.0's or .5's in Figure 5, variance components are defined that reflect genetic parameters as specified by theory.

The variance components, τ_1, τ_2, and τ_3, represent linear genetic effects that contribute to parent-offspring resemblance on a trait. The effects,

τ_4, τ_5, τ_6 reflect environmental influences on parental phenotypes. These are fixed at 1.0 in the present analysis and variance components are found from the square of the path values denoted by g_1, g_2, and g_3. The linear contribution of parental environmental influences on an offspring's phenotype is reflected in the path value of the offspring's phenotype (e.g. X_{ijk}) on parent's environment (τ_4, τ_5, or τ_6). Residual or specific environmental influences to an offspring's phenotype are represented by e's in Figure 5. Variance components τ_7 and τ_8 reflect non-additive gene effects (dominance) and/or non-transmissible, familial environmental effects that are assumed to contribute to the covariance of full-siblings but not half-siblings. Genetic covariance due to non-random mating is reflected in the covariance among linear genetic effects of the parents (e.g. $\sigma(\tau_1, \tau_2)$).

Table 5. Univariate statistics of age and sex standardized body mass index scores by vectors of parental (X_i, X_j, $X_{j'}$) or sibling (X_{ijk}, $X_{ijk'}$, $X_{ijk'''}$) scores.

Sib or parental vector	N	$\bar{X}$	s.d.	Skewness	Kurtosis
X_i	40	0.048	1.118	0.79	0.96
X_j	34	0.125	0.825	0.37	0.43
$X_{j'}$	33	0.192	0.853	0.03	-0.47
X_{ijk}	37	0.057	1.080	0.52	-0.68
$X_{ijk'}$	37	-0.278	0.958	1.16	0.59
$X_{ij'k''}$	37	0.119	0.888	0.71	0.25
$X_{ij'k'''}$	35	-0.258	1.039	0.62	-0.51

Results

Univariate statistics of the standardized body mass index scores by parent and sibling vectors are shown in Table 5. The sample age range is from 5 to 75 years. Body mass index scores after standardization by age and sex groupings range from -2.23 to 3.65.

The goodness-of-fit of the model represented in Figure 5 on body mass in the Pima is shown in Table 6 and labelled Model 1. The chi-square value of 19.94 for this model is less than the specified chi-square value of 29.14 at the .01 level with 14 degrees of freedom and the model is accepted as a plausible explanation of the observed variation of body build in the Pima. This model (depicted in Figure 5) contains various genetic and environmental sources of variation (e.g., dominance, transmissible environmental effects, assortative mating). We tested the significance of such genetic and environmental parameters through model comparisons. Results of these model comparisons are also shown in Table 6.

The first model comparison (Model 1 vs. Model 2) is a test of the significance of any covariance of linear genetic effects among parents (a possible consequence of non-random mating).

Significance of these covariance parameters is tested by constraining $\sigma(\tau_1, \tau_2) = \sigma(\tau_1, \tau_3) = \sigma(\tau_2, \tau_3) = 0$ and comparing the resulting chi-square value with the chi-square value of the less restricted model where these parameters are free. The chi-square difference for this model comparison (Model 1 vs. Model 2, Table 6) is not significant ($\chi^2 = 2.25$, d.f. = 3) and we accept these parameters as zero in the population.

We next tested the effect of dominance and/or familial non-transmissible environmental influences through constraining $\tau_7 = \tau_8 = 0$ and computing the chi-square difference for this model against the less restricted model where these parameters are estimated. The chi-square difference for this model comparison (Model 2 vs. Model 3, Table 6) is not significant at

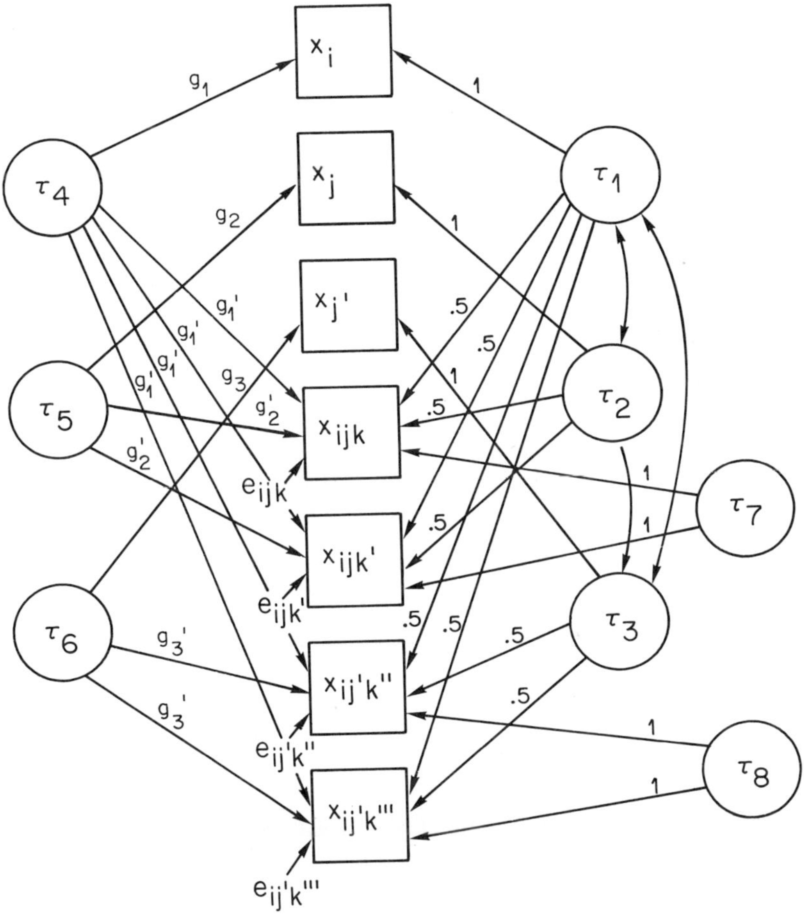

Figure 5. Illustration of full-sib, half-sib sampling with parental scores on a single trait (variable), X.

the .01 level (X^2 = .33, d.f. = 1) and the parameters are accepted as zero in the population.

Table 6. Model comparisons and goodness-of-fit statistics for body mass index scores among partent-offspring, full-sib and half- sib in the Pima Indians.

Model	X^2	d.f.	Prob.
(1) G, E_t, E_c, D, and Assort.	19.94	14	.132
(2) G, E_t, E_c & D	22.21	17	.177
(3) G, E_t	22.54	18	.209
(4) G	25.81	20	.172
Model Comparisons:			
No assort. mat. (1 vs. 2)	2.27	3	.4
No E_c and D (2 vs. 3)	.33	1	.5
No E_t (3 vs. 4)	3.27	2	.1

G = genetic effects
E_t = transmissible environmental effects
E_c = non-transmissible familial environmental effects
D = non-additive genetic effects (i.e., dominance)
Assort = assortative mating

The final comparison is a test of the hypothesis that the observed covariation of parent with offspring and sibling with sibling on body build among the Pima can be explained by a genetic model without transmissible environmental effects. The model comparison (Model 3 vs. Model 4) is a comparison of the restricted model where $g_1' = g_2' = g_3' = 0$ against the less restricted model where these parameters are free. Since the parameters g_1', g_2', g_3' reflect the regression of an offspring's phenotype on parental environment independent of genetic effects, constraining these parameters to zero and evaluating the chi-square difference (against the less restricted model where the parameters are free) is a test of the significance of one type of transmissible environmental influence. The chi-square difference for this model comparison is not significant at the 0.01 level (X^2 = 3.27, d.f. = 2) and the genetic model is accepted as a sufficient explanation of the covariation of body mass index values in the Pima. Parameter estimates based on this model (Model 4) are shown in Table 7.

Table 7. Parameter estimates based on the genetic model for body mass index scores in the Pima under full-sib, half-sib sampling with parental scores.

Parameters in the model	Parameter estimates (±s.e.)	Variance components	Variance component estimates
$\tau_1=\tau_2=\tau_3$	.283±.110	L	.283
g_1	1.032±.142	e_i*	1.065
g_2	.618±.132	e_j*	.382
g_3	.687±.130	$e_{j'}$*	.472
e_{ijk}	.878±.215	e_{ijk}	.878
$e_{ijk'}$	.812±.200	$e_{ijk'}$	.812
$e_{ij'k''}$	.583±.151	$e_{ij'k''}$	.583
$e_{ij'k'''}$	1.031±.249	$e_{ijk'k'''}$	1.031

L = linear genetic effects
e = environmental effects (non-transmissible, non-familial)
* = variance components found by squaring correspon-ding parameters (e.g., g_1)

The linear genetic variance is estimated to be 0.283 ± 0.110 with an environmental contribution (averaged over parents and offspring) of .746. The total phenotypic variance is equal to .283 + .746 = 1.029. The proportion of phenotypic variance due to additive gene effects based on these values is 27.5%.

Discussion

In contrast to our earlier findings based on full-sib, half-sib sampling without parental scores, the estimate of narrow heritability for body mass index in the present analysis is .275 compared to the earlier value of .526. It should be noted that any conclusions based on this second analysis should be considered with caution since the data set consists in part of estimated missing values. Nevertheless, the findings raise some interesting issues that should be addressed in future research using between and within generational data.

First, estimates of additive genetic variance (and subsequently heritability) may be larger under full-sib, half-sib sampling without parental scores than with parental scores if familial environmental effects due to a common parent increase the covariance of siblings but not parent-offspring. Falconer (1981) discusses this type of maternal (or parental) effect for tail length in mice and the relationship with nest temperature. In this example, nest temperature (a maternal effect) increases the covariance among siblings in tail length but does not influence the covariance between mother and offspring tail length. If such environmental covariances (due to a common parent) are present for body mass index among the Pima, the estimates of heritability derived from functions of the variance component estimates (under full-sib and half-sib sampling without parental scores) will be overestimated by four times this amount. Second, we know that major environmental changes, in nutritional as well as health care, have occurred among the Pima over the period covered by the ages of subjects in our sample. This could reduce parent-offspring covariances without reducing sibling covariances and lead to a difference in heritability estimates based on sibling sampling compared to parent-offspring sampling. Third, in the first application (full-sib, half-sib sampling), dominance and/or common environmental (non-transmissible) influences were indicated from the broad heritability estimate being greater than one. However, through model comparisons in our second application (using full-sib, half-sib sampling with parental scores), common environmental and/or dominance effects were not significant. This may, in part, be due to the estimation of missing data in the second application (which would tend to reduce full sibling covariance) and should be considered with caution. From consideration of the standard error of the variance component estimate representing common environmental and/or dominance under full-sib, half-sib sampling (i.e., $\sigma_{\tau_{ij}}$ = .594 ± .288), the presence of common environmental and/or dominance is indicated. Future applications of the present methodology to obesity data without missing values may clarify this issue.

SUMMARY

In this paper, we have presented a general covariance structure model for quantitative genetic research that incorporates measurement theory, components of variance, and regression theory for specification of structural relations among variance components. Each portion of the general model addresses specific issues important in delineating the genetic etiology of continuous traits. Through specification of a measurement model, genetic and environmental influences can be estimated independently of measurement error. Genetic and environmental sources of variance are defined from familial sampling designs through the components of variance model. Structural relationships among several traits at the genetic or environmental level can be specified through the regression model. The significance of parameters specified in each part of the model can be tested through model comparisons using a likelihood ratio chi-square test. We utilized the general model to test genetic covariance as a source of observed covariation of obesity and glucose tolerance in the Pima Indians. We initially applied the modeling approach using full-sib, half-sib sampling among the Pima with a second application including offspring as well as parental scores.

Our initial applications of the methodology suggest that the covariance structure model can be a useful tool in genetic epidemiological research. Through model comparisons, our findings suggest that the association of glucose tolerance and obesity in the Pima is not due to a common set of genes but rather due to non-familial environmental influences. In conclusion, one task important for future research, as we see it, is the application of covariance structure models to other familial sampling designs and the evaluation of the usefulness of this approach through further applications to data.

ACKNOWLEDGEMENTS

The authors wish to thank the members of the Gila River Indian Community for their patience and assistance in these studies. We thank the staff of the Southwestern Field Studies Section, National Institute of Arthritis, Diabetes, and Digestive and Kidney Diseases for making the field data available. These persons are not responsible for the interpretation, or possible errors, in the present study.

This research was supported in part by a grant from the U.S. Public Health Service, DA01070.

LITERATURE CITED

Bennett PH, Burch TA, Miller M (1971). Diabetes mellitus in American (Pima) Indians. Lancet ii:125.
Biomedical Computer Programs P-Series (1983). Berkeley, CA: University of California Press.
Browne MW (1984). Asymptotically distribution-free methods for the analysis of covariance structures. Brit J of Math & Stat Psych 37:62.
DeFries JG, Johnson RC, Kuse AR, McClearn GE, Polovina J, Vandenberg SG, Wilson JR (1979). Familial resemblance for specific cognitive abilities. Behavior Genetics 9:23.
Eaves LJ, Last KA, Young PA, Martin NG (1978). Model-fitting approaches to the analysis of human behavior. Heredity 11:249.
Eaves LJ, Gale JS (1974). A method for analyzing the genetic basis of covariation. Behavior Genetics 4:253.
Fisher RA (1918). The correlation between relatives on

the supposition of Mendelian inheritance. Trans Roy Soc Edinburgh 52:399.
Goldberger AS, Duncan OD (1973). Structural Equation Models in the Social Sciences. New York: Academic Press.
Jellinek EM (1960). The Disease Concept of Alcoholism. New Haven, Ct: College and University Press.
Jöreskog KG (1969). A general approach to confirmatory maximum likelihood factor analysis. Psychometrika 34(2):183.
Jöreskog KG (1974). Analyzing psychological data by structural analysis of covariance matrices. In Krantz DH, Atkinson RC, Luce D, Suppes P (eds): "Measurement, Psychophysics and Neural Information Proceedings," San Francisco, Ca: W.H. Freeman, p 1.
Jöreskog KG (1978). Structural analysis of covariance and correlation matrices. Psychometrika 43:443.
Jöreskog KG, Sörbom D (1981). LISREL V: Analysis of Linear Structural Relationships by the Method of Maximum Likelihood. Chicago: National Education Resources.
Kempthorne O (1957). An Introduction to Genetic Statistics. New York: Wiley and Sons.
Knowler WC, Pettitt DJ, Savage PJ, Bennett PH (1981). Diabetes incidence in Pima Indians: Contributions of obesity and parental diabetes. Am J Epid 113:114.
Langenbeck V, Jorgensen G (1976). The genetics of diabetes mellitus:A review of twin studies. In Creutzfeldt W, Köbberling J, Neel JV (eds):"Genetics of Diabetes Mellitus," Berlin: Springer-Verlag, p 21.
Li CC (1981). Half-sib analysis of quantitative data. In Mielke JH, Crawford MH (eds): "Current Developments in Anthropological Genetics," New York: Plenum, p 373.
Martin NG, Eaves LJ (1977). The genetical analysis of covariance structure. Heredity 38:79.
Morton NE (1974). Analysis of family resemblance I. Introduction. Am J Hum Genet 26:318.
Rao DC, Morton NE, Yee S (1974). Analysis of family resemblance. II. A linear model for familial correlation. Am J Hum Genet 26:331.
Rao DC, MacLean CJ, Morton NE, Yee S (1975). Analysis of family resemblance. V. Height and weight in Northeastern Brazil. Am J Hum Genet 27:509.

Ritenbaugh C (1974). The Pattern of Diabetes in Pima Community. Ph.D. Thesis, University of California, Los Angeles.
Roth G, Muggeo M (1981). Insulin receptors and hyperglycemia. In Rifkin H, Raskin P (eds): "Diabetes Mellitus," Vol V, New York: American Diabetes Association, p 63.
Rotter JI, Rimoin DL (1981). Etiology-genetics. In Brownlee M (ed): "Handbook of Diabetes Mellitus," New York: Garland STPM Press, p 3.
Smith C, Falconer DS, Duncan LJP (1972). A statistical and genetical study of diabetes:II. Heritability of liability. Ann Hum Genet 35:281.
Stern J, Johnson PR, Batchelor BR, Zucker LM, Hirsch J (1975). Pancreatic insulin release and peripheral tissue resistance in Zucker obese rats fed high and low carbohydrate diets. Am J Physiology 228:543.
Wiley DE, Schmidt WH, Bramble WJ (1973). Studies of a class of covariance structure models. J Am Stat Assoc 68:317.
Woodward JA, Bonett DG, Cullian L (1981). The generalizability of latent variables (unpublished manuscript). University of California, Los Angeles.
Wright S (1921). Correlation and causation. J Agricultural Res 20:557.

Diseases of Complex Etiology in Small Populations:
Ethnic Differences and Research Approaches, pages 97–102

Chapter 5

EFFICIENCY OF RECOMBINATION ESTIMATES USING TWO-AND THREE-POINT LINKAGE DATA

G.M. Lathrop and J.M. Lalouel

Laboratoire d'Anthropologie Biologique, Université de Paris 7, Paris, France

INTRODUCTION

The increasing number of identified DNA polymorphisms leads to new problems of multilocus estimation of recombination, gene mapping, and calculation of genetic risks. As illustrated with Duchenne muscular dystrophy (Wieacker et al., 1983), flanking markers increase the precision of risk calculations.

MULTIPOINT LINKAGE ANALYSIS

The utility of multipoint rather than pairwise linkage analysis to obtain estimates of the recombination fractions rests on the related question of statistical efficiency. This will depend on interference, penetrance of alleles at the marker loci, and order on the chromosome. Bailey (1961) discusses classical multipoint linkage analysis restricted to particular genetic systems and mapping types. Recently, Meyers et al. (1976) have introduced three-point linkage of family data in human genetics for inference of order of codominant allelic systems. The program LINKAGE, available from us upon request, implements multipoint linkage analysis for arbitrary genetic systems and pedigree data.

The relative efficiency of various strategies of analysis can be studied by comparison of the large-sample variances and covariances of the recombination estimates given by the inverse of the expected information matrix. In the absence of interference and when the order of the loci on the chromosome is known, it can be shown that the likelihood of family data for a triple backcross involving codominant genetic systems factorizes into two components: one of which is a function of the recombination only in the first segment flanking the center marker, while the other is a function of the recombination only in the second segment. The information matrix is then diagonal, and the efficiency is not increased by analyzing simultaneously the linkage in the two segments. A similar result holds when the order is unknown or interference occurs, but not generally for all mating types or when the central locus has a rare recessive allele or incomplete penetrance.

To illustrate the latter, we consider nuclear families with two children and two-allelic flanking markers with allelic frequencies 0.5. The test locus consists of a rare disease allele with zero penetrance in heterozygotes, and either complete or 0.5 penetrance in homozygotes. Complete ascertainment of families with affected children is assumed. The expected information matrix, over all mating types, has been calculated numerically under the supposition that recombination rates between the flanking markers and the disease locus are both estimated, and interference does not occur.

Table 1 shows that the efficiency of the two-point linkage estimates compared to the three-point estimates for various values of the recombination fraction for one test locus, with the recombination for the second test locus fixed at 0.1. We recall that the efficiency can be defined as the ratio of the large-sample variance of three-point linkage estimate to that of the two-point estimate. With a penetrance of 0.5, the three-point estimate is more than twice as efficient as the two-point estimate for values of recombination in the range 0.05 to 0.15.

Three-point estimates may also be more efficient when the phenotype for the center locus is a quantitative measurement. As an example, we present some results obtained for Duchenne muscular dystrophy (DMD) using creatine kinase for carrier detection. Two pedigrees, illustrated in Figure 1, were obtained from actual counselling situations, and two flanking markers (designated A and B) were simulated to match those reported by Murray et al. (1982), and Davies et al. (1983). Parameters at the DMD locus were chosen in agreement with reported figures (Vogel and Moltulsky, 1981): a gene frequency of 0.0003, a mutation rate of 0.0001, and means and standard deviations in normal and obligate carrier women of 1.57, 0.242 and 2.10, 0.409, respectively (Morton and Lalouel, 1979).

Table 1. Efficiency of two- and three-point linkage estimates where recombination with the first test locus is fixed at 0.1.

Penetrance at the main locus	Efficiency for the estimate of	Recombination with the second test locus		
		0.05	0.10	0.15
1.0	First Rec.	0.698	0.819	0.894
	Second Rec.	0.861	0.819	0.797
0.5	First Rec.	0.483	0.668	0.802
	Second Rec.	0.780	0.668	0.591

The phenotypes at the test locus were generated randomly assuming that the proband's mother was informative for recombination at the A locus (allelic frequencies 0.85 and 0.15). Allelic frequencies at the B locus were assumed to be 0.70 and 0.30. The frequency of recombination with DMD locus was 0.15 in both cases. For simplicity in presenting the results, we will suppose that the recombination fraction is known for DMD and the B locus, and the other recombination is estimated.

Five replicates of a simulation of the flanking markers were generated for both pedigrees. In the simulation, DMD genotypes were assigned in agreement with affection status and creatine kinase values.

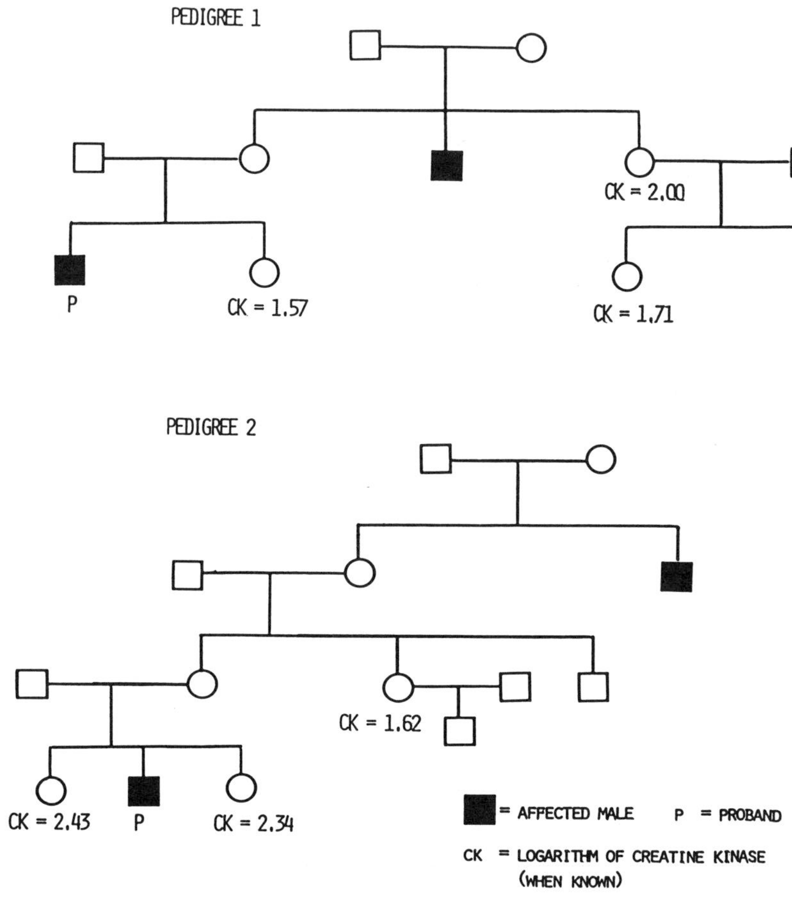

Figure 1. Duchenne Muscular Dystrophy pedigrees used for linkage analysis.

Table 2. Lod scores for five replicates of two pedigree types for Duchenne Muscular Dystrophy.

No. of Markers	Pedi-gree	Recombination Value 0.00	0.05	0.10	0.15	0.20	0.25	0.30	0.35	0.40	0.45
One	1	-0.96	0.65	0.94	0.98	0.92	0.82	0.68	0.53	0.36	0.19
	2	-6.06	-1.12	-0.22	0.20	0.41	0.49	0.50	0.44	0.34	0.19
	Total	-7.02	-0.47	0.71	1.18	1.33	1.31	1.18	0.97	0.70	0.38
Two	1	1.68	1.91	2.02	1.95	1.78	1.55	1.28	0.99	0.68	0.35
	2	-6.06	-0.82	0.06	0.50	0.71	0.79	0.77	0.67	0.50	0.28
	Total	-4.38	1.09	2.09	2.45	2.50	2.34	2.05	1.66	1.18	0.63

Thereafter, they were treated as unknown, and the recombination with the A locus was estimated with and without information from the B locus. The results are presented in Table 2. The inclusion of the B locus provides substantial information increasing the lod-score from a maximum of 1.33 to a maximum of 2.45 in the interval 0.15 to 0.20.

The results presented in this note show that in certain circumstances multipoint linkage analysis can be more efficient than two-point linkage analysis for the estimation of recombination rates. Treatment of multipoint linkage data for estimates of interference, and the order of genes on the chromosome will be considered elsewhere.

LITERATURE CITED

Bailey NTJ (1961). "Introduction to the Mathematical Theory of Genetic Linkage." Oxford: Oxford University Press.

Davies KE, Pearson PL, Harper PS, Murray JM, O'Brien T, Sarfarazi M, Williamson R (1983). Linkage analysis of two cloned DNA sequences flanking the Duchenne muscular dystrophy locus on the short arm of the human X chromosome. Nucleic Acid Res 11: 2303.

Murray JM, Davies KM, Harper PS, Meredith L, Mueller CR, Williamson R (1982). Linkage relationship of a cloned DNA sequence on the short arm of the X chromosome to Duchenne muscular dystrophy. Nature 300:69.

Morton NE, Lalouel JM (1979). Genetic counselling in sex linkage. Birth Defects: Original Article Series XV:9.

Meyers DA, Conneally PM, Lovrien EW, Magenis RF, Merritt AD, Norton JA, Palmer CG, Rivas ML, Wang L, Yu PL (1976). Linkage group 1: Simultaneous estimation of recombination and interference. Birth Defects: Original Article Series XII: 335.

Vogel F, Motulsky A (1981). "Human Genetics: Problems and Approaches." Berlin: Springer-Verlag.

Wieacker P, Davies K, Pearson P, Ropers HH (1983). Carrier detection in Duchenne muscular dystrophy by use of cloned DNA sequences. Lancet i:1326.

SECTION II
ETHNIC DIFFERENCES, RISK OF DISEASE, AND ROLE OF MIGRATION

Diseases of Complex Etiology in Small Populations:
Ethnic Differences and Research Approaches, pages 105–117

SECTION II. INTRODUCTORY REMARKS

E.J.E. Szathmary and R. Chakraborty

Ideas concerning the causes of different chronic diseases give rise to models that need to be tested. Epidemiologists are therefore interested in studying "natural experimental" situations, wherein the distribution of groups of people approximates a particular research design. For example, to detect whether environmental factors are important in the onset of a specific disease, one may wish to control the effect of genes. Increased or decreased disease incidence in a group compared to its genetic "control" could be attributed to environmental factors, if the latter are the only factors free to vary. This sort of rationale has led to the study of migrant populations, and to comparisons of morbidity rates between migrants, their hosts and the nonmigrants from which the migrants are derived (e.g. Reed et al., 1970; Syme et al., 1975; Beaglehole et al., 1977; Hanna and Baker, 1979). Traditionally it has been assumed that the migrants and nonmigrants are not heterogeneous on the critical variables, that is, in genotype, in morphology and in lifestyle associated traits which influence phenotype. Differences in morbidity between migrants and nonmigrants accumulate because of the effects of the altered environment in which the migrants reside, and eventually morbidity of and mortality from a given chronic disease in the migrants approximates that found in the host population. The appropriateness of the assumptions in such a research design have been challenged (e.g. McGarvey, 1983) and found wanting in some (e.g. Carter et al., 1984) though not in other instances (e.g. Stanhope and Prior, 1976). Hence studies of migrant populations continue to be regarded as an extremely useful research approach (e.g. DEW, 1981).

Population isolates, or ethnic minorities in certain geographic regions, comprise another category of "natural experiments" in which models of disease causation can be tested. For example, association of a particular chronic disease with a particular genetic marker could indicate that the allele, or an unknown allele at a closely linked locus confers some susceptibility to the disease (Thomson, 1981). Such an association, if it recurs consistently, at minimum identifies individuals at risk for the disease, and also serves to strengthen the validity of the causal hypothesis. One of the best known examples of such an association is that of ankylosing spondylitis with the B27 allele of the HLA region within the Major Histocompatibility Complex (MHC). The association is seen in unrelated Amerindians such as the Pima (Calin, 1982), Haida and Bella Coola (Gofton et al., 1975), Japanese, American Blacks, East Indians, and a variety of Caucasian ethnic groups (Ryder et al., 1979).

Population isolates that are undergoing the cultural transition loosely referred to as "Westernization" are also desirable units for epidemiological investigation. Chronic diseases prevalent in technologically complex societies, for example, non-insulin dependent diabetes mellitus (NIDDM), appear to be linked with "Western" lifestyles. Obesity in particular, a consequence of increased caloric intake in association with reduced physical activity is thought to be a very important risk factor for NIDDM (West, 1978). However, tests of this hypothesis in population isolates do not give it unequivocal support and in some cases suggest other causal models may be more appropriate. Zimmet et al. (1981) for example, find that obesity and age are insufficient to explain rural-urban differences in NIDDM prevalence in Samoans, and that the influence of psychosocial stress in abetting disease onset requires investigation. Knowler et al. (1981) have found that in the Pima, duration of obesity, rather than the occurrence of obesity, is predictive of disease. Studies on Dogrib Amerindians, on the other hand, indicate it is not general obesity that is associated with elevated blood sugar level, but upper trunk, or "centripetal" adiposity (Szathmary and Holt, 1983), a finding that has also been observed in Caucasians

(Kissebah et al., 1982; Feldman et al., 1969).

As all the foregoing examples indicate, populations rather than being incidental to a particular research design, are sometimes integral parts of the research strategy used to elucidate further a particular hypothesis, or test a particular etiological model. The papers in this section have in common such a population centered approach, and serve to illustrate the complexities involved and advances made in such investigations.

Two of the papers in this section, those by Szathmary and by Mayer, Bonaïti and Benoist concentrate on finding evidence for a genetic involvement in the onset of two different conditions in two very different populations. The three remaining papers by Kirk, Serjeantson, King and Zimmet, by Ward and by Weiss each focus on evidence for gene-environment interaction, again by examining different diseases in different societies.

Kirk et al. deal with the issue of heterogeneity in diabetes mellitus, a disease that occurs at minimum in two different forms: the insulin dependent (IDDM: Type I diabetes: juvenile-onset diabetes) and the non-insulin dependent (NIDDM: Type II diabetes: maturity-onset diabetes) varieties (NDDG, 1979; WHO, 1980). Their review of the evidence for genetic susceptibility to IDDM shows that the disease is more common among European (or European-derived) populations than in other groups. However, when IDDM does occur among the latter societies, it occurs with a higher frequency in individuals who possess particular HLA haplotypes. Interestingly, different HLA associations occur with IDDM in different populations and this is also the case for antigens encoded at other loci in the MHC (e.g. Complement components C2, C4A and C4B, and Properdin Factor B (BF)). Recent research on the role of extended haplotypes in IDDM, that is genes at loci in the MHC plus others on chromosome 6 suggests the existence of further genetic heterogeneity in IDDM, with possibly more than two HLA-region genes involved in susceptibility (Rich et al., 1984). This may account for the population differences Kirk et al. have noted.

On the other hand, analysis of the HLA DR antigens indicates that antigens DR3 and DR4 do not directly predispose individuals to IDDM, but that antigen DR2 has a protective effect, at least in Caucasians (Thomson, 1984).

Kirk and coworkers also review the distribution of NIDDM, concentrating their attention on populations of Oceania. Environmental factors, such as those that exist between rural and urban populations, clearly influence NIDDM prevalences. However, comparisons of different ethnic groups occupying apparently similar environments indicate that in some groups genetic factors may be particularly important. For example, rural and urban Fijians have much lower prevalence rates than rural or urban Indians residing in Fiji. Comparisons among indigenous ethnic groups of Oceania show that the Micronesian Nauruans not only have higher prevalence of NIDDM than either Polynesians or Melanesians, but they also display the second highest prevalence in the world. The existence of indigenous "susceptibility" genes in the Nauruans is a possibility, for individuals who carry HLA haplotypes of European origin have significantly reduced risk of developing NIDDM. These "susceptibility" genes are, however, unknown. The restriction fragment length polymorphism associated with the 5' flanking region of the insulin gene, thought by some to identify individuals at risk for NIDDM (Rotwein et al., 1983), is not associated with diabetes in Nauruans. Nor are the weak associations seen between some genetic markers and NIDDM in some Oceanic groups present in Nauruans. For example, there is a very significant excess of $\underline{Gc^1}$ in Polynesians, though not in other Oceanic peoples, and there is some evidence that some Polynesian diabetics may carry a susceptibility allele that is close to or part of the MHC. To date there is no known explanation for the differential associations seen between specific genes and NIDDM in different Oceanic populations. Nevertheless, that genetic factors are implicated <u>within</u> each group is suggested by multivariate analysis of marker genes in diabetics, in persons with impaired glucose tolerance (IGT) and in normals: Diabetics are significantly different from controls among Polynesians and Melanesians, but not among Micronesians. The latter observation suggests that the susceptibility gene(s) occurs in very high frequency in Micronesians, and may explain the extremely high prevalence of NIDDM in Nauruans specifically.

Ryk Ward's discussion of the etiology of high blood pressure focuses on gene-environmental interactions. He presents a complex etiological model that includes major gene, polygenic, random environmental and household-environmental components. Critical to the testing of this model are longitudinal data on a population in cultural transition, and the definition of an adequate measure of the phenotype that can be subjected to genetic analysis. Ward's "transitional" population is Polynesian, drawn from the Tokelauan Islands. Detailed biomedical and behavioral information on this group of people was collected before a sizeable proportion of the population migrated to New Zealand (Prior et al., 1977), and characteristics of migrants upon arrival in New Zealand were compared with those remaining on the home atolls (Stanhope and Prior, 1976). The migrants in New Zealand and nonmigrants on the Tokelau Islands were again surveyed in 1975/76 and 1977, respectively.

A persistent problem in migrant studies is how to define variables that can be subjected to genetic analysis. For example, to attribute measured blood pressure responses in migrants to new environmental influences alone is misleading, because migrants had been exposed to influences of the old environment prior to migration. However, to attribute the difference between blood pressure response in migrants and nonmigrants to the effects of the new environment only is equally misleading, for this assumes the nonmigrants have not changed over time on their atolls. Ward solves this problem elegantly through a series of linear regression equations, made possible by his having longitudinal data, and he derives several different residuals that serve as appropriate blood pressure response measures for genetic analysis.

Ward found that both migrants and nonmigrants have undergone change in blood pressure values from those seen in premigrants, and furthermore the changes were in opposite directions. Much of the change could be attributed to an altered relationship of blood pressure response to age. It is worth emphasizing that had comparisons been restricted to migrants with nonmigrants (as in cross-sectional studies), not only would the difference in blood pressure have been large, but it would have been attributed solely to factors operating in the new environment. In fact, Ward shows that genetic factors are involved in blood pressure response. Firstly, there is strong evidence for gene-environmental interaction as indicated by the altered relationship of blood pressure with age. Secondly, both systolic and diastolic blood pressure responses are influenced approximately equally by polygenic factors and two components. Genetic analysis of the distribution of the components suggests different mechanisms are operating on systolic and on diastolic blood pressure responses, respectively. For the former, non-genetic factors best explain the familial clustering of the minor component in migrants. For systolic blood pressure, however, a major gene controlling blood pressure response and transmitted as an autosomal recessive may explain familial clustering of the minor component in migrants.

Kenneth Weiss explores further the notion that gene-environmental interaction is responsible for the occurrence of some chronic diseases, as well as for certain classes of diseases that do not share any obvious etiological connection to a given chronic disease except that the same organ may be affected. Weiss notes that it is often very difficult to make inferences about the cause of a chronic disease from the analysis of familial data. Similarly, elucidation of the genetic causal factor involved in the appearance of an acute, non-infectious disease in families is equally difficult. However, if the second disease (acute) is actually a product of the first (chronic), then understanding of the causal mechanisms involved in the onset of both diseases could be achieved by the examination of the chronic disease in a particular population context.

Central to Weiss' idea is the notion that genes express themselves differently in different environments, and that alteration of gene expression is age or time dependent. Mutant alleles that arose in an "old" environment, for example, do not necessarily have to have deleterious consequences in that environment. However, with environmental shift these mutants could give rise to pathological states in the new environment. Moreover, the initial pathology could be expressed either at a younger age, or after a shorter exposure time to the new environment. Weiss calls this model of causation "phenotype amplification".

The populations within which Weiss explores his thesis are Native American. The disease of direct interest is gallbladder cancer (GBCA), which is approximately 2-6 times as common in these groups as in the remaining US population. The rarity of GBCA in families precludes formal genetic analysis of causation, yet the occurrence of the disease in Native populations as diverse as those of Alaska and Bolivia indicates there is no consistent environmental factor to which the disease might be attributed. On the other hand a genetic component is suggested by the increased risk to people of Native American origin, and by the fact that disease risk in Mexican Americans increases with the proportion of Amerindian ancestry. Weiss argues that to understand the cause of GBCA in Native Americans one needs to shift attention from GBCA to the occurrence of gallbladder disease, and especially to the appearance of cholesterol gallstones. While the latter are known to constitute a risk factor for GBCA (Lowenfels, 1980), in Native Americans this risk is considerably increased because cholesterol gallstones themselves aggregate in families, indicating a possible genetic component in etiology (Weiss et al., 1984a).

In Amerindians, gallbladder disease appears to have been rare before the onset of World War II, but has become increasingly more common since and occurs at an earlier age, especially in women (Weiss et al., 1984a). This epidemiological pattern fits well with the model of phenotype amplification. Indeed, Weiss and coworkers have defined a "New World Syndrome" of chronic diseases that may be explained by this model (Weiss et al., 1984b). With respect to the etiology of GBCA in New World people, this disease may result almost entirely from a genetic lesion that either affects a bile component that then becomes carcinogenic, or may influence the formation of "silent" gallstones that are carcinogenic. Whatever the precise cause, a genetic factor influencing the onset of GBCA would not have been suspected without examination of gallbladder disease data under the model of phenotype amplification.

In her chapter Szathmary brings together two themes introduced in previous papers in this section: the issue of the cause of non-insulin dependent diabetes mellitus (Kirk et al.), where the genetic factors involved may manifest themselves in a precursor state prior to the onset of clinical disease in an Amerindian population (Weiss). Dogrib Indians of the Canadian Northwest Territories are uniquely suited to pursue these themes. Firstly, clinically recognizable diabetes was not diagnosed in a member of the Band until 1981, in spite of the fact that the Dogrib have had access to local medical care for over 30 years. Secondly, Dogrib over the age of 35 years represent a group that underwent within their lifetimes, a major cultural transition from a predominantly trapping-hunting-fishing subsistence pattern to sedentism and increasing dependence on a wage economy. Dogrib also claim that a gradient in westernization currently exists among their settlements. Accordingly, the population is "ideal" for examining the role acculturation may have in the onset of diabetes. The group is also "ideal" from a genetic perspective because non-Indian admixture is low--indeed in the sample studied, it is not more than 8.5% (Szathmary et al., 1983) -- and people in all settlements are linked genetically (ties of blood) and socially (ties of marriage) (Szathmary, 1983).

There is no evidence among adult Dogrib for bimodality in the distribution of plasma glucose level, a finding that differs markedly from expectations based on long-term studies of diabetes in the Pima (e.g. Knowler et al., 1983). Bimodality is interpreted by many, though not all (e.g. Neel, 1976) as perhaps indicating the existence of a major gene, the presence of which can then be tested by complex segregation analysis (e.g., Elston et al., 1974). The

Dogrib data clearly did not warrant this approach. Nevertheless, there is evidence within the group for the operation of genetic factors. Szathmary pursues different lines of evidence, including searching for clustering of hyperglycemic individuals in pedigrees, seeking association between hyperglycemia and a wide range of genetic markers, and assessing intrafamilial correlations in plasma glucose levels. The first two of these approaches are suggestive of some genetic involvement, but only the last is particularly strong. Szathmary found that of the 3 sets of intrafamilial correlations she computed (parent-child, husband-wife, siblings) only the sib-sib intraclass correlation was substantial and differed significantly from zero. The genetic interpretation of such a finding is that variation in glucose level is influenced by genetic and environmental components, the genetic elements consisting of additive and dominant genes. Szathmary argues that the environmental component cannot represent intrafamilial variables because siblings in her sample (mean age 42.1 ± 13.4 years) have not shared common homes for decades. Rather, what is common to them is an extrafamilial, intragenerational environment that underwent rapid changes within their lifetimes. Future research on the etiology of NIDDM in Indians needs to focus on clarifying the nature of these intragenerational environmental factors. In addition, to test the etiological model of pre-morbid plasma glucose regulation in Indians suggested by this study, new statistical approaches need to be devised. Existing methods to partition covariance, for example, assume independence of individuals and large sample sizes, attributes that are precluded by the complex interrelationships and absolutely small population sizes found in most Amerindian isolates.

Mayer, Bonaïti and Benoist contribute the last paper in this section. Like the others, it is population-specific, but its methodology deviates considerably from those in the other chapters. Mayer and coworkers describe a genealogical approach in an ongoing study to identify common ancestors of individuals suffering from severe deafness in a Caribbean isolate of French origin. While the problem appears straightforward, the situation is exceedingly complex because of the high frequency of hypoacusia on the island, difficulties in the interpretation of audiograms that constitute the phenotype, and the greatly intertwined relationships among individuals in the population.

The current inhabitants of St. Barthélemy descend from a colonizing group that settled the island over 300 years ago. Except for minor perturbations in its history, the island was a French possession and received minimal infusion of genes from "outside" after initial settlement. Among the white inhabitants there has been a great deal of endogamy within two population components that represent windward and leeward sides of the island. Indeed, St. Barthélemy can be characterized as an isolate divided into two sub-isolates, each of which is characterized by some degree of socio-cultural, linguistic and biological differentiation.

Genealogies encompassing the past 150 years have been reconstructed for all individuals exhibiting profound deafness and the patterns of exchange among the genealogies have been identified. Assuming there is a founder responsible for the hypoacusia measured in both of the subisolates of the island, that founder must have introduced the pathology prior to the 150 years covered by the genealogical investigation. Other studies, not detailed by Mayer et al., are currently attempting to elucidate the hereditary nature and mode of transmission of hypoacusia through segregation analysis. When completed the two approaches will complement each other and clarify the genetic components involved in the onset of this disease in this isolate.

As the papers in this section attest, population specific studies allow the assessment of different models of causation in the onset of different chronic diseases. While specific research approaches will differ, all require adequate definition of the variable of interest for genetic analysis. In addition in some instances it may be more fruitful to look at precursor variables rather than the disease endpoint itself. However, this approach as well as that employed in migrant studies requires carefully designed, longitudinal investigation to identify causal components in disease onset. Such studies to date have been rare, but their scarcity belies their importance. It is time now to let the authors of the chapters in this section address the matter of chronic disease causation themselves.

LITERATURE CITED

Beaglehole R, Salmond CE, Hooper A, Huntsman J, Stanhope J, Cassel JC, Prior IAM (1977). Blood pressure and social interaction in Tokelauan migrants in New Zealand. J Chronic Dis 30:803.

Calin A (1982). High risk of sacroiliitis in HLA-B27 positive Pima Indian men. Arthritis Rheum 25:236.

Carter, C, McGee D, Yano K (1984). Morbidity and mortality rates in Okinawan Japanese vs. mainland Japanese: The Honolulu heart program. Hum Biol 56:339.

DEW (Diabetes Epidemiology Workgroup, National Conference on Diabetes) (1981). Research needs in the epidemiology of diabetes. J Epidemiol 113:105.

Elston RC, Namboodiri KK, Nino HV, Pollitzer WS (1974). Studies on blood and serum glucose in Seminole Indians: Indication for segregation of a major gene. Am J Hum Genet 26:13.

Feldman R, Sender AJ, Siegelaub AB (1969). Differences in diabetic and nondiabetic fat distribution patterns by skinfold measurements. Diabetes 18:478.

Gofton JP, Chalmers A, Price EE, Rave CE (1975). HL-A27 and ankylosing spondylitis and BC Indians. J Rheum 2:314.

Hanna JM, Baker PT (1979). Biocultural correlates to the blood pressure of Samoan migrants in Hawaii. Hum Biol 51:481.

Kissebah AH, Vydelingum N, Murray R, Evans DJ, Hartz AJ, Kalkhoff RK, Adams PW (1982). Relation of body fat distribution to metabolic complications of obesity. J Clin Endocrin and Metab 54:254.

Knowler WC, Pettitt DJ, Bennett PH, Williams RC (1983). Diabetes mellitus in Pima Indians: Genetic and evolutionary considerations. Am J Phys Anthrop 62:107.

Knowler WC, Pettitt DJ, Savage PJ, Bennett PH (1981). Diabetes incidence in Pima Indians: Contributions of

obesity and parental diabetes. Am J Epidemiol 113:144.
Lowenfels A (1980). Gallstones and the risk of cancer. Gut 21:1090.
McGarvey ST (1983). Premigration differences in stature, weight, skinfolds and blood pressure between migrant and non-migrant Samoan adults. Am J Phys Anthrop 60:223.
NDDG (National Diabetes Data Group) (1979). Classification and diagnosis of diabetes mellitus and other categories of glucose intolerance. Diabetes 28:1039.
Neel JV (1976). Diabetes mellitus -- a geneticist's nightmare. In Creutzfeldt W, Köbberling J, Neel JV (eds): "The Genetics of Diabetes Mellitus," New York: Springer-Verlag, p 1.
Prior IAM, Hooper AB, Huntsman JW, Stanhope JM, Salmond CE (1977). The Tokelau Island migrant study. In Harrison GA (ed): "Population Structure and Human Variation." Cambridge: Cambridge University Press, p 165.
Reed D, Labarthe A, Stallones R (1970). Health effects of Westernization and migration among Chamorros. Am J Epidemiol 92:94.
Rich SS, Weitkamp LR, Barbosa J (1984). Genetic heterogeneity of insulin dependent (Type I) diabetes mellitus: Evidence from a study of extended haplotypes. Am J Hum Genet 36:1015.
Rotwein PS, Chirgwin J, Province M, Knowler WE, Pettitt DJ, Cordell B, Goodman HM, Permutl MA (1983). Polymorphism in the 5' flanking region of the human insulin gene: A genetic marker for insulin dependent diabetes. New Eng J Med 308:65.
Ryder LP, Anderson E, Svejgaard A (eds) (1979). "HLA and Disease Registry." Third Report. Copenhagen: Munksgaard.
Stanhope JM, Prior IAM (1976). The Tokelau Island migrant study: Prevalence of various conditions before migration. Int J Epidemiol 5:259.
Syme SL, Marmot MG, Kagan A, Kato H, Rhoads G (1975). Epidemiologic studies of coronary heart disease and stroke in Japanese men living in Japan, Hawaii, and California: Introduction. Am J Epidemiol 102:477.
Szathmary, EJE (1983). Dogrib Indians of the NWT, Canada: Genetic diversity and genetic relationship among subarctic Indians. Annals Hum Biol 10:147.

Szathmary EJE, Ferrell RE, Gershowitz H (1983). Genetic differentiation in Dogrib Indians: Serum protein and erythrocyte enzyme variation. Am J Phy Anthrop 62:249.

Szathmary EJE, Holt N (1983). Hyperglycemia in Dogrib Indians of the Northwest Territories, Canada: Association with age and a centripetal distribution of body fat. Hum Biol 55:493.

Thomson G (1984). HLA DR antigens and susceptibility to insulin-independent diabetes mellitus. Am J Hum Genet 36:1309.

Thomson G (1981). A review of theoretical aspects of HLA and disease associations. Theor Popul Biol 20:168.

Weiss KM, Ferrell RE, Hanis CL, Styne PN (1984a). Genetics and epidemiology of gallbladder disease in New World native people. Am J Hum Genet 36:1259.

Weiss KM, Ferrell RE, Hanis CL (1984b). A New World syndrome of metabolic diseases with a genetic and evolutionary basis. Yearbook of Physical Anthropology 27:153.

West KM (1978). "Epidemiology of Diabetes and Its Vascular Lesions." New York: Elsevier.

WHO, Expert Committee on Diabetes Mellitus (1980). WHO Technical Report Series, No. 646. Geneva: World Health Organization.

Zimmet P, Faaiuso S, Ainuu J, Whitehouse S, Milne B, De Boer W (1981). The prevalence of diabetes in the rural and urban Polynesian population of Western Samoa. Diabetes 30:45.

Diseases of Complex Etiology in Small Populations:
Ethnic Differences and Research Approaches, pages 119–146

Chapter 6

THE GENETIC EPIDEMIOLOGY OF DIABETES MELLITUS

R.L. Kirk[1], S.W. Serjeantson[1], H. King[2], and P. Zimmet[2]

[1]Human Biology Department, John Curtin School of Medical Research, Canberra, Australia, and [2]Royal Southern Memorial Hospital, Melbourne, Australia

INTRODUCTION

It is a truism now to describe diabetes mellitus as a heterogeneous group of disorders. All diabetics share in common an inability to metabolize glucose normally, an inability which manifests itself with various degrees of clinical severity and other biochemical disturbance. However, the widespread distribution of diabetes, the varying prevalence of its various types in populations of different geographic and ethnic background and its long established familial basis make it an excellent model for the study of gene-environment interactions. Such studies in human populations are being complemented by many elegant investigations of diabetic syndromes in other species of mammals.

Records of diabetes as a clinical disorder date back at least two thousand years in India and also in China (Bose, 1907; Jiang, 1982) but most work in recent times has been focused on diabetes in persons of European descent. Only relatively recently has detailed attention, other than the compilation of prevalence and incidence data (excellently summarized by West, 1978) been given to diabetes in persons of different ethnic background. Studies of indigenous peoples as well as of migrant and hybrid populations are now beginning to give valuable clues to the complexity of this group of disorders.

Recent classifications (National Diabetes Data Group, 1979; WHO, 1980) recognize insulin-dependent (IDDM: Type 1: Juvenile Onset) and non-insulin dependent (NIDDM: Type 2: Mature Onset) forms of diabetes mellitus together with a miscellaneous category where the diabetes is secondary to other disease entities. These latter include hormonal disturbances, drug-induced pancreatic damage, insulin receptor anomalies, certain genetic syndromes as well as nutritional disturbances giving rise to secondary diabetes (Rimoin, 1976; Podolsky and Viswanathan, 1980). Related to NIDDM is a relatively mild non-insulin dependent form of the disease which frequently becomes manifest between ages 20-40 in persons of European descent and which is inherited under simple dominant control (Tattersall, 1974) and referred to as Mature Onset Diabetes of Young People (MODY; Tattersal and Fajans, 1975).

The classification into the two major categories of IDDM and NIDDM gains considerable support both from clinical and laboratory based investigations. In IDDM, for persons of European descent, onset is predominantly during the first two decades of life. Islet cell function is severely impaired and islet cell antibodies are commonly present at the time of diagnosis. Weight loss occurs and proneness to the production of ketones is a frequent feature. Endogenous insulin production is very low or zero. It has been considered that onset is usually precipitate, but whilst this may be true for the emergence of the final clinical picture, a number of recent studies have shown that islet-cell antibodies frequently are detectable for many years before the onset of syndromes (Gorsuch et al., 1981; Srikanta et al., 1983).

In NIDDM the disease becomes manifest over a longer period of time, clinical symptoms occurring normally above age 40. Insulin production may be either above or below normal and the hyperglycemia can be controlled by restricting the diet or by oral drugs. As the disease progresses it may be necessary to give exogenous insulin in some cases. NIDDM has a strong familial pattern and concordance in MZ twins is high (90%) in contrast to IDDM where multiple-case families are less common and the concordance rate among MZ twins approximates 50 percent. Islet-cell antibodies are not a striking feature in NIDDM but pre-clinical indications are manifest by above normal levels of blood glucose and increased time of decay following an oral load of glucose. Such impaired glucose tolerance can be demonstrated for many years, sometimes in childhood, before the onset of clinically recognized NIDDM.

One of the most striking contrasts between IDDM and NIDDM is the association between HLA and IDDM and the lack of such association with NIDDM. Some exceptions to this will be discussed in further detail below.

INSULIN-DEPENDENT DIABETES (IDDM)

The original HLA associations with IDDM in Europeans was reported by Singal and Blajchman (1973) and by Nerup et al. (1974) and Cudworth and Woodrow (1974). These groups found an increase in the antigens HLA B8 and HLA B15 among patients. Subsequent studies have shown also an increase in HLA B18 and a decrease in HLA B 5 and B7. Stronger associations have now been demonstrated with the HLA D or DR locus. Svejgaard et al. (1980) have summarized results for IDDM obtained for the 8th International Histocompatibility Workshop. Among IDDM patients of European origin the Relative Risk ratios and corresponding probabilities for the HLA DR antigens are given in Table 1. There are highly significant increases in DR3 and DR4, with decreases in DR2, DR5 and DR7. Further analysis of the data indicates that the increases of HLA B8 and B18 are secondary to the increase in HLA DR3, with which both B8 and B18 are in linkage disequilibrium. Similarly, the increase in HLA B15 is secondary to the increase in HLA DR4, with which it is in linkage disequilibrium.

The 8th International Histocompatibility Workshop had data for IDDM patients from a number of other ethnic groups and the results indicated some similarities with, as well as some differences from, those in European patients. DR1 showed no significant deviation in any population but DR2 was decreased in all populations, although the decrease was not significant for Japanese. DR4, on the other hand, was significantly increased in all populations, including Japanese.

Table 1. IDDM in persons of European Descent Relative Risks for HLA DR antigens.[1]

	Relative Risk	Probability
DR 1	0.72	0.04
2	0.25	$<10^{-10}$
3	3.30	$<10^{-10}$
4	6.36	$<10^{-10}$
5	0.39	10^{-6}
7	0.51	10^{-4}
8	1.19	>0.05

[1]Source: Svejgaard et al. (1980).

Additional HLA data for Asian IDDM patients has been provided by the 2nd Asia-Oceania Histocompatibility Workshop in 1981. Despite heterogeneity between laboratories it seems clear that DR3 is increased in Chinese and Indians (R.R. 3.1 and 11.3 respectively) that DR4 is increased in some, but not all, Japanese and Indian series and DRw9 is increased in Chinese and Japanese. DR2 is significantly decreased in Chinese, Japanese and Indian IDDM patients.

The contrast between Chinese and Japanese with respect to DR3 clearly requires further study but could be related to the fact that DR3 has a low frequency in the normal Japanese population (0.3%) compared to China, where it has a frequency of approximately 20%. Such heterogeneity between neighboring populations is not without precedent. Among Europeans DR3 is increased in all diabetic series studied, but the relative risk for DR3 is particularly high for Basques, Yugoslavians and non-Ashkenazi Jews, being 123.7, 47.4 and 114.3 respectively (Svejgaard et al., 1980).

The importance of linkage disequilibrium in relation to the HLA results for IDDM has focused attention on the products of other genes in the MHC region on the short arm of Chromosome 6 (Figure 1). Of those which can be tested easily and for which polymorphism occurs in the population, data have been accumulated for the enzyme Glyoxalase (GLO) and for the complement components C2, C4A and C4B and for Properdin Factor B (BF). The latter has yielded the greatest amount of information so far but studies of C2 and C4B also have shown significant associations.

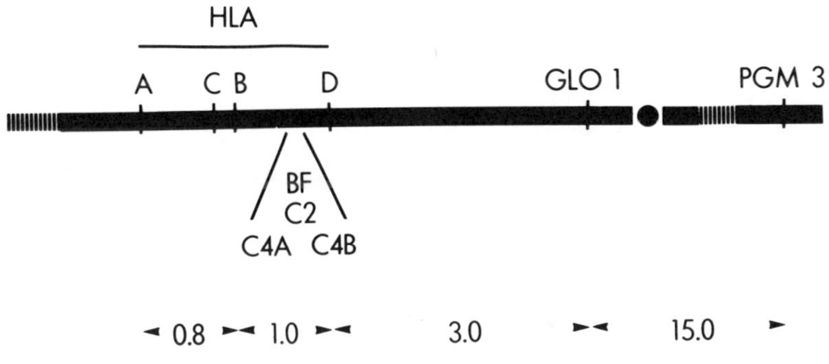

Figure 1. The MHC region of chromosome 6. Map distances are in centimorgans.

No significant association with GLO alleles has been demonstrated presumably because the map distance between GLO and HLA (2 cm) does not permit close disequilibrium with a putative susceptibility allele(s) in the HLA D region.

In European IDDM patients BF*S and BF*F1 are significantly increased (Raum et al., 1979, 1981, 1982; Kirk et al., 1979a; Bertrams et al., 1979a, 1980; Dornan et al., 1980; Dyer et al., 1981; McCloskey et al., 1983) and there is evidence for heterogeneity of these increases both with the population studied and with age at time-of-onset of the disease (Kirk et al., 1979b; Barbosa et al., 1979; Bertrams et al., 1979b, 1981).

In other populations varying results have been obtained for BF alleles in IDDM. BF*F appears to be increased in Japanese (Bashir et al., 1983). Tokunaga et al. (1981) report a novel BF allele, BF*FTokyo, is significantly increased in IDDM (3.1% vs. 0.2% phenotype frequency). In north Indians, on the other hand, the rare allele BF*S1 is significantly increased in IDDM, with a relative risk of 14 (Kirk et al., 1982a) but in South India, where BF*S1 is very rare it is BF*F which is increased (Kirk et al., 1983).

The complement component C2 also shows allele association with IDDM in Europeans, the C2*2 allele being significantly increased (Kirk et al., 1980). In many parts of the world, however, C2 is monomorphic and, in such situations, can contribute no information on associations.

Perhaps the most informative of the non-HLA markers are the closely linked loci C4A and C4B. This system is highly polymorphic and therefore offers a greater chance of detecting a disease association. For IDDM in Europeans several studies have found a significant association between the disease and particular C4 alleles. Complement C4 is controlled, by genes at two closely linked loci, C4A (Rodgers) and C4B (Chido) (O'Neill et al., 1978). Electrophoresis, after desialation of the protein, gives rise to a large number of phenotypes and in Europeans at least 12 structural variant alleles and a null allele are recognized at the A locus and at least 20 structural variant alleles and a null allele at the B locus (Mauff et al., 1983). Various reports have indicated increased frequency of C4B types in IDDM, particularly of C4B3 and C4BQ0 (Q0 is a null allele; Bertrams et al., 1982; Awdeh et al., 1980; Raum et al., 1982). The most striking increase in C4B*Q0 has been observed in IDDM patients among Basques. Here Mouzon et al. (1979; 1982) found that the C4B*Q0 allele greatly increased in diabetics (55% vs. 19%) and this contrast was even greater for IDDM patients with age-of-onset less than 20 years.

Because all the loci being discussed here are on the short arm of chromosome 6, attention is being given now to extended haplotypes, including alleles at the loci for GLO; HLA A, B, C, D (DR); BF; C2; C4A, C4B. The number of possible combinations, of course, is very large but, in fact, certain combinations occur relatively frequently. Awdeh et al. (1983) have investigated the extended haplotypes in members of 151 families of European descent in the Boston area of the U.S.A. Haplotypes for healthy members of these families, including the GLO types, numbered 295.

Table 2. The seven most common extended haplotypes in Europeans.[1]

Locus						Frequency (in %)
HLA B	BF	C2	C4A	C4B	HLA DR	
8	S	1	0	1	3	9.3
7	S	1	3	1	2	5.9
44	F	1	3	1	7	3.7
44	S	1	3	0	4	3.4
57	S	1	6	1	7	2.8
61	S	1	0	2	6	1.1
62	S	1	3	3	4	0.9

[1]Source: Awdeh et al. (1983).

Excluding the GLO and HLA A loci, Table 2 gives the frequencies of the seven most common extended haplotypes. The B, DR, BF, C2, C4A and C4B haplotypes shown in Table 2 account for 27.1% of the total. One third of these (9.3% of the total) are accounted for by B8 : DR3 : BF*S : C2*1 : C4A*Q0 : C4B*1.

In European IDDM persons this latter haplotype with HLA A1 is increased in frequency but, in addition, two other haplotypes become prominent (Rittner and Bertrams, 1981; Raum et al., 1982; McCluskey et al., 1983). These are:

B15(62) : DR4 : BF*S : C2*2 : C4A*3 : C4B*2.9
B18 : DR3 : BF*F1 : C2*1 : C4A*3 : C4B*Q0

It is of interest that the first of these extended haplotypes is increased also in patients with rheumatoid arthritis. This could be a factor in explaining the familial association of RA and IDDM (Barbosa et al., 1983; Dawkins et al., 1983).

Focusing attention on particular elements in the haplotypes, Raum et al. (1982) studied 14 IDDM persons with BF*F1. All but one were associated with DR3 and most were HLA B18. In all cases BF*F1 was associated with C2*1 : C4A*3 : C4B*Q0. Raum et al. conclude that the "protective" effects of HLA B7 and DR2 from IDDM is due probably to the absence of a susceptibility allele from the haplotype A3 : B7 : DR2: BF*S : C2*1 : C4A*3 : C4B*1. Similarly, Mouzon et al. (1982) show that the common extended haplotype in IDDM patients among Basques is: Aw30 : B18 : DR3 : BF*F1 : C4B*Q0 and that the haplotype most frequently found in controls is never found in patients. Recently, Acton et al. (1983) have noted a significant increase in C4B*Q0 in Black Americans with IDDM and in 5 of 6 cases this was associated with BF*F1. They conclude this adds further support to the hypothesis that the increase in IDDM in Black Americans may be partially due to admixture with European genes.

Discussion at present is focused on the implications of the extended haplotype associations for understanding the genetic susceptibility to IDDM. Greatest significance is attached to the increased frequency of HLA DR3 and DR4 and to the apparent excess of DR3/4 heterozygotes among affected individuals. Claims have been made that this supports a single recessive gene model of susceptibility (Falk and Rubinstein, 1980; Falk et al., 1983) or is not compatible with a dominant, recessive or intermediate model (Svejgaard and Ryder, 1981; Hodge et al., 1980; Rotter et al., 1983). More complex models involving susceptibility alleles at more than one locus have been invoked also (Thomson, 1980) and have received support from segregation and linkage analysis (Green et al., 1982; Morton et al., 1983). So far, however, the analysis of extended haplotypes does not permit an unequivocal answer to the question whether the susceptibility allele(s) in the HLA region is either or both the HLA DR3 or DR4 alleles themselves or is in linkage disequilibrium with another susceptibility allele at a closely linked locus. Dawkins et al., (1983) believe that the relatively increased frequency of certain extended haplotypes within the DR3 or DR4 categories is evidence for a functional significance of the extended haplotype itself. Clearly, further data on the distribution of extended haplotypes, particularly in families with affected persons, is required urgently.

NON-INSULIN-DEPENDENT DIABETES (NIDDM)

In all populations NIDDM is far more prevalent than is IDDM. Among Europeans the former is about ten times as prevalent as the latter whilst, in India and many parts of Asia and the Pacific, the disproportion is even greater. Whilst NIDDM appears to be increasing in prevalence in many of these populations, IDDM is relatively rare.

Epidemiologic studies of NIDDM reveal prevalence rates ranging from 1% to 35% (Table 3), the highest figure being for the Pima Indians in the USA and close to it, with an age-standardized prevalence rate of 30.4% are the Nauru Islanders in the Central Pacific.

Closer study shows also that even within a single geographic area significant differences in NIDDM prevalence rates exist between populations with different ethnic background (Table 4). Among the more striking of these differences are those between Indians and Fijians in Fiji or between Indians, Malays and Black Africans of South Africa.

Table 3. Prevalence rates for NIDDM in selected populations.[1]

Country	Ethnic Group	Age group (yrs)	Diagnostic criteria 2hr plasma glucose (m. mol.)	Diabetes prev.
Japan	Japanese	20+	≥ 8.3 (50g)[2]	1.0
Indonesia	Indonesian	14+	≥ 7.8 (50g)	1.5
India	Rural Indian	15+	≥ 7.8 (75g)	1.2
USA	Eskimo	20+	≥ 8.9 (100g)	1.9
USA	Cherokee Indian	34+	≥ 9.4 (1g/kg)	29.0
USA	Pima Indian	15+	≥ 8.9 (75g)	35.0
Singapore	Chinese	15+	≥ 8.9 (50g)	1.6
Australia	European	20+	≥ 8.3 (50g)	2.3
Cook Isls.	Polynesian (rural)	20+	≥ 8.3 (100g)	2.4
S. Africa	Black African	15+	≥ 7.8 (50g)	3.6
Nauru	Micronesian	20+	≥11.0 (75g)	30.4

[1]Source: Zimmet (1982).
[2]The figure in parentheses is the oral load of glucose administered initially.

However, detailed epidemiological studies of diabetes prevalence reveal striking differences for populations of the same ethnic group living in different environmental situations. Table 5 provides some contrasts for urban and rural communities in several Pacific Islands taken from Zimmet et al. (1982). In each case the rural prevalence rate is lower than the urban rate. However, Indians in both rural and urban areas in Fiji have prevalence rates higher than urban Fijians.

These differences in prevalence rates demand careful examination to determine the contributory factors and our work during the last few years has been aimed at such an examination.

Obesity has long been considered a risk factor for diabetes (West, 1978), and there is a correlation between relative body weight and diabetes prevalence in populations in various parts of the world (West and Kalbfleisch, 1971) and the WHO Expert Committee on Diabetes stated that obesity is the most powerful risk factor for diabetes (WHO, 1980). However, as Zimmet and King (1982) point out there are some exceptional cases. Barnett et al. (1981) have shown than that MZ twins concordant for NIDDM may differ considerably in weight: in some cases this is true even when neither twin is over-weight.

Table 4. Prevalence rates for NIDDM among persons of different ethnic groups in the same country.[1]

Country	Ethnic Group	Age Group (yrs)	Prevalence (%)
Fiji	Melanesian	20+	7.0
	Indian		14.0
Singapore	Chinese	15+	1.6
	Malay		2.4
	Indian		6.1
Trinidad	Black	20+	2.5
	Indian		4.5
New Zealand	European	20+	2.8
	Maori		7.5
New Caledonia	Melanesian	20+	2.0
	Polynesian		5.8

[1]Source: Zimmet (1982).

Zimmet and King (1982) explored further the relationship between obesity (measured as body mass index, BMI) [Weight (kg) / Height $(m)^2$] and diabetes as determined by 2 hour glucose tolerance tests on individuals in Pacific Island populations. For each age group, in both sexes, the mean BMI was lower in rural than in urban samples, the difference being highly significant ($P<0.001$). The corresponding age-standardized diabetes prevalence rate overall was 3% in the rural and 9% in the urban populations. Prevalence was then calculated separately for low, medium and high BMI tertiles in three ethnic groups, namely, Fijians in Fiji, Indians in Fiji and Micronesians in Kiribati.

Table 5. Rural and urban age-standardized diabetes prevalence rates for persons aged 20 or over in selected Pacific populations.[1]

Population	Male		Female	
	N	%	N	%
Western Samoa				
Rural	358	1.3	387	4.1
Urban	325	7.1	419	6.8
Wallis Islands				
Rural	274	1.5	305	3.3
Urban	257	12.8	315	11.2
Fiji (Fijians)				
Rural	242	1.5	235	1.6
Urban	401	4.6	452	8.6
Fiji (Indians)				
Rural	214	12.6	238	13.0
Urban	384	14.8	452	13.4

[1]Source: Zimmet et al. (1982).

Figure 2, taken from Zimmet and King's (1982) paper, reveals an interesting set of relationships. For Fijians in Fiji, increasing BMI had little effect on diabetes prevalence, particularly in urban males. For Indians in Fiji, however, prevalence increases with obesity in both males and females and there is no striking difference between the rural and urban environments. Still another pattern emerged from Kiribati. Here diabetes prevalence increases with BMI in both males and females and, in both, there is a higher prevalence rate among urban dwellers. These authors point out that obesity and other factors resulting from urbanization are interacting to result in high diabetes prevalence rates which, in Micronesian Nauruans, gives crude prevalence rates of 24% for persons aged 20 years and over, rising to 46% in those aged 35 years and over. They conclude that, although urbanization is always associated with increased prevalence of diabetes, obesity itself in some cases seems to have little relationship with the disease whilst, in others, it remains an important factor. Further studies are aimed at elucidating what other factors associated with urbanization may play a role in increasing the prevalence of diabetes. These factors include reduced physical activity, altered dietary habits (increase in calorie intake and decrease in dietary fiber) and psychosocial factors such as stress or alcohol intake.

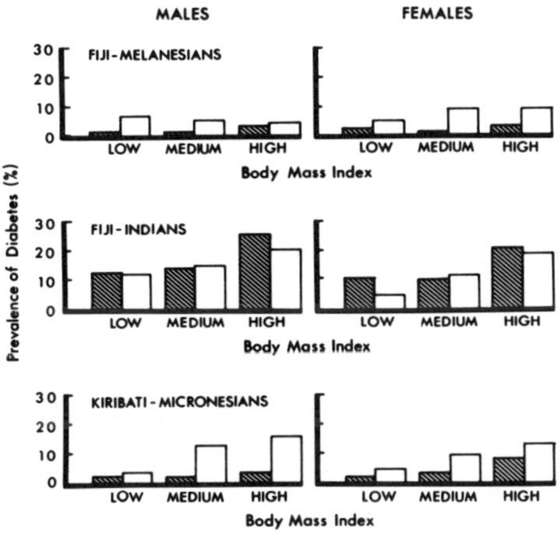

Figure 2. Age-standardized diabetes prevalence in three Pacific populations by tertiles for body mass index. Shaded rectangles - rural; open rectangles - urban.

Some of these factors have been investigated by King et al. (1983) using a multiple logistic regression model. Nine of 24 estimates were found to have significantly increased risk factors for diabetes. These increased risk factors were: physical inactivity in Fijian and Indian males, high body mass index in Indian females, increased BMI in both male and female Micronesians and urbanization in male Micronesians. The risk figures differ between populations and between sexes within populations. Obesity was strongly associated with risk in some cases but, in others, the chief risk factor appeared to be physical activity. More than one risk factor was found in Micronesians and in Micronesian males there was evidence of interaction between obesity and urbanization. Further refinement of the factors investigated undoubtedly will lead to greater insights into the real nature of the risk factors. For example, King and his colleagues point out that the urbanization factor is complex, one facet of which may be a change from traditional home-grown foods to imported processed foods. In the case of Indians in Fiji, food habits were similar in both rural and urban groups and their diabetes prevalence was also similar. By contrast urban and rural Micronesians differ markedly in their food habits and also in diabetes prevalence.

GENETIC INTERACTIONS IN NIDDM

Not only are the environmental interactions complex but the complexities are likely to be compounded by factors affecting genetic susceptibility, which themselves may vary from population to population. Our attempts to understand the genetic basis of susceptibility to NIDDM have made use of two approaches; pedigree analysis on the one hand, and the amassing of data on genetic markers in diabetic and nondiabetic groups on the other.

In a recent paper, Serjeantson and Zimmet (1984) have made an intensive study of family data for more than 1,300 Nauruan adults of known glucose tolerance. The pedigrees were verified using genetic marker data. Using maximum likelihood solutions and two lognormal distributions, each individual's liability for hyperglycemia was calculated as a function of the observed two-hour plasma glucose and age. They found that most of the variation in the glucose tolerance can be attributed to a major autosomal gene. This gene is probably inherited in a dominant fashion, with a frequency of 0.31 and pentrance of 95%, although the alternative possibility of a recessive gene could not be entirely ruled out.

From our studies of genetic markers in diabetic and nondiabetic groups in the Pacific, let us consider firstly, evidence based on HLA and other chromosome 6 markers. Among Indians in Fiji, Serjeantson et al. (1981) found a significant increase in HLA Bw61 among diabetics. This increase in Bw61 was reported also for Indian diabetics in South Africa by Hammond and Asmal (1980) but it has not been observed in any other population in the Pacific that we have investigated. Serjeantson et al. (1982) have shown an increase for HLA Bw22 in Polynesians with diabetes and impaired glucose tolerance and also among diabetics on the island of Nauru, but the effect is slight and, when corrected for the number of antigens tested, it is not significant. These authors showed also by another method that HLA is not contributing in any significant way to susceptibility to diabetes. They carried out a multivariate analysis of the HLA data and showed that, in each population, the diabetics and persons with impaired glucose tolerance (IGT) cluster together with the controls for that population.

Two other non-HLA markers on chromosome 6 also show significant differences between diabetics and controls for Polynesian populations but not for Micronesians or Melanesians, although for the latter the number of diabetics is relatively small (Table 6). The BF*S gene in Polynesians is significantly decreased (P = .01 - .001). The Melanesians and Micronesians show a shift in the same direction but the difference is not significant. Similarly, in Polynesians, the GLO*1 gene is decreased (P<0.001), but the decrease of GLO*1 in Micronesian diabetics is not significant. In the small series of Melanesian diabetics the GLO*1 gene is increased but, again, the difference is not significant. One other chromosome 6 marker, complement factor 2, revealed no significant

Table 6. Percent gene frequencies for Properdin factor B (BF), Glyoxalase (GLO) and complement factor 2 (C2) in various Pacific population groups.

Populations Groups	N	BF*S	$X^2_{(1)}$	N	GLO*1	$X^2_{(1)}$	N	C2*1	$X^2_{(1)}$
Polynesians									
Diabetic	418	14.35		405	12.84		288	99.48	
Control	638	19.36		490	18.67		277	100.00	
(C - D)		5.01	9.33		5.83	11.56		0.52	
Micronesians									
Diabetic	238	2.94		236	5.93		152	99.67	
Control	259	4.05		295	7.63		103	98.54	
(C - D)		1.11	0.91		1.70	1.21		- 1.13	1.58
Melanesians									
Diabetic	56	9.82		52	14.42		55	100.00	
Control	241	12.45		212	9.57		238	99.58	
(C - D)		2.63	0.68		- 4.85	1.69		- 0.42	
Fiji Indians									
Diabetic	66	38.64		64	28.91		64	95.31	
Control	50	37.00		49	20.41		49	96.94	
(C - D)		- 1.64	0.06		- 8.50	2.21		1.63	0.08

differences in any of the groups studied.

The significant change of frequency of BF and GLO genes among Polynesian diabetics adds support to the increased frequency of HLA Bw22 among Polynesians reported by Serjeantson et al. (1982). It suggests that a proportion of diabetics among Polynesians have a susceptibility allele close to, or part of the MHC region of chromosome 6.

We have investigated also a series of non-chromosome 6 genetic markers. Those which revealed polymorphism in one or more of the populations studied include: Hb, PGM-1, PGM-2, ACP, 6PGD, AK, ADA, PHI, GPT, PGP, ESD, Gc, Hp, Tf and complement factor 6 (C6). The differences in frequencies for selected alleles between diabetics and controls in the various groups (Table 7) are significant in only four of the 52 comparisons made and three of these differences are significant at the 0.05 level. One of these, for the 6PGD*A allele in Melanesians, may warrant further investigation. The increase in 6PGD*A in diabetics is consistent in Polynesians, Micronesians and Fiji Indians as well as in the Melanesians, even though the increase does not reach the formal level of 0.05 probability in these other groups.

One other change in gene frequency is also worthy of further study. In the grouped Polynesian results the Gc*1 allele in the Vitamin D-binding protein is very significantly increased (P=0.001). This has been noted in a previous report (Kirk et al., 1982b) where we pointed out that two previous studies by Cleve (1966) and Jorgensen and Hopfer (1967) reported an increase in Gc*1 in diabetics. Berg et al. (1967) however found no significant increase in Gc*1 among diabetics aged 14-86 years in Oslo. In the present study the results show a non-significant increase in Gc*1 for diabetics among Fiji Indians and non-significant decreases for diabetes in the Micronesians and Melanesian groups.

Finally, we have addressed the question whether diabetics in the various populations covered by our epidemiological studies are genetically distinct from non-diabetics in a general way rather than through some specific locus difference. That this may be the case for diabetics in Nauru has been indicated by work reported by one of us (Serjeantson et al., 1983) on Nauruans with some proportion of foreign admixture, as

Table 7. Percentage difference in gene frequencies for selected alleles in various Pacific populations (Control vs. diabetic).

Allele	Poly-nesians	Micro-nesians	Mela-nesians	Fiji Indians
PGM1*1	-0.75	-3.73	4.07	- 2.85
PGM2*1	0	0	1.28	- 1.02
ACP*A	-1.93	-3.68	-0.09	11.62
6PGD*A	-1.37	-0.55	-9.94*	- 1.74
AK*1	0.58	-0.34	0	- 3.41
PHI*1	0	0	0	- 2.04
GPT*1	4.17**	-2.92	1.35	- 0.52
PGP*1	0	-0.13	-2.36	- 1.74
ESD*1	-1.94	1.91	-5.02	-13.00*
GC*1	6.64***	-0.39	-3.82	4.55
Hp*1	1.49	1.29	-7.01	2.58
Tf*C	0.83	0	0	0.76
C6*A	-1.74	-6.70*	-3.18	- 0.90

*P < 0.05 **P < 0.001 ***P < 0.001

evidenced by possessing characteristic foreign HLA haplotypes. Of diabetic Nauruans aged 60 years and over, only 5% of non-diabetics had foreign HLA haplotypes whereas 56% of non-diabetics had foreign HLA haplotypes. The differences in diabetes prevalence could not be attributed to any differences in life-style. Table 8 shows also that the pure-Nauruans and part-Nauruans do not differ significantly in body mass index. Superficially, these two groups differed only in the proportion of non-Nauruan genes which they possessed and, as this extends to frequencies of alleles at many other loci, it might lead to identification of a sub-set of the population particularly susceptible to diabetes.

Table 8. Body Mass Index (kg/m^2) for Nauruans with and without "foreign" admixture as judged from HLA data.

	Males			Females		
	N	BMI	S.D.	N	BMI	S.D.
Pure-Nauruan	93	32.5	5.0	111	34.5	6.7
Part-Nauruan	17	34.4	5.8	10	33.2	4.4

We have carried out a multivariate analysis utilizing all the information available from the genetic marker studies of diabetics and controls in the various Pacific populations surveyed. We have included in this analysis also persons with impaired glucose tolerance, i.e. those with 2 hour plasma glucose values between 7.8 and 11.0 m. equivalents after a 75g oral glucose load. Genetic distance matrices were generated using the method of Nei (1972). Dendrograms or eigenvector diagrams were constructed using the computer program ARBOR and PHEIGEN (Lalouel, 1973) or a maximum likelihood program (Felsenstein, 1973).

Populations were considered either separately or grouped according to the broad ethnic relationships used already, that is, Polynesian, Micronesian and Melanesian. Since no consistent patterns were evident in the analysis of separate populations the analysis given here refers to data for the three broad groupings.

The distance matrix is given in Table 9 and the dendrogram and eigenvector representations are displayed in Figures 3 and 4. Although each triad of diabetics, impaired glucose tolerance and normals cluster together in each ethnic group the distance values between diabetics and normals are significant at the conventional level of twice the standard deviation for Polynesians and Melanesians whilst, for Micronesians, it just falls short of significance. This is true also for the distance values between

Table 9. Nei's distance values ($D \times 10^3$) for diabetics, impaired and normals in three major ethnic groups in the Pacific.

	Polynesian			Melanesian			Micronesian	
	Diab-etic	Imp-aired	Nor-mal	Diab-betic	Imp-aired	Nor-mal	Diab-etic	Imp-paired
Polynesian								
Impaired	3.2 ±1.7							
Normal	0.8 ±0.3	1.3 ±0.6						
Melanesian								
Diabetic	3.8 ±2.7	7.6 ±4.3	5.0 ±3.3					
Impaired	2.4 ±1.1	7.4 ±3.9	4.1 ±1.7	3.1 ±1.3				
Normal	3.2 ±1.9	6.6 ±3.2	4.0 ±2.2	1.4 ±0.6	3.1 ±1.4			
Micronesian								
Diabetic	7.6 ±3.4	8.6 ±3.1	8.0 ±3.1	16.5 ±9.8	12.6 ±6.2	13.3 ±7.6		
Impaired	7.6 ±3.9	10.1 ±3.7	8.5 ±3.5	17.6 ±11.5	13.5 ±7.4	14.7 ±9.2	1.1 ±0.6	
Normal	8.9 ±5.0	9.4 ±4.0	9.0 ±4.5	17.3 ±10.1	14.5 ±7.3	14.2 ±8.1	0.5 ±0.3	1.2 ±0.6

normals and persons with IGT.

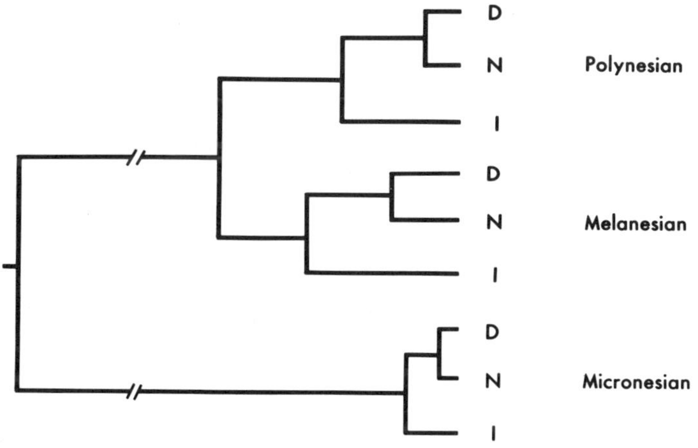

Figure 3. Dendrogram based on Nei's genetic distances for diabetics, persons with impaired glucose tolerance and normals in Pacific populations. D = diabetic; I = Impaired; N = normal.

The multivariate analysis suggests, therefore, that diabetics and persons with IGT are a genetically distinct subgroup of the populations in each ethnic group. However, the magnitude of the difference is small compared to that which distinguishes the ethnic groups from each other.

In conclusion, therefore, we have to admit that so far the study of genetic markers has not enabled us to identify any specific genetic factor, or constellation of factors which markedly increase the chance that Pacific Island individuals will develop diabetes of the non-insulin dependent type. There are some tantalizing bits of evidence indicating that some genetic predisposition is involved, particularly the chromosome 6 markers HLA, BF and GLO in Polynesians.

As well the Vitamin-D binding protein system may be involved in Polynesians.

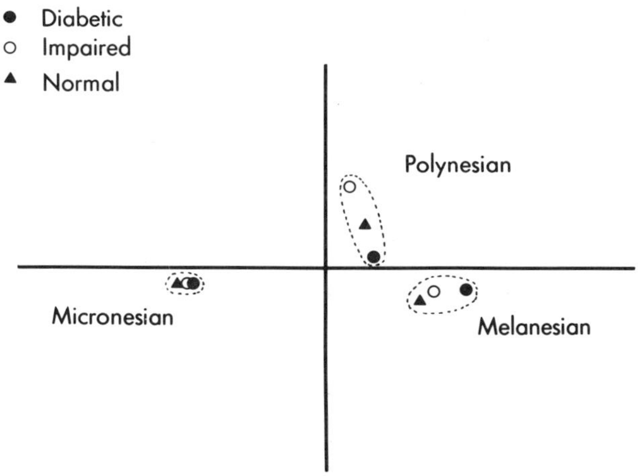

Figure 4. Eigenvector diagram using the first two principal components from Nei's genetic distances. The groups are the same as those in Figure 3.

The evidence that the introduction of foreign HLA haplotypes significantly reduces the risk of becoming diabetic in Nauru is so far the best evidence for genetic susceptibility for NIDDM. Together with the evidence from pedigree studies of Nauruans carried out by Serjeantson and Zimmet (1984) which shows that susceptibility to NIDDM is under the control of a single autosomal dominant gene, we are not carrying out further investigations to determine whether similar factors are present in other Pacific populations.

ACKNOWLEDGEMENTS

We are especially indebted to N.M. Blake,

Carolyn Hawes and Pam Ranford for carrying out the genetic marker tests and for critical comments on the manuscript, to Michelle Reid for assistance with the computations and to Robbie Williams for typing the manuscript.

We are indebted also to the Australian National University and NIH grant (R01 AM 25446-01) for financial assistance.

LITERATURE CITED

Acton RT, Roseman JM, Go RCP, Barger BO, Budowle B (1983).The association of complement C4 with Type 1 diabetes in Black Americans. Diabetes 32 (Supp 1): 46A.

Awdeh ZL, Raum D, Gabbay KH, Alper CA (1980). C4 genetics in normals and insulin-dependent diabetes mellitus patients. J Immunol 124:1513.

Awdeh ZL, Raum D, Yunis EJ, Alper CA (1983). Extended HLA/Complement allele haplotypes: evidence for T/t-like complex in man. Proc Natl Acad Sci USA 80: 259.

Barbosa J, Weitkamp L, Guttormsen S, Johnson S, Szalpski E (1979). Bf in early-onset insulin-dependent diabetes. Lancet ii:1239.

Barbosa J, O'Neill G, Nerl C, Rich S (1983). New genetic marker for Type 1 diabetes is shared by rheumatoid arthritis: complement C4B 2.9. Diabetes 32 (Supp 1):45A.

Barnett AH, Eff C, Leslie RDG, Pyke DA (1981). Diabetes in identical twins: a study of 200 pairs. Diabetologia 20:87.

Bashir H, Juji T, Moffitt P (1983).Joint report - Diabetes Mellitus. In Simons MJ (ed): "Proceedings Second Asia-Oceania Histocompatibility Workshop," Melbourne: Immunopublishing, p 332.

Berg K, Aarseth S, Lundevall J, Reinskon T (1967). Blood groups and genetic serum types in diabetes mellitus. Diabetologia 3:30.

Bertrams J, Baur MP, Grüneklee D, Gries FA (1979a). Association of Bf F1, HLA-B8 and insulin-dependent diabetes mellitus. Lancet ii:98.

Bertrams J, Sodemann P, Grüneklee D, Gries FA (1979b). Bf in early-onset insulin-dependent diabetes.

Lancet ii:1240.
Bertrams J, Baur MP, Grüneklee D, Hintzen U (1980). Association of Bf F1 and haplotype HLA-B8, Bf F1 with insulin-dependent diabetes mellitus. Immunobiol. 158:129.
Bertrams J, Baur MP, Grüneklee D, Gries FA (1981). Age-related association of insulin-dependent daibetes mellitus with Bf F1 and HLA-B18, Bf F1 haplotypes. Diabetologia 21:47.
Bertrams J, Hintzen U, Schlicht V, Schoeps S (1982). C4: Another marker for Type 1 diabetes. Lancet i: 41.
Bose RKC (1907). Comments on diabetes in the tropics. Brit Med J 2:1053.
Cleve H (1966). Die verteilung der Gc-typen und Gc-allele bei kranken mit diabetes mellitus und chronischer polyarthritis. Humangenetik 2:355.
Cudworth AG, Woodrow JC (1974). HLA antigen and diabetes mellitus. Lancet ii:1153.
Dawkins RL, Christiansen FT, Kay PH, Garlepp M, McCluskey J, Hollingsworth PN, Zilko PJ (1983). Disease associations with complotypes, supratypes and haplotypes. Immunological Rev 70:5.
Dornan J, Allan P, Noel EP, Larsen B, Farid NR (1980). Properdin factor B (Bf) allele Bf-F1 specifies an HLA-B18 diabetogenic haplotype. Diabetes 29:423.
Dyer PA, Klouda PT, Harris R (1981). HLA antigens associated with properdin factor B allotype Bf F1. Tissue Antigen 17:362.
Falk CT, Rubenstein P (1980). The effect of association of genetic factors on relative risk. Ann Hum Genet 43:295.
Falk CT, Mendell NR, Rubenstein P (1983). Effect of population associations and reduced penetrance on observed and expected genotype frequencies in a simple genetic model: Application to HLA and insulin-dependent diabetes mellitus. Ann Hum Genet 47:161.
Felsenstein J (1973). Maximum-likelihood estimation of evolutionary trees from continuous characters. Amer J Hum Genet 25:471.
Gorsuch AN, Spencer KM, Lister J, McNally JM, Dean BM, Bottazzo GF, Cudworth AG (1981). Evidence for a long prediabetic period in Type 1 (insulin-dependent) diabetes mellitus. Lancet ii:1363.
Green A, Morton NE, Iselius L, Svejgaard A, Platz P,

Ryder LP, Hauge M (1982). Genetic studies of insulin-dependent diabetes mellitus: segregation and linkage analysis. Tissue Antigen 19:213.

Hammond MG, Asmal AC (1980). HLA and insulin-dependent diabetes in South African Indians. Tissue Antigen 15:244.

Hodge SE, Rotter JI, Lange KL (1980). A three allele model for heterogeneity of juvenile onset insulin-dependent diabetes. Ann Hum Genet 43:399.

Jiang GY (1982). Diabetes mellitus in China, past and present. In Mimura G, Baba S, Goto Y, Köbberling J (eds): "Clinico-genetic Genesis of Diabetes Mellitus," Amsterdam: Excerpta Medica, p 27.

Jörgensen G, Hopfer A (1967). Die verteilung der Gc-Phänotypen und Gc-allele bei einigen Krankheiten (Diabetes Mellitus, Leberparenchymschaden, Psoraisis vulgaris). Humangenetik 3:273.

King H, Zimmet P, Raper LR, Balkau B (1983). Risk factors for diabetes in three Pacific populations. Amer J Epidemiol 119:396.

Kirk RL, Theophilus J, Whitehouse S, Court J, Zimmet P (1979a). Genetic susceptibility to diabetes mellitus: The distribution of properdin factor B (Bf) and glyoxalase (GLO) phenotypes. Diabetes 28:949.

Kirk RL, Serjeantson SW, Theophilus J, Zimmet P (1979b). Age relationship between insulin-dependent diabetes and rare alleles of Properdin factor B. Lancet i:537.

Kirk RL, Ranford PR, Court J, Zimmet P (1980). Distribution of complement C'2 and C'6 types in Australian cases of diabetes mellitus. Med J Australia 2:614.

Kirk RL, Ranford PR, Theophilus J, Ahuja MMS, Mehra NK, Vaidya MC (1982a). The rare factor BF S1 of the properdin system strongly associated with insulin-dependent diabetes in north India. Tissue Antigens 20:303.

Kirk RL, Serjeantson SW, Zimmet P (1982b). Genes and diabetes in the Pacific. In Mimura G, Baba S, Goto Y, Köbberling J (eds): "Clinicogenetic Genesis of Diabetes Mellitus", Amsterdam: Excerpta Medica, p 34.

Kirk RL, Ranford PR, Viswanathan M, Mohan V, Ramachandran A, Snehalatha C, Chetty SMM, John L (1983). Another association between the properdin

system (BF) and insulin-dependent diabetes in south India. Tissue Antigens 22:170.
Lalouel JM (1973). Topology of population structure. In NE Morton (ed): "Genetic Structure of Populations," Honolulu: Univ. Hawaii Press, p 139.
Mauff G et al. (1983). Statement on the nomenclature of human C4 allotypes. Immunobiol 164:184.
McCluskey J, McCann VJ, Kay PH, Zilko PJ, Christiansen FT, O'Neill GJ, Dawkins RL (1983). HLA and complement allotypes in Type 1 (insulin-dependent) diabetes. Diabetologia 24:162.
Morton NE, Green A, Dunsworth T, Svejgaard A, Barbosa J, Rich SS, Iselius L, Platz P, Ryder LP (1983). Heterozygous expression of insulin-dependent diabetes mellitus (IDDM) determinants in the HLA system. Amer J Hum Genet 35:201.
Mouzon AC-de, Ohayon E, Ducos J, Hauptmann G (1979). Bf and C4 markers for insulin-dependent diabetes in Basques. Lancet ii:1364.
Mouzon AC-de, Ohayon E, Hauptmann G, Sevin A, Abbal M, Sommer E, Vergnes H, Ducos J (1982). HLA-A, B, C, DR antigens, Bf, C4 and glyoxalase 1 (GLO) polymorphisms in French Basques with insulin-dependent diabetes mellitus (IDDM). Tissue Antigens 19:366.
National Diabetes Data Group (1979). Classification and diagnosis of diabetes mellitus and other categories of glucose tolerance. Diabetes 28: 1039.
Nei M (1972). Genetic distance between populations. Amer Nat 105:385.
Nerup J, Platz P, Anderson OO, Christy M, Lyngsoe J, Poulsen JE, Ryder LP, Nielson LS, Thomson M, Svejgaard A (1974). HLA antigens and diabetes mellitus. Lancet ii:864.
O'Neill GJ, Yang SY, Dupont B (1978). Two HLA-linked loci controlling the fourth component of human complement. Proc Natl Acad Sci USA 75:5165.
Podolsky S, Viswanathan M (eds) (1980). "Secondary Diabetes: The Spectrum of the Diabetic Syndromes." New York: Raven Press.
Raum D, Alper CA, Stein R, Gabbay KH (1979). Genetic marker for insulin-dependent diabetes mellitus. Lancet i:1208.
Raum D, Awdeh Z, Alper CA (1981). Bf types and the mode of inheritance of insulin-dependent diabetes mellitus (IDDM). Immunogenetics 12:59.

Raum D, Awdeh ZL, Gabbay K, Yunis EJ, Alper CA (1982). Extended MHC haplotypes in juvenile onset insulin-dependent diabetes mellitus (IDDM). Amer Diabetes Assoc, Boston, 1982. Abstract.

Rimoin DL (1976). Genetic syndromes associated with glucose intolerance. In Creutzfeld W, Köbberling J, Neel JV (eds): "The Genetics of Diabetes Mellitus," Berlin: Springer-Verlag, p 43.

Rittner C, Bertrams J (1981). On the significance of C2, C4, and Factor B polymorphisms in disease. Hum Genet 56:235.

Rotter JI, Anderson CE, Rubin R, Congleton JE, Terasaki PI, Rimoin DL (1983). HLA genotypic study of insulin-dependent diabetes: The excess of DR3/DR4 heterozygotes allows rejection of the recessive hypothesis. Diabetes 32:169.

Serjeantson SW, Ryan DP, Ram P, Zimmet P (1981). HLA and non-insulin dependent diabetes in Fiji Indians. Med J Australia 1:462.

Serjeantson SW, Ryan DP, Zimmet P, Taylor R, Cross R, Charan M, Le Gonidec G (1982). HLA antigens in four Pacific populations with non-insulin dependent diabetes mellitus. Ann Hum Biol 9:69.

Serjeantson SW, Owerbach D, Zimmet P, Nerup J, Thoma K (1983). Genetics of diabetes in Nauru: Effects of foreign admixture, HLA antigens and the insulin-gene-linked polymorphism. Diabetologia 25:13.

Serjeantson SW, Zimmett P (1984). Diabetes in the Pacific: evidence for a major gene. In Baba S, Gould MK, Zimmet P (eds): "Diabetes Mellitus: Recent Knowledge on Aetiology, Complications and Treatment," New York: Academic Press, p 23.

Singal DP, Blajchman WA (1973). Histocompatibility (HLA) antigens, lymphocytotoxic antibodies and tissue antigens in patients with diabetes mellitus. Diabetes 22:429.

Srikanta S, Ganda OP, Eisenbarth GS, Soeldneu JS (1983). Islet-cell antibodies and beta-cell function in monozygotic triple and twins initially discordant for Type 1 diabetes. New Eng J Med 308:322.

Svejgaard A, Platz P, Ryder LP (1980). Insulin-dependent diabetes. In Terasaki PI (ed): "Histocompatibility Testing 1980," Los Angeles, U.C.L.A. Tissue Typing Lab, p 638.

Svejgaard A, Ryder LP (1981). HLA genotype

distribution and genetic models of insulin-dependent diabetes mellitus. Ann Hum Genet 45:293.
Tattersall RB (1974). Mild familial diabetes with dominant inheritance. Q J Med 43:339.
Tattersall RB, Fajans SS (1975). A difference between the inheritance of classical juvenile onset and maturity-onset type diabetes among young people. Diabetes 24:44.
Thomson G (1980). A two locus model for juvenile diabetes. Ann Hum Genet 43:383.
Tokunaga K, Omoto K, Maeda H, Juji T, Ishiba S, Maruyama H (1981). Bf and C2 polymorphism in Japanese patients with juvenile onset diabetes mellitus: Existence of a variant Bf allele. Tissue Antigen 18:365.
West KM, Kalbfleisch JM (1971). Influences of nutritional factors on prevalence of diabetes. Diabetes 20:99.
West KM (1978). "Epidemiology of Diabetes and Its Vascular Complications". New York: Elsevier.
WHO: World Health Organization Expert Committee on Diabetes Mellitus (1980) Second Report. Tech Rep Ser 646. Geneva: WHO.
Zimmet P (1982). Type 2 (Non-insulin-dependent) diabetes: An epidemiological overview. Diabetologia 22:399.
Zimmet P, King H (1982). The role of obesity in the high prevalence of diabetes in Pacific populations. Proc Nutri Soc Australia 7:69.
Zimmet P, Taylor R, King H (1982). Diabetes in the Pacific-an epidemiological perspective. In Eschwege E (ed): "Advances in Diabetes Epidemiology," Amsterdam: Elsevier Biomedical Press, p 75.

Diseases of Complex Etiology in Small Populations:
Ethnic Differences and Research Approaches, pages 147–177

Chapter 7

ISOLATES IN TRANSITION:A RESEARCH PARADIGM FOR GENETIC EPIDEMIOLOGY

R.H. Ward

Medical Genetics, University of British Columbia, Vancouver, British Columbia, Canada

INTRODUCTION

The past decade has seen the rapid proliferation of a relatively new field, genetic epidemiology, the existence of which provides a challenging stimulus to many areas of biological anthropology. While slightly different definitions of "genetic epidemiology" have been emphasized by various practitioners, the following definition is likely to meet with some general consensus.

> "Genetic epidemiology aims to identify the distribution of genetic risk, in terms of the underlying etiology of disease, by analyzing the distribution of diseases, and associated risk factors, in groups of related individuals."

As Morton has observed (Morton, 1980), the degree of biological relationship between the groups of individuals under study may be as close as twins or as distant as large ethnic groups. While there is a clear implication that genetic factors will play some role in the underlying etiology of disease, or risk factor, the magnitude of this may not be discernable until after the investigation has been concluded.

The challenge that this field presents to biological anthropology stems from two conceptual consequences. First, as explicitly denoted by the definition, the field of genetic epidemiology has a focused emphasis on the distribution of disease, or risk factors for disease, in traditional societies which often form the main target for the biological anthropologist. By focusing attention on attributes that have relevance to the functional adaptation of the population, rather than restricting attention to polymorphic variability, a genetic epidemiology study is likely to yield some pertinent insight into the possible action of selective forces in the population. Such selective forces are not likely to be readily discerned for single genes. However, evaluating the overall impact of mortality and morbidity of disease that has a genetic component, within a given cultural melieu, will enable more realistic estimates of the operation of selection in human populations. Secondly, the study of genetic epidemiology in traditional societies allows an investigation of a manner in which cultural evolution has interacted with biological evolution to yield the spectrum of adaptations that are currently recognized in different traditional societies scattered around the globe.

Neither should an additional reason be ignored. While it is difficult, if not impossible, to define the relevance of a study of genetic polymorphisms to the day to day concerns of the population being studied, the opposite is true for a genetic epidemiology study. Many traditional societies correctly perceive that the trade-off involved in their participation in an anthropological study should not be solely to the anthropologist's benefit. A focus on genetic epidemiology not only gives rise to a more deserving set of scientific questions, but also provides an opportunity for the investigation to benefit the people being studied. There are numerous situations where a genetic epidemiology study of a traditional society can be established within the context of the development of an appropriate community based health care program (in the broadest sense). Elsewhere I have advocated (Ward, 1983b) that this should be the norm rather than the exception.

The Etiological Spectrum

One requirement for a successful study in genetic epidemiology is an appreciation for the manner in which diseases, and their associated risk factors, are distributed in different etiological categories. Although it is often supposed that etiological components can be dichotomized into the genetic and non-genetic, a more realistic, and heuristically appropriate, concept is to consider etiology as a spectrum ranging from the wholly genetic to the wholly environmental (Ward, 1980a) - a view shared by others (e.g. McKeown, 1979). Originally, I suggested that three major categories could be recognized along the etiological continuum, each category being somewhat arbitrarily subdivided into two subcategories.

In the first category, representing the traditional "genetic diseases", the proximal cause of pathology tends to be genetic in origin, though the ultimate etiology may not be. When the genetic dysfunction is qualitative, as in the case of the Mendelian disorders, transmission of disease, and disease risk, can be deduced from the well-established principles of statistical genetics. When the genetic dysfunction is due to a quantitative aberration at the gene level, as is often the case with chromosomal aberrations, the distribution of risk will not necessarily follow Mendel's law, nor can stable patterns of transmission be assumed.

In the second category, both genetic and environmental factors operate to give a multifactorial etiology. While an arbitrary subdivision can be made on the basis of the relative importance of genetic factors compared to environmental factors (high heritability versus low heritability), a single formulation can be used to specify the general etiological concept in this category (see below). For the past decade it has been recognized that multifactorial etiology can incorporate both major genes displaying Mendelian segregation along with polygenic factors (Morton and MacLean, 1974). Similarly, it is now recognized that environmental components may have a random distribution and display marked familial aggregation.

These two conceptual developments -- non-random environments and a mixture of genetic distributions - suggest the following general linear model of etiological components. If the ith individual in the population is considered, that individuals's phenotype, or liability to disease, can be represented as a sum of individual deviations, thus:

$$Y_i = \mu_o + G_f + G_m + \tfrac{1}{2}g_f + \tfrac{1}{2}g_m + \Delta_f + \Delta_m + \lambda_i + e_i \qquad (1)$$

Here, μ_o represents the population mean; G_f and G_m the genetic contributions to the major locus from the father and mother respectively; g_f and g_m the polygenic deviations of the father and mother; Δ_f and Δ_m the non-random environmental deviations transmitted by (or associated with) the father and mother; λ the segregation deviation of the polygenic components; e the random environmental deviation.

Such a linear model allows specification of the constituent etiological components and, following the principles laid down by Elston and Stewart (1971), allows estimation and hypothesis testing in a number of situations. Equally importantly, this model, which tends to embody the parameters of interest for analyzing traits in the second (or central) etiological category, also serves to represent the general concept of the etiological spectrum. When the deviations, G, are of paramount importance, Mendelian patterns will occur and the disease will fall into the first etiological category. Conversely, when the deviations Δ and e have the predominant influence, diseases of the third category will occur. Lastly, as indicated below, such a model readily yields a representation of the various parametric forms of genotype-environmental interaction.

The third category is represented by those diseases where the primary etiological component is due to some environmental insult. Here an arbitrary division can be made between diseases initiated by biological agents, such as infections or parasitic diseases, and those diseases caused by non-biological agents, often culturally derived. In terms of the model above, this implies that the deviations G, g, and λ are small, though they may still play an important role in determining genetic susceptibility to an environmental factor. It will be noted that in this model the distribution of environmental influences may exhibit strong cultural transmission in which case the Δ will be appreciable, and diseases will show familial (or cultural) clustering.

Changing Contribution of Etiologies Following Cultural Evolution

One important point of this concept is that the contribution of each etiological category to the population's burden of morbidity and mortality will vary markedly as a consequence of the biological and cultural environment of that population. Hence, the gradient imposed by cultural evolution will tend to result in differing contributions of each etiological category, by age group, as well as in total. Simple traditional tribal societies, whose subsistence depends on hunting and gathering or primitive agriculture, will have their major burden due to diseases of the third etiological category, such as infections. However, as evidenced by studies on the Yanomama (Neel, 1980) and other South American Indians (Salzano, this volume), the total burden caused by infectious diseases tends to be relatively evenly distributed over all age groups. Thus the survivorship function decreases fairly steadily throughout the entire age range. With the advent of centralized societies, where population crowding increases and the ecological resource base often becomes minimal for many in the population, the toll taken by infectious diseases becomes more substantial (McNeill, 1980). In such societies both mortality schedules and fertility schedules are raised, with an appreciable proportion of deaths occurring in childhood.

Diseases of the first two etiological categories only become important when the stage of modern urbanized society is reached. This is attributable to the great abundance of resources available for the bulk of individuals in such societies (partly due to technological development and partly due to exploitation of other less developed populations).

Following the overall decline of childhood mortality evidenced in most industrial societies during the past 100 years, genetic disorders (both Mendelian and chromosomal) currently represent an appreciable portion of all illnesses (McKeown, 1979). Even more notable is the substantial increase in diseases belonging to the second etiological category, to the extent that they are now termed the "common diseases." Conversely, the profile of mortality and morbidity caused by cardiovascular disease and cancer, which preoccupies our society, appears insignificant or absent in more traditional societies. Our society's disease burden is likely to be attributed to relative affluence, rather than "bad" genes.

Given this different distribution of disease burden by etiological category at different cultural levels, it is apparent that the present cultural gradient from simple traditional societies to complex urban societies is likely to be accompanied by a similar gradient in the changing distribution of type of disease. Consequently, societies which find themselves undergoing the transition from a traditional cultural environment to a westernized environment are likely to exhibit markedly changing risk of disease. Since such societies are well nigh ubiquitous (because of the mad scramble to become "westernized"), the study of such societies in their transition may shed light on the processes underlying the onset of those diseases which are of considerable concern to our own society.

Strategies of Research

It also needs to be emphasized that the classification of disease by etiological category has considerable implication for the strategy required to elucidate the underlying mechanism. Geneticists have long been familiar with a variety of analytic methods designed to evaluate the mode of transmission of Mendelian disorders, and their co-segregation with linked markers. Similarly, epidemiologists weaned on the tradition of William Farr and John Snow have also successfully developed strategies for study design and data analysis applicable to identifying etiological factors, especially when they are infectious. However, in the second etiological category, where both genes and environment are important, the situation is less clear cut. It is this area which has formed the primary focus for genetic epidemiology, but there is still lack of agreement as to the most effective approach.

On the one hand there are investigators, predominantly geneticists, who emphasize the utilization of complex genetic analysis in an attempt to resolve which etiological components are genetic. These investigators stress the adoption of complex pedigree analysis in order to test hypotheses about complex genetic models. Unfortunately, elementary epidemiological and biological principles are sometimes sacrificed in order to accomplish this. The rather simple and straightforward sampling procedures which the early geneticists could adopt in their analysis of simple Mendelian traits is no longer appropriate for more complex forms of disease. On the other hand there is a minority group of genetic epidemiologists who take a broader perspective by emphasizing the integration of genetic and epidemiological principles. This group would argue that as much attention should be paid to the distribution of environmental factors as is normally paid by the geneticist to the distribution of genetic factors. Consequently, issues of study design and measurement of concomitants should be carried out in an epidemiologically defensible manner (Ward, 1980a; Schull and Weiss, 1980).

My sympathies clearly lie with this latter group - not merely out of a chivalrous regard for the underdog, but because of a belief that we are unlikely to learn anything of value about causation unless we take account of both genetic and environmental influences on the distribution of disease. This concern may be less important when either extreme of the etiological spectrum is under consideration. If a major etiological force is either genetic or environmental, the failure to recognize the minor etiological component will only lead to inconsequential perturbations in the definition of disease risk. However, when the focus is on the middle of the etiological spectrum, adoption of an overly simplistic approach can only lead to inappropriate conclusions.

The issue of defining an appropriate strategy is most starkly brought into focus when the problem of genotype environmental interaction is considered. As noted above, the current models allow discrimination between two conceptually distinct kinds of genetic influence - major genes whose effects segregate in nuclear families according to the dictates of Mendel's law, and polygenic components. Similarly, environmental attributes may be partitioned into a random component and a component which aggregates in families and thus increases the covariance between relatives. The form that this covariance structure will have will depend on the form of relationship between the coefficient of genetic kinship between individuals and their probability of sharing common familiar environments. When genotype-environmental interactions are considered, as they must be, a new set of concerns must be considered.

INTERACTION BETWEEN GENOTYPE AND ENVIRONMENT

One of the clearest descriptions of genotype environmental interaction is Haldane's classic paper on the subject (Haldane, 1946). By using a simple model of two genetic strains and two environments, he identified the six unique configurations that would result, in terms of simple 2 x 2 tables. Of these, four represent interactions in the sense most commonly used. The remaining two patterns indicate superiority of one genotype over all environments, or maximum desirability of one environment, irrespective of genotype. Although Haldane couched his discussion in terms of different genetic strains, and thus was referring to a polygenic model, it is equally instructive to consider these patterns of interaction as if they applied to distinct genotypes of the major locus, coexisting in the same population.

As indicated in Figure 1, the four interactions are all characterized by a differential response of the two genotypes. However, in two of the four

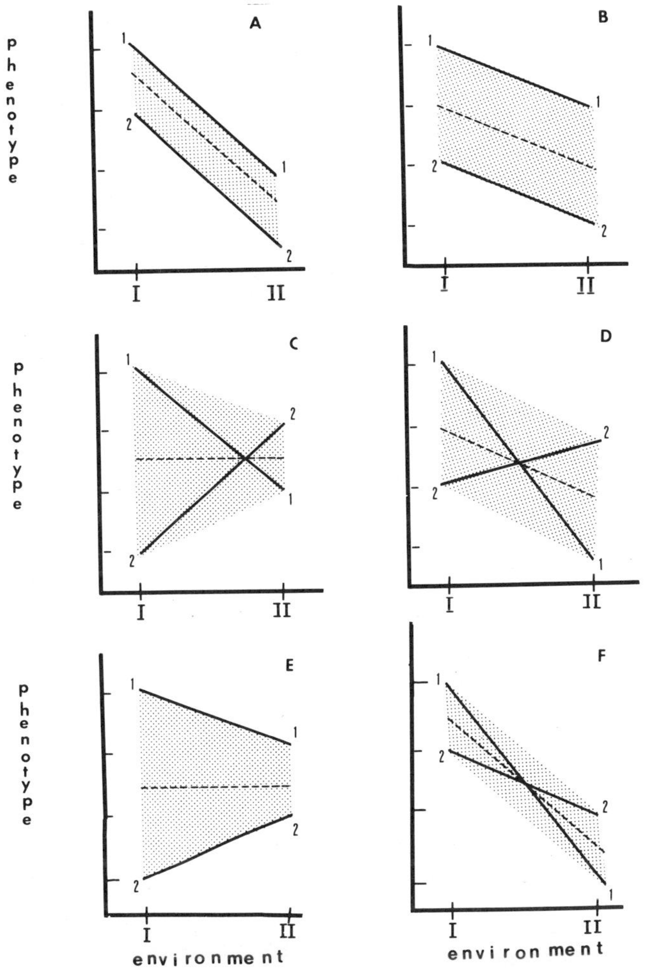

Figure 1. Depiction of Haldane's (1946) concept of the phenotypic response of two strains (or genotypes) to environmental change. By convention, strain "1" is assumed superior to strain "2" in environment "I", which is optimal. Genotype-environment interactions may reverse this relationship in the inferior environment, "II". Assuming additivity of effect, and equal proportions of each strain (or genotype), the population mean can be depicted by the dashed line, and the phenotypic variance by the shaded band.

interaction patterns, the population mean may remain unchanged, assuming additivity of response and equal frequencies of the two genotypes in the population. In one instance (IE) the relative position of the two genotypes is maintained (though the phenotypes have converged), while in the other (IC), the phenotypic values are reversed. Under the same assumption of additivity of effect and equal genotypic frequency, the remaining two patterns result in a changed population mean, though both genotypes may display a similar trend in response - though with different rates (1F), or inversely related trends (1D). Lastly, it will be noted that with these same assumptions, the two interactions exhibiting a change in population mean in response to environmental change (1D, 1F) maintain a constant phenotypic variance (represented by the shaded band), whereas the two interactions with stable means (1C, 1E) display a change in phenotypic variable. This latter situation is likely to have been a fairly common occurrence in human evolution. Thus, the concept of "phenotypic amplification" (Weiss, this volume) is but one example of a genotype-environmental interaction in which greatly increased phenotypic variability results from environmental change, with consequent appearance of a "notably deleterious genotype".

The complexity of the situation will be correspondingly increased when three (or more) genotypes are considered; when gene action is not additive (i.e. where the phenotypic response can be transformed onto a linear scale); when the genotypes displaying differential response to environmental change have markedly different gene frequencies in the population. Also, by reference to the model displayed in Equation 1, it will be noted that the interaction of genotypes with environmental change could involve either the polygenic component (as envisaged by Haldane), or a major locus contributing to an individual's deviation from the population mean (see below). As a consequence, the covariance structure of phenotypic response will need to be critically examined in order to discriminate between substantially different types of genetic involvement.

While it can be presumed that genotypic

frequencies will also change as a consequence of differential response to fluctuating environments, this is unlikely to be a critical factor in most human studies. Even in the situation depicted by Figures 1C and 1D where the contrasting response of different genotypes is most marked, the magnitude of selective differentials will not tend to be large enough to yield a noticeable change in allele frequencies in the time frame experienced by most human populations. In general, the time period that it takes most isolates to undergo substantial cultural and environmental transition is of the order of two generations or less. While this may cause a substantial perturbation in the equilibrium between selective differentials and allele frequencies, these are not likely to be of sufficient magnitude for any appreciable shift in allele frequencies to have occurred during the time period since the transition was initiated - at most four generations. For the same reason, shifts in allelic association (or linkage disequilibrium) are unlikely to result from environmental perturbations, in contrast to the consequences of small population size and population fission and fusion (Smouse et al., 1981).

As indicated by Equation (1), some consideration must be given to the form of distribution of environmental factors that interact with the genotypes within the population. The traditional model assumes that environmental factors are randomly distributed within the specified environmental zone. When polygenic influences only are considered, this leads to the standard analysis of variance model. However, it is well known that in human populations, environmental factors are often non-randomly distributed and tend to cluster in households with similar aggregations of biologically related individuals. This leads to the situation where culturally transmitted environments which interact with genetic traits may themselves cluster within nuclear families (Eaves, 1982; Rao et al., 1983). When such situations are analyzed by standard methods of path analysis, biased estimates of genetic heritability can result, if the situation is not explicitly controlled (Lathrop et al., 1984). Since the non-random environmental component can interact with either the major gene component, or the polygenic component, the final model for genotype-environmental interaction is remarkably complex.

Using the deviations defined by (1), the general model that includes genotype-environmental interaction can be given by the following equation:

$$Y_i = \mu_o + (1 + G_f + G_m + \tfrac{1}{2}g_f + \tfrac{1}{2}g_m)(1 + \Delta_f + \Delta_m + e_i) + \lambda_i - 1 \qquad (2)$$

This allows the definition of four distinct kinds of interaction: 1) the traditional interaction component represented by terms involving g.e; 2) interaction involving major locus susceptibility and random environment, G.e, as is likely to be important in infectious disease susceptibility; 3) interaction involving the polygenic component and culturally transmitted environmental component, g.Δ, as envisaged by Lathrop et al. (1984); and 4) interaction involving a major gene and culturally transmitted environment, G.Δ. Each kind of interaction will normally require a distinct set of contrasts to be set up for this estimation. However, as suggested by the results of the Tokelau study discussed below, there is suggestive evidence for the existence of interactions of the first two kinds in blood pressure response, while interactions of the third kind are likely to occur for a host of behavioral traits. In many cases, the study of isolates in transition will allow detection of any of these kinds of interactions, especially if an appropriate measure of response is defined.

ISOLATES IN TRANSITION

Earlier (Ward et al., 1979; Ward, 1980b) it has been emphasized that isolates in transition form an ideal study design for the estimation of etiological factors involved in the distribution of disease. Since such a study represents a "quasi-experimental study design", it is often possible to make inferences about underlying causal relationships. When dealing with traits in which genotype-environmental interactions play a role, such a study design has appreciable advantages, which are only surpassed by those studies which are analogous to a clinical trial - yielding the strongest level of epidemiological inference. Studies of isolates in transition rank alongside the classical epidemiological studies of migrants, in terms of their strength of inference - for many similar reasons. Elsewhere, the relative strengths and weaknesses of such study designs have been tabulated (Ward, 1980b). In the present context, it suffices to emphasize the following three advantages of studying isolates in transition, especially where genotype-environmental interactions are concerned.

First, even more than the case of migrant studies, analysis of disease risk in isolates in transition ensures that there is minimal misinterpretation of genetic effects and environmental factors. Since the gene pool of isolates is relatively homogeneous, any changes in the distribution of disease that follow, or accompany, the cultural transmission can be attributed to the action of environmental factors, with or without genotypic interaction.

Second, the transition experienced by many isolates tends to be relatively rapid and usually involves quite marked environmental contrasts. The existence of a strong environmental gradient, often with sharp discontinuities, tends to ensure that a phenotypic response will definitely occur. As a consequence, those isolates experiencing transition are usually faced with the onset of a new distribution of disease. Consequently, an appropriate study by the genetic epidemiologist can help alleviate at least a portion of the increased burden suffered by such societies - the price they pay for entry into the "western club". Given a broad distribution of environmental variables, the experimental contrasts that can be set up will lead to a moderately powerful test of hypothesis.

Third, in many cases, it is possible to set up contrasts to test specific hypotheses by evaluating the phenotypes of closely related individuals who inhabit measurably different environments. For example, if a fixed cluster approach is to be taken (Schull et al., 1970; Chakraborty and Schull, 1979), with relatives of a given type distributed across distinct environments (or stages of transition), the covariance structure can be set up to allow an explicit test of genotype-environment interactions. More complex fixed clusters can also be defined, with increased ability to identify the parameters of the model given by (2). When the situation does not permit sampling fixed clusters, analyses of complex pedigrees may allow similar hypotheses to be tested - provided the appropriate environmental measures are made. Since the genealogical structure of most traditional societies tends to be both extensive and all-encompassing (Huntsman et al., no date), the definition of complex pedigrees with members distributed throughout the environmental gradient is usually feasible for many isolates undergoing transition. The only significant disadvantage to this approach is the daunting complexity of the likelihood expression that is required to resolve the parameters of the model in an unambiguous manner.

From the above it will be apparent that when isolates in transition form the study design for an investigation of the impact of interaction between genotype and environment, the focus will necessarily be on the measurement of response. However, when the issue of genotype-environmental interaction can safely be ignored, the measurement of response may be less critical. Before examining some of the issues that need to be considered when defining response, it should first be stressed that measuring response alone is not sufficient to test a genetic hypothesis. The distribution of response amongst related individuals must also be assessed in terms of a genetic model. Such a study requires complete integration of both genetic and epidemiological techniques. In general, the definition of response is not possible without a comprehensive epidemiological analysis. Conversely, failure to accomplish an adequate genetic analysis will not permit any inference about presumptive genetic etiology. Thus, it is the integration of sampling methods and analytic designs from both fields which provides the real challenge to genetic epidemiology - unfortunately this challenge is still largely ignored.

DEFINING RESPONSE

One of the primary requirements in accomplishing a genetic epidemiological study of an isolate in transition, is to consider the manner in which "response" should be defined and measured. Given the objective of drawing genetic inference from the study, an *a priori* definition of response that takes account of the biological characteristics of the disease and the importance of making inference about causation becomes a necessity. In many instances, the manner in which the investigator chooses to define response will dictate the form of the study. Usually it will not be possible to define an adequate measure of response, leading to any strong inference, from an opportunistic survey of a population undergoing transition.

In this regard it is important to give consideration to the time required for an adequate response to develop. This time period will be a function of the characteristics of the biological variable being studied as well as of the magnitude of environmental change. For the "common diseases", such as cardiovascular disease or cancer, an appreciable time must elapse between the initiation of environmental change and the onset of a well defined physiological, or clinical, end point. Hence, studies of such diseases, and their associated risk factors, will normally require an appreciable longitudinal component. By contrast, when the response being investigated is represented by differential genetic susceptibility to an acute insult, such as an infectious disease, a properly executed cross-sectional study may be equally informative.

Thus, when investigating chronic diseases, or their associated risk factors, in a traditional isolate, a longitudinal study will be required. The variable of interest will be the changes in a risk factor such as blood pressure, after exposure to the novel environment over a period of time. These changes must also be evaluated in terms of the changed, and changing, distribution of relevant concomitants. As indicated below, an analysis of residuals may represent the most appropriate definition of response. Such a strategy requires a long term commitment to evaluating the distribution of a number of relevant concomitant variables in the population isolate over an appreciable period of time. The epidemiological investment in such a study can be extensive. For example, the Tokelau study has followed the fortunes of a small Polynesian atoll population over a 20 year period, during which they have migrated to New Zealand and adjusted into that environment.

On the other hand, the investigation of immediate differences in genetic susceptibility to a new environmental challenge such as an infectious agent can proceed more rapidly. For genetic analysis the variable being measured should be as close to a gene product as possible. Given the advances in immunology which allow the specification of products of immune response genes, it is now possible to investigate the interaction between components of the immune system and new environmental challenges. With well defined measures in cellular immunology being rapidly developed, this may soon prove to be a powerful area of investigation. Similarly, one can evaluate the changed relationship between a defined genotype, such as an HLA haplotype, and the onset of disease that shows marked association with that genotype, following environmental transition. Hence, the study of autoimmune diseases in isolates which are experiencing environmental transition may represent an equally useful paradigm.

DEFINING RESPONSE - ANALYSIS OF RESIDUALS

When dealing with a quantitative risk factor such as blood pressure, some measure of response is required before genetic analysis can be undertaken. Presuming that the transition experienced by an isolate results in two or more discernable environments, the distribution of the trait in the changed environment needs to be evaluated in terms of the distribution of the original environment. In a truly longitudinal study, observed changes in the trait that follow the environmental transition represent a crude but unsatisfactory measure of response. The altered distribution may be due to changes in other concomitants, such as age, that have little to do with the advent of a new environmental challenge. Accordingly, an analysis of residuals can be used to define a more realistic measure of response.

The response variable will be defined by using information from both the original environment and the new environment. The objective is to partition the distribution of the trait in the new environment into three specific and identifiable components. The first component represents changes in the trait due to changes in concomitants, such as age, that would occur irrespective of the environmental change. This first component will be of little interest to the geneticist - though it may be of considerable interest to the epidemiologist. The second component identifies changes in the relationship between the originally defined set of concomitants and the trait in the new environment. This changed relationship can be viewed as an interaction component due to the influence of environmental transition, though a genetic analysis is required to determine whether the interaction involves genetic factors. The third component represents changes in the trait that cannot be attributed to a changed relationship with the original concomitants, and is therefore attributed to new factors which were not present in the old environment. This third component is also a candidate for interpretation as a genotype-environment interaction effect.

By analogy with analysis of covariance, we have set up a simple linear model which allows identification of these three components in blood pressure response in Tokelauans (Ward, 1983a; Ward et al., 1985a). The model can be used in a truly longitudinal survey or in a mixed cross-sectional longitudinal study design.

It is assumed that in the original environment, the relationship between a trait, Y, and an epidemiologically defined set of concomitants can be represented by the following linear equation.

$$Y_1 = f(\text{concomitants}) + \text{residual} \quad (3)$$

In the new environment the distribution of the trait will normally be changed. It can be represented as due to a relationship between the original set of concomitants, though the relationship may well be altered, plus the relationship with a new set of concomitants in the new environment. This is represented by:

$$Y_2 = h(\text{old concomitants}) + y(\text{new concomitants}) + \text{error} \quad (4)$$

However, the new functional relationship between the trait and the original set of concomitants can be split into two parts. The first will represent the original functional relationship, while the second identifies the new functional relationship. This is represented by:

$$Y_2 = f(\text{old concomitants}) + g(\text{old concomitants}) + y(\text{new concomitants}) + \text{error} \quad (5)$$

Given this simple system, it is clear that response in the new environment can be specified in terms of the deviation of the observed trait from the value predicted in terms of the relationship between the trait and the concomitants in the original environment. Thus, if the original relationship between the trait and the epidemiologically defined concomitants is defined by the function f, the full response can be defined as follows.

$$R_1 = Y_2 - f(\text{concomitants}) \quad (6)$$

This residual represents the "full response" since it incorporates both the changed relationships with the concomitants plus the influence of new concomitants, not present (or measured) in the old environment. If the relationship between the full response and the original set of concomitants is investigated by regression, this will define g. As seen below, the form of this function will identify the extent of the changed relationship between the trait and the original concomitants in the new environment. This functional form can then be subtracted from the first residual, as indicated below, to give a second residual, which measures the effect of new concomitants in the new environment.

$$R_2 = R_1 - g(\text{concomitants}) \quad (7)$$

The advantage of this kind of model is twofold. First, it allows a simple partition of the factors influencing the changed distribution of the trait in the new environment. In particular, it allows identification of secular changes that would have occurred anyway (e.g. increase in blood pressure due to increased age) and which will not normally be of interest for a genetic analysis. Secondly, the model can be used for a truly longitudinal study, as well as for a mixed cross-sectional longitudinal study. In the latter case, where there is not a complete set of measurements on each individual for the complete time period, the model is used as indicated by the equations specified above (Ward et al., 1985; Altman et al., 1985). However, in the event that a truly longitudinal survey exists, the increased information can be utilized by regressing directly on the changes in concomitants in order to identify the functional form g. Similarly, in a longitudinal study the original residual from (3) can be subtracted from the second residual defined by (7) in order to develop an unbiased estimate of the interrelationship given by the new concomitants, specified by function y. These principles are illustrated in more detail in Ward (1983) and Ward et al. (1985).

In terms of defining genotype-environmental interaction, the estimation of the changed relationship between the trait and the concomitants, as given by g, will form an important part of interpreting the data. Since the distribution of concomitants is likely to change in the new environment, identifying the components of such changed relationships without such a procedure will be difficult. The importance of being able to do this is illustrated by the change in age-specific rates, and age-specific relationships of traits as environments change. Age is one of the most ubiquitous concomitants for chronic disease and the change in the age-specific relationship as a consequence of environmental transition is suggestive of the existence of genotype-environmental interaction. Elsewhere in this volume Weiss elaborates on this specific representation of genotype-environmental interaction under the term "phenotype amplification." Parenthetically, it can be noted that if the relationship between concomitants differs for different genotypes, and can be properly defined, estimation of genotypic specific risk can be accomplished by procedures analogous to multiple logistic regression (Bucher et al., n.d.).

BLOOD PRESSURE RESPONSE IN TOKELAUAN MIGRANTS

As indicated elsewhere, the Tokelau Island migrant study affords a good example of a genetic epidemiology study based on an isolate in transition (Ward et al., 1979; 1980). Initiated in 1967/68, the study aimed to follow the distribution of cardiovascular risk factors in this small Polynesian population as they underwent migration from their traditional atoll environment in Tokelau, to the modern environment of New Zealand. At the present time, the total population numbers approximately 4,000 individuals of which some 1,600 still remain in their traditional atoll environment while the remaining 2,400 now reside in New Zealand. The bulk of the migration to New Zealand occurred between the period 1968 and 1972, though some sporadic migration (and back-migration) still occurs.

In their traditional environment, the Tokelauans inhabit three atolls which may be regarded as three distinct sub-populations, though genetically these are remarkably similar (Ward et al, 1980). A single pedigree has been constructed for the entire population, numbering some 8,000 individuals, and stretching back to 10 to 15 generations. By analyzing genetic markers determined on a subset of the population, the accuracy of this pedigree for the past 4 generations was found to be remarkably high (Lathrop et al., 1983).

Although blood pressure and other cardiovascular risk factors have actually been collected from this population over the period 1963 to 1982, we shall focus on three surveys only. The first, accomplished in 1968/71 defines the "premigrant" population. The distribution of blood pressure in this premigrant population indicated that, at that time, there were no substantial differences in blood pressure of other cardiovascular risk factors between those individuals who would migrate and those who would choose to remain at home. We shall use the distribution of blood pressure, and concomitants of blood pressure, in this survey population to define the baseline relationship of Equation 3.

In order to define the impact of environmental transition, we shall analyze the response of blood pressure in two subsequent surveys. The first is the survey of migrant Tokelauans living in New Zealand, carried out in 1975/77. The distribution of blood pressure in the population will reflect the impact of the new environment over a 5 to 8 year time period. The second is the 1976 survey of nonmigrant Tokelauans living in their home atolls. This will serve as a comparison point, against which to evaluate the results for migrants. It will also serve to identify the existence of secular change that has occurred in the atolls. Even though migration is a readily defined environmental change, a number of environmental transitions have occurred in the home atolls. Over 850 adults form the premigrant survey, while the nonmigrant survey comprises 640 adults, and the migrant survey 980.

In order to first define the original relationship between baseline concomitants and blood pressure in the original environment, as depicted by Equation 3, we used step-wise regression procedures as well as an all-subsets regression. The concomitants defined for blood pressure were: atoll of origin, sex, height, weight, fat index, body mass index, serum cholesterol, and age (expressed as a third degree polynomial). The blood pressure response was then calculated for both the nonmigrants and migrants, according to Equation 6 above. For comparison, the change in age standardized blood pressure was also calculated for these two populations.

These results are presented in Table 1 for both

systolic and diastolic blood pressure, separately by sex. It will be noted that both change in age standardized blood pressure and blood pressure response is negative for the nonmigrant populations. However, it will be seen that the blood pressure response is more negative than the change in standardized blood pressure. This suggests that the incremental change in blood pressure is somewhat less than would have been predicted by changes in the concomitants. For the migrants, observed blood pressure has increased, relative to the premigrant baseline blood pressure, however blood pressure response is only positive for males. It will be noted that the separation between migrants and nonmigrants is similar, irrespective of whether age standardized change in blood pressure is used, or blood pressure response. However, note that these results show that the migrant and nonmigrant populations have both diverged from the original premigrant values - in opposite directions. Hence, the presently observed difference in blood pressure between migrants and nonmigrants cannot be attributed entirely to factors in the New Zealand environment.

Table 1. Distribution of blood pressure change and blood pressure response in Tokelauans.

	Blood pressure change		Blood pressure response (full)	
	Nonmigrants	Migrants	Nonmigrants	Migrants
Systolic				
Males	-1.5	7.0	-5.0	5.6
Females	-1.8	3.4	-6.9	-4.0
Diastolic				
Males	-0.8	5.8	-2.9	6.6
Females	-2.9	-0.9	-4.7	-0.6

Having defined a simple measure of blood pressure response, it is relevant to investigate which factors contributed to the change in blood pressure over this time. This was accomplished by regressing blood pressure change against the set of concomitants for both the cross-sectional data (Ward, 1983; Ward et al., 1985) and the longitudinal data (Ward et al., 1985). In general, changes in blood pressure were highly associated with changes in weight as well as with the initial blood pressure, the initial age, and the initial body mass. Hence, as indicated by other epidemiological studies, the rate of blood pressure change in either environment is not evenly distributed within the population, but is influenced by factors such as age, relative obesity and so forth.

Having defined blood pressure response, it was of interest to determine to what extent blood pressure response was a function of a changed relationship with the original concomitants. This analysis was carried out by regressing the full blood pressure response against the set of original concomitants in step-wise fashion. The results are presented in Table 2. It will be noted that except for nonmigrant females, the changed relationship between blood pressure and the original concomitants made a significant contribution to blood pressure response. Further, despite the _a priori_ assumption that the biggest change in slope would be with variables such as weight and body mass, this was not generally observed. Body mass, and to a lesser extent cholesterol and weight, did exhibit significant changes in slope in most of the populations, but these were not as marked as the evidence for a changed relationship with age.

As indicated by Table 2, by far the greatest contribution to the R^2 for the full response came from the changed relationship with age, either singly or in interaction with the atoll of origin. Thus, in this population the full blood pressure response in both the migrant and nonmigrant environment is substantially influenced by the changed relationship with age. Inspection of the data indicates that the consequence of environmental transition has been to increase the slope of blood pressure with age. This is consistent with the general observation that in traditional societies blood pressure does not rise appreciably with age in adulthood, while in highly urbanized societies increasing age usually results in a sharp rise in blood pressure. Hence, the transition experienced by Tokelauan migrants, and to a lesser extent nonmigrants, is to result in a changed relationship with age. These results suggest that the concept of "phenotypic amplification" (Weiss, this volume) will have general validity for most isolates in transition, and is likely to denote genotype-environmental interaction.

Table 2. Blood pressure response in postmigrant Tokelauans defined by changed relationships with original concomitants. Successive contributions to R^2 by regressing baseline concomitants against residuals in postmigrants, where residuals result from original baseline (premigrant) regression. Variables enter in the order indicated.

		Weight	Body Mass	Choles- terol	Age	Atoll	Total
Migrant							
Male	SBP	0.0	2.9**	0.7	2.3**	6.4**	12.3**
Female	SBP	1.6**	0.2	3.5**	6.0**	2.1**	13.4**
Male	DBP	0.2	0.1	0.9*	1.4**	4.5**	7.1**
Female	DBP	1.3*	0.2	0.4	2.1**	3.0**	7.0**
Nonmigrant							
Male	SBP	0.3	6.8**	1.1	12.0**	5.0**	25.2**
Female	SBP	0.2	0.0	0.0	2.2**	0.1	2.5
Male	DBP	0.4	2.9**	2.4*	3.0*	5.3**	14.0**
Female	DBP	0.7	0.1	0.1	1.1	1.5*	3.5

* $.01 < p < .05$
** $p < .01$

Having identified response in terms of a significant change in the relationship between blood pressure and concomitants, it remains to determine whether genetic factors are implicated in this response. This analysis was carried out by complex segregation analysis using the mixed model of Morton and McLean (1974) and the program POINTER (Lalouel and Morton, 1981). The results are depicted in Table 3. For all populations there is significant evidence for the existence of two distributions of response - a major component and a minor component - with the mixture contributing about 30% of the total variance in response, except for nonmigrant diastolic response.

There is also consistent evidence for the existence of a polygenic component in response which contributes 17 to 27% of the total variance. It is noteworthy that the magnitude of the variance component attributed to polygenic factors in response is approximately the same as the contribution of additive genetic factors to the blood pressure variability in these populations. There is thus reasonable evidence that genetic factors are involved in the response, and hence that genotype-environmental interactions play a role in the altered distribution of blood pressure.

Table 3. Genetic analysis of full blood pressure response in Tokelauans.

	% Variance attributed to:		Minor component		
	Polygenic component	Mixture distri-putions	Fre-quency	Deviation from major component	Interpre-tation
Nonmigrants					
Systolic	20.8	30.1	0.198	2.83	Non-familial
Diastolic	27.5	17.1	0.122	3.42	Non-familial
Migrants					
Systolic	17.6	29.2	0.201	2.74	? Recessive
Diastolic	22.3	29.5	0.072	4.14	Familial

However, there is little evidence for the existence of major genes. In the nonmigrant population there is no familial aggregation of the minor component and the presumption is that those individuals who are "high responders" are those who have been exposed to a particular constellation of environmental factors. In the migrant population there is some evidence for familial aggregation of the minor component, but in the case of diastolic blood pressure, evaluation of the transmission parameters indicates that the mode of transmission is not Mendelian. For the systolic blood pressure response, the likelihood associated with transmission parameters consistent with a Mendelian hypothesis is not significantly different from the likelihood where the parameters are jointly estimated from the data. This could be interpreted as possible evidence for the existence of a major gene influencing blood pressure response. However, since this is not observed in the other analyses, some caution must be exercised in accepting this conclusion.

The analysis indicates that the distribution of blood pressure response in both Tokelauan populations is influenced approximately equally by polygenic factors, and the existence of two components ("high responders" and "low responders"). Collectively, these two components account for about half of the total variability in response. Since the response has been shown to be largely a function of changed relationships with original concomitants (especially age), the estimate of a significant polygenic component gives some credence to the concept of genotype-environmental interaction of the type originally envisaged by Haldane. In this Polynesian population a changed distribution of environmental variables results in a markedly different distribution of a cardiovascular risk factor such as blood pressure, which is partly attributable to underlying genetic differences in the response to the new environment.

The apparent existence of a small population of "high responders" is more difficult to interpret. The evidence from the nonmigrant population, and from the distribution of diastolic response in the migrants, is more suggestive of the introduction of a new set of environmental factors, which appear to cluster in the migrants. Clarification of this issue can only be attained by further analysis of response, especially the definition of the contribution made by new concomitants to response by evaluating the distribution of the difference in residuals, for those individuals measured at both points in time. This analysis is currently being carried out, with evaluation of the change in blood pressure over a 19 year period.

CONCLUSION

This paper has aimed to stress the importance of studying isolates in transition, as a means of identifying underlying etiological components for many diseases, It has been pointed out that the specification of both major gene components and polygenic components, in conjunction with randomly distributed environments and environments which aggregate in households, results in a complex etiological model. In general, while such a model is realistic it is not amenable to analysis unless a quasi-experimental study design is adopted. Isolates in transition have a number of advantages in this respect.

However, one of the critical assumptions in such a study is that an adequate measure of response can be defined and then subjected to genetic analysis. In general, little attention is paid to the proper definition of a response variable. As indicated by the Tokelau study, this can be effectively done by considering variously defined "residuals" and subjecting these residuals to genetic analysis. It should be stressed however that this approach usually requires a fairly extensive longitudinal study when appreciable time is needed for a physiological response to become manifest. If response is more immediate, or a defined gene product can be identified, it may be more efficient to attempt to identify genotype-environmental interactions directly, in terms of the distribution of disease risk amongst identifiable genotypes.

Based on the analysis of blood pressure response in Tokelau, plus a similar analysis on response of lipoprotein fractions (Ward, in preparation), it appears that genotype-environmental interactions may be a common occurrence in the epidemiology of isolates in transition. This imposes a number of restrictions on the study designs, and analytic strategies, that can be used to properly identify such contributions to etiology. Usually a simple cross-sectional analysis of data will not suffice. This is indicated by the Tokelau data, where a simple comparison of migrant and nonmigrant populations suggests that migrants exhibit a substantial increase in blood pressure as a consequence of entering the new environment. As indicated by the response model, not only is this false but, more importantly, there has been a marked change in the relationship between blood pressure and concomitants such as weight and age. Thus increments of weight result in a smaller rise of blood pressure than would have been formerly predicted, while increments of age result in a larger rise.

If the response to the new environment is not properly identified, there is little point in carrying out a genetic analysis. Hence, it appears that for the majority of common diseases, such as cardiovascular disease and cancer, without a properly designed longitudinal study there is little chance in realistically identifying genetic components of etiology, especially where genotype-environmental interactions are involved. Given the importance of this type of study, and the current interest amongst genetic epidemiologists in these issues, it appears imperative that such longitudinal study designs be given increased emphasis. In some instances, it will be possible to resurrect old studies and convert them into longitudinal studies of the type required. However, in the majority of instances, new studies will have to be devised and given the time required for completion.

There appears little time to be lost. Twenty years ago a warning note was sounded that unless the genetic structure of tribal societies was studied immediately, the onset of acculturation would result in this information being lost forever (Neel and Salzano, 1964). Ten years later the field of genetic epidemiology struggled into existence, but even today properly designed and executed genetic epidemiology studies of isolates are a rarity. Today the situation for physiological traits is much more acute than Neel and Salzano envisaged for the genetic polymorphisms. Not only have we lost twenty years, but genetic markers are much more immutable than physiological traits such as blood pressure, obesity, and serum glucose. There is an urgent need to identify those few traditional isolates that are currently undergoing the transition from a traditional environment to a more acculturated, westernized environment, and than to execute a properly designed study. Thus the current major challange to biological anthropology is to identify such populations and carry out appropriate studies which focus on the identification of etiological components before this information is lost forever. In so doing, biological anthropologists may also begin to repay the debt they owe to traditional societies, by helping to alleviate the burdens caused by the changing patterns of disease as societies adjust to new environments.

ACKNOWLEDGEMENTS

Supported by Grant HL26829 from the U.S. National Institutes of Health.

LITERATURE CITED

Altman NS, Ward RH, Prior IAM (1985). Patterns of blood pressure response in migrant and non-migrant Tokelauans. II. Factors influencing blood pressure reponse in adults. J Chron Dis (submitted).

Bucher KD, Moll PP, Davignon J, Sing CF (n.d.). Multivariate genetic models for risk of developing a common disease: Major gene models. (manuscript).

Chakraborty R, Schull WJ (1971). Fixed cluster designs. In Sing CF, Skolnick MH (eds): "Genetic Analysis of Common Disease," New York: Alan R. Liss, p 343.

Eaves LJ (1982). The utility of twins. In: Anderson VE, Hauser WA, Penry JK, Sing CF (eds): "Genetic Basis of Epilepsies," New York: Raven Press, p 249.

Elston RC, Stewart JA (1971). A general model for the genetic analysis of pedigree data. Hum Hered 21:253.

Haldane JBS (1946). The interaction of nature and nurture. Ann Eugen 13:197.
Huntsman JW, Hooper AB, Ward RH (n.d.). Genealogies as culture and biology: A Tokelau case study. Amer Anthropol (submitted).
Lalouel JM, Morton NE (1981). Complex segregation analysis with pointers. Hum Hered 31:313.
Lathrop GM, Huntsman JW, Hooper AB, Ward, RH (1983). Evaluating pedigree data. II. Identifying the cause of error in families with inconsistencies. Hum Hered 33:389.
Lathrop GM, Lalouel JM, Jacquard A (1984). Gene-environment interactions in the path analysis of family resemblance. Biometrics (in press).
McNeill WH (1980). "The Human Condition." New Jersey: Princeton.
Morton NE (1980). Diseases determined by major genes. Soc Biol 26:94.
Morton NE, MacLean CJ (1974). Analysis of family resemblance. III. Complex segregation of quantitative traits. Am J Hum Genet 26:489.
Morton NE, Gulbrandsen CL, Rao DC, Rhoads GG, Kagan A (1980). Determinants of blood pressure in Japanese-American families. Hum Genet 53:261.
Neel JV, Salzano F (1964). A prospectus for genetic studies of the American Indian. Cold Spring Harbor Symp Quant Biol 29:85.
Rao DC, Williams WR, McGue M, Morton NE, Gulbrandsen CL, Rhoads GG, Kagan A, Laskarezewski P, Glueck Cj, Russell JM (1983). Cultural and biological inheritance of plasma lipids. Am J Phys Anthropol 62:33.
Schull WJ, Harburg E, Erfurt JC, Schork MA, Richard R (1972). A family set method for estimating heredity and stress. J Chron Dis 23:83.
Schull WJ, Weiss KM (1980). Genetic epidemiology; Four strategies. Epidemiologic Rev 2:1.
Smouse PE, Vitzthum VJ, Neel JV (1981). The impact of random and lineal fission on the genetic divergence of small human groups: A case study among the Yanomama. Genetics 98:179.
Ward RH (1980a). Genetic epidemiology: Promise or compromise? Soc Biol 27:87.
Ward RH (1980b). Genetic epidemiology in an anthropological context. Med Anth 4:293.
Ward RH (1983a). Genetic and sociocultural components

of high blood pressure. Am J Phys Anth 62:91.
Ward RH (1983b). Culture, Genes and Disease: Physical Anthropology in a Community Setting. Auckland University Centenary Symposium "Anthropology and the Community", Auckland, May 1983, p 1.
Ward RH, Chin PG, Prior IAM (1979). Genetic epidemiology of blood pressure in a migrating isolate: Prospectus. In Sing CG, Skolnick MH (eds): "Genetic Analysis of Common Diseases." New York: Alan R. Liss, p 675.
Ward RH, Raspe PD, Ramirez ME, Kirk RL, Prior IAM (1980). Genetic Structure and Epidemiology: The Tokelau Island Study. In Eriksson A et al. (eds): "Population Structure and Genetic Disorders," Academic Press, p 301.
Ward RH, Altman N, Prior IAM (1985). Patterns of blood pressure response in migrant and nonmigrant Tokelauans. I. Defining response. J Chron Dis (submitted).

Diseases of Complex Etiology in Small Populations:
Ethnic Differences and Research Approaches, pages 179–198

Chapter 8

PHENOTYPE AMPLIFICATION, AS ILLUSTRATED BY CANCER OF THE GALLBLADDER IN NEW WORLD PEOPLES

K.M. Weiss

Center for Demographic and Population Genetics, University of Texas Graduate School of Biomedical Sciences, Houston, Texas

INTRODUCTION: SOME PROBLEMS IN GENETIC EPIDEMIOLOGY

Many diseases may be thought of as having point sources. That is, one may be able to identify a specific point in time and space at which the disease was caused. This is the case for infectious diseases, the 'point' being the occurrence of exposure to a pathogen. In the case of those genetic diseases which are present from birth, the 'point' is effectively the time of conception, at which inheritance of the deleterious allele occurs. The analysis of diseases of point etiology has occupied much attention in epidemiology and anthropological approaches to disease have largely been concerned with such diseases.

Interest has shifted in recent years to diseases which do not have point etiology but which instead seem to be caused by the continual operation of pathogenic processes over a period of time. Such processes neither instantaneously produce disease nor do they by themselves imply that disease will occur in a specific exposed individual. For a variety of reasons, generally not yet understood, only a subset of the exposed individuals in a population will ever manifest a clinical disease as a result of that exposure. Degenerative diseases of this type have come to dominate the attention of epidemiology in places where the impact of infectious diseases has been relieved. Among them are cancer, circulatory diseases, chronic inflammatory and autoimmune diseases, and metabolic diseases like diabetes. These seem to be the result of long-term exposure to many different causal factors (including genes), and each victim may not need to be exposed to the same specific factors. A term frequently used for such etiology is 'multifactorial'. Where the infectious disease epidemiologist seeks coincidence between an exposure and disease, his chronic disease counterpart evaluates the correlation between disease rates (or phenotype measures, like blood pressure) and levels of exposure to risk factors. Similarly, where a geneticist traditionally has searched for segregation proportions, we now search for correlations between relatives. However, we no longer expect the correlations to resemble those of purely genetic inheritance. By analogy with environmental dose-response relationships, genetic epidemiology invokes 'incomplete penetrance' in various manifestations to explain the deviation from pure Mendelian expectations in family members (e.g., Vogel and Motulsky, 1979).

ETIOLOGY OF CHRONIC DISEASE

Environmental interaction is usually necessary, even among the genetically susceptible, to produce chronic disease. The incomplete effect of exposure on susceptible genotypes is a major source of incomplete penetrance, though this concept has generally been used in a black-box way to account for all sorts of errors and problems, including misdiagnosis, competing causes of disease, and various gene-environment interactions. To compound the problem, it is generally considered that some, perhaps most, cases of chronic disease are not genetic in origin, but are sporadic occurrences of the same pathology that are totally environmentally produced.

For quantitative traits, especially ones for which a polygenic etiology is hypothesized, one can treat the problem of gene-environment effects by including appropriate terms in the equations which decompose the variance in the measure of the trait, or risk of exceeding a phenotypic threshold, into components due to environment, genes, or both. However, such approaches cannot identify a causal genotype, nor do they characterize the genes involved, since the epidemiological models (e.g., path diagram) are explicitly agnostic. For example, they often postulate that the disease-related genes are indeterminate in number and have equal effects.

For a trait in which one suspects that a major gene is involved, however, one may hope to detect and characterize an actual gene product involved in risk, namely, an allelic variant at a specific, mappable locus. In this circumstance, incomplete penetrance is frequently a devastating phenomenon. A very 'non-Mendelian' disease pattern can be taken as statistical evidence for the existence of a Mendelian locus if the data are much more likely to arise that way than from an environmental or polygenic model, but this is often found only in some data sets. Even if there is statistical support for a major locus, if relatively few individuals in a pedigree are affected--due to age, sex, or other forms of incomplete penetrance--the attempt to identify genotypes often fails. The effort to find a linkage map location can be thoroughly frustrated, because one may not be able to differentiate between true recombinants and the effect of incomplete penetrance. As a result, many diseases which consistently seem to be familial have eluded definitive determination of the kinds of genes involved and where they are located. Heart disease, adult-onset diabetes, and many of the major cancers are examples.

An improved ability to assess the role of genes in the etiology of chronic disease might be gained by reconsidering the biological models which underlie the analysis. In particular, more careful thought might be given to the means by which deleterious alleles alter or affect human physiology. For some diseases, single genes may underlie what appear superficially to be very complex processes, and a discrimination between single and polygenic control may be possible by refining the biological analysis of the data.

IMPROVEMENT OF EXISTING MODELS: PHENOTYPE AMPLIFICATION

Degenerative diseases, by and large, were probably quite rare through most of human evolution. During that time, loss of teeth, physical dangers, and biological parasites probably prevented most individuals from living long enough to suffer serious degenerative deterioration. Variants arising which improved, or did not alter, physiological function could have persisted whether or not they had deleterious effects only in old age.

Similarly, genetic variants may arise in environments in which their phenotypic expression is only slightly different from that of genes already present. In particular, such genes may be clinically 'silent' producing no ill effects, or may even have some positive effects under the conditions in which they arose. Major environmental change, however, could serve to exaggerate the phenotypic differences expressed by different genotypes to the point that some became pathological.

The essential point of this paper is the thesis that many degenerative disease phenotypes may have a genetic basis which is the result of the exaggerated, or amplified, expression of otherwise normal genetic variants under new, or substantially changed, environments. Such genes may only be partially or indirectly related to the disease which ultimately results from that change. This phenomenon can be referred to as 'phenotype amplification'.

The concept of phenotype amplification can help provide a working model for the understanding of the biology underlying many degenerative diseases. This concept is similar to that of gene-by-environment interaction in quantitative genetics (Falconer, 1981), and, though widely recognized in general, it is less often put to practical use in human genetics.

Substantially new environments are typical of our time, as shown by (1) the rapid and comprehensive relief from acute causes of death early in life, especially from biological pathogens, (2) the great increase in the amount, variety, and predictability of nutrients, (3) great improvements in hygiene accompanied, however, by long-term exposures to new chemicals of various kinds, and (4) the rapid and often overwhelming changes which have accompanied the acculturation of native peoples around the world to modern ways.

In most degenerative diseases of interest, the salient facts usually include exposure to substantial amounts of some pathogenic agent(s), and long enough survival for the cumulative effects of that exposure to be expressed in the form of disease. In general, it appears that degenerative diseases can arise in almost any individual given enough time and the relevant exposure. A common characteristic of phenotype amplification in genetics is that the expression of the susceptible genotype occurs at an earlier age, or after a shorter exposure time, than in the normal genotypes. However, while age effects are generally to be expected, they need not be so large as to be the defining difference between genetic and sporadic cases.

We are used, in genetics, to look for genes directly related to a phenotype of interest--for example, genes 'for' blue eyes or cystic fibrosis. However, when there is phenotype amplification, there may be many steps in the pathogenic process, and the genetic variant which leads some individuals to be susceptible to a particular clinical outcome may not be directly related to that outcome. Thus, some breast cancer may be 'genetic' in that certain individuals are susceptible, but there may not be genes 'for' breast cancer in the usual sense. For example, a genetically-based increase in the production of normal hormones causing the cells lining the breast ducts to divide may lead to an increased probability that a mutated cell will proliferate and become malignant--but such a hormone-related gene is not, in any direct sense, related to cancer itself. Indeed, the final disease may be randomly distributed among those at risk, for example, the result of a chance mutation in a ductal stem-cell. Familial polyposis of the colon, a familial cancer precursor, may produce cancer merely by increasing the number of at-risk cells in the colon as a result of extensive polyp growth. To consider a disease like cancer to be the phenotype of interest in genetic epidemiology, just because we are interested in cancer epidemiology, may be to misunderstand the nature of the disease process.

When phenotype amplification occurs, there may be so many events or so much time between the processes leading to disease and their final expression as disease that only a fraction of the susceptibles ever manifest the disease. Even though there may appear to be an excess of cases in family members, there may not be enough cases to segregate in clear Mendelian fashion, and the familiality may be attributed to low heritability, very incomplete penetrance, or common exposures among family members--with little ability to resolve the issue among these and other 'explanations'. The effect of such genes might only be to raise the absolute risk by a few percent or less. In what sense can we say, then, that they are genes 'for' the disease? By what physiological mechanism do they work?

With improved biological models, and the biological data to support them, diseases thought to be of low heritability or low penetrance may be discernible as due to major genes at single loci. This is because the underlying genetic variant, if it could be identified, is probably expressed early--even from birth--its pathologic effects only appearing much later. The earlier one can examine the pathogenic process, the more likely is this variant to be detected, and as a result, the more likely is a truly Mendelian pattern to be identifiable. This can open the way to effective efforts to identify genetic linkage, map variant proteins, or to improved counseling, prevention, or treatment.

Many of the concepts of phenotype amplification can be illustrated by the example of an important disease problem in peoples native to the New World and their genetic relatives. The following is based partly on our own work in Mexican-Americans and on a synthesis of reports taken from many unrelated studies of Amerindians.

METABOLIC RESPONSE TO NEW ENVIRONMENTS: GALLBLADDER CANCER IN NEW WORLD PEOPLES

Cancer of the gallbladder (GBCA) is about 2-6 times as frequent in Amerindians and peoples related to them as it is in the rest of the US population. This has been found in groups ranging from Amerindians in Alaska to Bolivia (Weiss et al., 1984a,b; Henson, 1983). Clearly, one might suspect that this is a genetic disease (Mack and Menck, 1982; Diehl, 1980). But is it? There are in the literature only 3 families in which it has been suggested that there is genetic risk for gallbladder cancer (Devor and Buechly, 1979; Sperling, 1964). In none of them does the disease occurrence resemble a clear Mendelian pattern.

GBCA may be one late-stage amplification product of exposure to recent environmental change. The evidence suggests that the high frequency of this disease pattern is largely a post-war phenomenon (Heaton, 1972; 1981) due probably to some elements of diet interacting with the genetic substrate present in some New World peoples. In this instance we can identify an earlier, and more highly penetrant, phenotype that is itself not a primary lesion. It is known that cholesterol gallstones are a common precursor of cancer of the gallbladder (Devor, 1982; Diehl, 1980) and they may even be a necessary prodromal state.

In Amerindian populations studied without regard to non-Amerindian admixture, the cumulative risk of gallstones by age 85 or so is very close to 90%, especially in women (Sampliner et al., 1970). If this disease has a genetic basis, the gene frequency in aboriginal Americans may have been virtually 1.0. That cholelithiasis has a genetic basis in the New World has strong support from a variety of evidence (Weiss et al., 1984a). Gallstones appear to be part of a New World 'syndrome' which also includes obesity, adult-onset diabetes, and possibly several digestive system cancers other than GBCA (Weiss et al., 1984b).

Genes responsible for cholesterol gallstones seem also to be expressed in admixed populations with some

Amerindian ancestry. It has been estimated that the admixture rate of Amerindian genes in Mexican-Americans in Colorado is 40% (Gottlieb and Kimberling, 1979), in California 32% (Reed, 1974), and in San Antonio, 18-46% (Relethford et al., 1983). If at a single locus, there were genes with frequency nearly 1.0 in pre-contact Amerindians, and as low as .20 in Mexican- Americans, with random mating with respect to this gene about 36% of individuals in the latter populations will have one or more copies of the gene at any relevant locus (the probability of at least one copy of the gene under Hardy-Weinberg assumptions). This is consistent with estimates derived from our own work in two communities, Laredo and Starr County, on the Texas-Mexican border. In Laredo we estimate a 32% rate of cholecystectomies in women who live to age 75 or so, and in Starr County a prevalence survey found the cumulative incidence of symptomatic gallbladder disease by age 55 to be about 29% in females (Weiss et al., 1984a). Males also are at elevated risk, but less so than females, for various reasons, one being that in men the exacerbating effects of pregnancy do not occur.

What is the Fraction of Mexican-American Sibships that is Expected to Show Familial Gallbladder Cancer?

Let us consider a demographically typical family of Mexican-Americans, and the probability that they would come to our attention by virtue of having more than one case of GBCA. The relevant members of such a family will largely be restricted to sibs born around 1900-1910: their parents will generally have died before the routine diagnosis of GBCA was possible (whether or not the disease was actually common), that is, before World War II (Weiss et al., 1984a), and their children will be too young to manifest the disease, which rarely strikes before age 60. To approximate the experience of such a sibship, we can use the mortality rates taken from the Laredo data up through 1940 (Badzioch, 1982), and the 1970 Texas Mexican-American rates thereafter (Buchanan and Weiss, in preparation). From this the survivorship of members of a cohort born about 1900 to their mid 60s in age is about 30-35% (Table 1). This is due largely to increased mortality rates, especially in infants, in the earlier part of the century, and is about a third lower than in the US as a whole (Moriyama and Gustavus, 1972). Of a typical family with a sibship size of roughly 4, only 1.44 will have survived to age 65 or more.

Table 1. Estimated survivorship for circum-1900 and projected survivorship for 1970 Cohort of Mexican-Americans.[1]

Age	1900		1970	
	Male	Female	Male	Female
0	1.00	1.00	1.00	1.00
5	0.70	0.71	0.96	0.97
10	0.69	0.70	0.96	0.97
15	0.67	0.69	0.96	0.97
20	0.64	0.66	0.95	0.97
25	0.59	0.59	0.93	0.96
30	0.53	0.52	0.92	0.96
35	0.50	0.49	0.91	0.95
40	0.48	0.46	0.89	0.94
45	0.47	0.45	0.88	0.93
50	0.45	0.45	0.85	0.91
55	0.43	0.43	0.81	0.88
60	0.40	0.41	0.75	0.84
65	0.36	0.38	0.66	0.78
70	0.30	0.34	0.56	0.69

[1]Source: 1900 values computed using actual data from deaths and the decennial censuses in Laredo, Texas up to 1930 and projecting the 1930 rates through 1940; subsequently, 1970 rates are used. This slightly overestimates survival, as the major changes since 1940 have to do with the infant mortality rate. 1970 cohort is based on 1970 rates, projected as if there were no change during the lifetime of the cohort (i.e., it is the 1970 period life table). 1970 data based on Texas 1970 census and state death certificates analyzed by Buchanan and Weiss (in preparation).

From age-specific incidence rates for Hispanics taken from the New Mexico tumor registry, using life table techniques (Elandt-Johnson and Johnson, 1980), the cumulative incidence of gallbladder cancer in an 85 year old is about 0.0085 for males and 0.0173 for females (Table 2). Although gallbladder cancer is usually quickly fatal, its incidence prior to age 60 is quite low and has been ignored here.

Table 2. Cumulative incidence of cancer of the gall-bladder in Mexican-Americans and Amerindians in New Mexico, based on 1975 rates.[1]

Age	Hispanic		Amerindians	
	Males	Females	Males	Females
60	0.0004	0.0017	0.001	0.007
65	0.0006	0.0035	0.002	0.011
70	0.0022	0.0076	0.008	0.021
75	0.0048	0.0095	0.013	0.026
80	0.0061	0.0136	0.013	0.036
85	0.0085	0.0173	0.013	0.041

[1]Source: Waterhouse et al. (1982). Computed as probability of disease by age x for survivors to age x. Based on population incidence rates, so does not account for the individuals who do not have a gallbladder at-risk. The Amerindian population is relatively small so that rates, such as in older males, are difficult to estimate without large standard errors.

From the survivorship and disease-risk figures, the probability that a sibship born around 1900 contains more than one member affected with gallbladder cancer can be computed. This is only about 0.000007. In 1975 in New Mexico there were about 437,000 Hispanic people, of whom 34,864 were over the age of 60 (Waterhouse et al., 1982). Ignoring migration and assuming that all of these individuals were descended from typical 4-child families, there are 24,211 such sibships currently represented. At the expected risk of multiple-affection just given, in the entire state, of nearly a half million people, one would expect only about .17 multiply affected sibships. Put another way, one would have to survey about 6 states the size of New Mexico to expect even one such sibship. Amerindians comprise a higher-risk population in the Southwest, and in New Mexico there are about 81,000 of them, but only about 5,000 over age 60, so they do not add much to the likelihood of discovering multiply affected families.

It is, hence, not surprising to find only three reports of familial gallbladder cancer (1 from Arizona, 2 from New Mexico, all Amerindians) in the literature. Efforts to associate gallbladder cancer with chromosomal markers (Hecht, et al., 1983), or with the common blood groups or family membership in Mexico (Henson, 1983), have also failed. Of course, populations contain pedigrees, not just sibships, but the narrow window of diagnostic reliability, the effect of competing causes, and the rarity, per person, of GBCA make 'familiality', in the usual sense, difficult to detect or characterize.

Yet, several lines of evidence suggest that here is genetic risk for GBCA (Weiss et al., 1984a):

(1) GBCA, though rare in absolute terms, is nonetheless relatively much more frequent in many different and widely dispersed Amerindian populations in a way not easily attributable to environmental factors;

(2) there is a gradient of risk which roughly corresponds to the degree of Amerindian admixture in New World populations like Mexican-Americans;

(3) there is evidence for familial risk of precursor gallbladder disease in Mexican-Americans.

The relative increase in the frequency of GBCA in Amerindian populations is considerably less than it might be, because a sizeable fraction of the population is not actually at risk, as a result of having had their gallbladder removed to treat the symptoms of gallstones. Based on the Laredo and Starr County data, between 30 and 40% of women and 10% of men over age 75 have lost their gallbladder through surgery for gallstones (Weiss et al., 1984a). The true incidence rates for GBCA, to those at risk, should be altered accordingly, roughly yielding the values given in Table 3 (for a more detailed assessment of the effect of cholecystectomy, see Weiss et al., 1984a). Indeed, if only a subset of New World populations are actually at risk, because not all individuals carry genes for susceptibility, then those who do carry such genes are at correspondingly higher risk (Weiss et al., 1984a).

Table 3. Age-standardized incidence of cancer in racial groups in New Mexico.[1]

	Racial Group					
	Male			Female		
Site	Amind	Hispan	Anglo	Amind	Hispan	Anglo
Lung	8.1	20.6	62.5	2.9	12.8	20.2
Breast	--	--	--	19.3	42.2	78.7
Colon	5.6	10.9	23.5	6.7	13.3	22.6
Cervix	--	--	--	18.1	21.5	12.5
Prostrate	31.6	38.7	54.6	--	--	--
Gallbladder	8.6	3.4	2.4	34.1	12.9	1.7

[1]Amerindian and Hispanic male gallbladder cancer rates adjusted by 1.0/0.90, and females by 1/0.65.
Source: Waterhouse et al.(1982).

In New World peoples gallbladder cancer risk, per individual at risk, is comparable to the more common and important cancers. Its importance is increased by the fact that, in comparison with the other sites, GBCA is much less often successfully treated. GBCA has frequently been reported to be one of the leading cancers in Latin America and in Amerindians (Creagan and Fraumeni, 1972; Henson, 1983; Mack and Menck, 1982; Rios-Dalenz et al., 1983).

Impact of GBCA on New World Peoples

The absolute risk of GBCA, even to a NW person, is small, but the disease is not unimportant in its total impact. Using the current crude incidence rates for New Mexico, and assuming that all Mexican-American and Amerindian populations in the US have roughly similar age distributions, we can expect an annual incidence of about 267 cases. Roughly speaking, among those individuals now age 50 and above, there will be about 1,279 cases. This is a young population, with current survivorship similar to those of the rest of the US, so that, in the lives of individuals now under 40, there will be many more cases: assuming survivorship to age 70 of 70%, about the current value, there will be about 18,000 cases, and several thousand after age 70 (poor data make it difficult to derive an estimate). These figures are derived using the census data given in Tables 4 and 5 and the age-specific incidence rates given in Table 6. It is worth noting that there is much dispute about the degree of underestimation involved in these census figures, especially in regard to Mexican-Americans, who have been estimated to number about 7 million (Stern et al., 1981). The amount of disease will be greater than suggested above in proportion to the increase in the census estimate one uses.

In individuals who undergo cholecystectomy for clinical cholelithiasis, there is undetected cancer or pre-cancer in about 0.5% of Anglos, but from 1-3% in New World peoples. The rate of cancer in subclinical gallstone cases (where gallbladder cancer usually arises), may be at the upper end of this 1-3% range. This would be consistent with the cumulative incidence of gallbladder cancer in those who have not undergone cholecystectomy. If the population incidence rates for gallbladder cancer are adjusted for the fraction of the population actually at risk (not having undergone previous cholecystectomy), the risk by age 85 is about 3-5% in Mexican-American women. This is very nearly the risk of lung cancer in the heaviest of lifelong smokers (which is roughly 5-10%). Therefore, gallstones are as clear-cut and important a risk factor for cancer as are cigarettes, and greater than, say, beef-fat may be for colon cancer.

Table 4. Table of 1970 census, by age and sex, of Spanish surnamed individuals in 5 southwestern US states (Texas, California, Arizona, New Mexico, Colorado).[1]

Age	Male	Female
0- 1	58,010	55,299
0- 4	278,814	270,693
5- 9	310,135	303,927
10-14	297,030	290,043
15-19	253,413	253,897
20-24	178,305	201,705
25-29	151,826	160,555
30-34	133,911	141,187
35-39	127,803	132,302
40-44	124,933	126,631
45-49	107,528	106,089
50-54	74,285	77,814
55-59	61,964	66,276
60-64	51,515	53,392
65-69	42,096	44,529
70-74	26,805	27,900
75-79	15,893	18,309
80-84	9,602	10,862
85+	6,038	7,690
Total	2,251,896	2,293,801

[1]Source: US Census, Persons of Spanish Surname. Washington, 1973.

This disease, were it not for cholecystectomy, would be a fairly common tumor. The risk factor, if the genetic hypothesis is correct, has a frequency which apparently ranges from 0.15 in Mexican-Americans to 1.0 in Amerindians. In every meaningful epidemiological sense, gallbladder cancer is a genetic disease. Yet it is virtually impossible to find this disease segregating in families and, of course, it is not possible to map the genes involved in its manifestation with the usual linkage techniques.

In the current environment, it is apparent that formerly neutral, or possibly even advantageous metabolic genotypes in New World peoples have led to

Table 5. Table of 1970 census, by age and sex, of Amerindians in the United States.[1]

AMERINDIANS IN THE UNITED STATES		
Age	Male	Female
0- 1	9,315	9,571
0- 4	46,017	45,439
5- 9	51,043	51,062
10-14	49,088	49,041
15-19	41,963	42,142
20-24	31,934	33,213
25-29	25,693	26,185
30-34	22,665	23,926
35-39	18,833	20,653
40-44	17,624	18,520
45-49	15,337	16,485
50-54	13,300	14,622
55-59	11,627	13,359
60-64	9,558	10,463
65-69	8,242	8,997
70-74	5,260	5,861
75-79	3,507	3,961
80-84	2,037	2,197
85+	1,656	2,084
Total	375,384	388,210

[1]Note: Includes states with 10,000 or more Amerindians only. From U.S. 1970 Census Subject Report: American Indians, Washington, 1973.

a high rate of pathology. This environment, of as-yet unknown nature, has amplified the phenotype in some genotypes to a clinically meaningful point. If the process is allowed to continue for decades amplification proceeds occasionally to a deadly cancer. By understanding this, one need not search for 'cancer' genes; the New World genes probably have nothing to do with cellular differentiation or oncogenes. Cancer is probably randomly distributed among those with gallstones. If some gallstone cases are purely environmental in nature, for example, in the fraction of Mexican-Americans not bearing a New

World gene at the relevant locus, it will be very difficult to find evidence in intra-population family data for genetic risk for GBCA On the other hand, the study of the genetic epidemiology of the prodromal states may have a reasonable probability of success.

Table 6. Age-specific incidence rates for cancer of the gallbladder in New World peoples of New Mexico, 1973-77, by sex.

Age	Hispanic Male	Hispanic Female	Amerindian Male	Amerindian Female
40-44	4.1	0.0	0.0	0.0
45-49	2.1	6.1	0.0	0.0
50-54	0.0	11.6	0.0	54.7
55-59	2.7	15.7	19.1	89.3
60-64	3.4	36.5	23.5	73.9
65-69	31.7	83.2	128.0	209.3
70-74	51.4	38.6	86.4	96.9
75-79	27.6	82.2	0.0	213.5
80-84	47.1	76.3	0.0	100.0
85+	0.0	178.4	94.3	410.3
Total	2.4	6.3	4.8	13.0

[1]Source: Waterhouse et al. (1982). Rates are incident cases/100,000 population.

CONCLUSION

The simple concept of phenotype amplification can be very useful in genetic epidemiology. It is based on biological consideration of what a chronic disease might be, and not on the arbitrary definition of the end point of interest as the direct genetic event. The importance of precursors is widely utilized, but not as widely recognized as the states of <u>primary</u> interest.

There are several specific consequences of using the phenotype amplification model, rather than simple end-point genetic models which derive from point-origin epidemiological concepts. These go beyond the simple consideration of environmental interaction. In particular, under a model of phenotype amplification: (1) It is recognized that disease causation is a continual process, which may biologically involve many pathologic, physiologic, or metabolic phenomena, some of which may be undetectable or even obliterated by later stages. (2) The end-point disease of interest may be only one of many late-stage amplification products, perhaps even randomly distributed among those manifesting earlier stages. (3) The phenotype of primary interest is the earliest variant physiology, which should manifest clear genetic patterns, but which may be difficult to detect after phenotype amplification has gone on for a long enough time to alter homeostatic mechanisms, tissue architecture, and the like. (4) The frequency of precursor states should usually be much higher than that of later-stage disease. (5) The approximations and assumptions usually employed on the assumption that gene frequencies are small may not be justified, for example, that most affected families are derived from Aa x aa matings. (6) Environmental dose-response relationships will change as one looks earlier in the pathogenic chain. These relationships may be very nonlinear, and specific environmental factors may only be involved in part, perhaps only a later part, of the process. (7) Neither the final disease, nor its relationships to the environment need be related to the physiology of the risk gene. Familial susceptibility to cancer, for example, may not have anything to do with oncogenes, kinases, or incorporated viruses-- they may be final 'causes' randomly imposed on a prepared tissue bed. (8) The apparent penetrance of alleles at a major locus should approach 1.0 as one moves earlier in the amplification process, ultimately appearing more classically Mendelian. In instances of polygenic risk, as one moves earlier in the process of pathogenesis, bi- or tri-modality should not arise, but a continuous distribution, shifted between parents and offspring, should persist with a clearer pattern of correlations of phenotypes among relatives reflecting theoretical genetic predictions. (9) Genetic linkage will be possible, in the same family data, relative to precursor stages rather than to the final end-point disease, when etiology is monogenic. (10) Data transformations by methods chosen suitably relevant to a suggested underlying biological process should help sharpen the significance and interpretation of statistical tests and estimation from family data. For example, if a gene product is expressed on the surface of a cell in which it is produced, the activity level of that enzyme may be related to the square of the gene dose (i.e., homozygote vs. heterozygote). This may occur, for instance, with a genetic variant for a cell-surface receptor or membrane-transport molecule.

Simple concepts can often be quite helpful. In the case of phenotype amplification, as we have termed it here, careful thinking before the collection of data can be at least as important as the use of powerful statistical methods. Those methods rely on one's ability to define the phenotype of interest meaningfully. Otherwise, some parameter like penetrance must bear the burden of the inaccuracy thus introduced.

In populations of interest to anthropologists, the conditions are often favorable for the occurrence of phenotype amplification, because such groups have evolved under conditions of high early mortality and small population size. Alleles which may be expressed pathologically under the conditions of recent acculturation may exist. It is often such groups which have (1) very isolated geography in which specific risk factors may be present in some local groups and absent in others, (2) genetically different neighboring demes sharing highly idiosyncratic environments, (3) rapid and well-documented acculturation of all or part of the group, or (4) estimable admixture with other groups, which may help identify the genetic epidemiology of precursor states. The use of anthropological data in this context may help to solve problems which are intractable in the vague, migrating, mixed populations of the large major racial groups.

ACKNOWLEDGEMENTS

This work was supported by grant CA 19311 from the US National Cancer Institute, which is gratefully acknowledged. This is Demographic Epidemiology of Aging and Disease, Paper No. 18.

LITERATURE CITED

Badzioch MD (1982). A study of mortality in a Mexican-American community--Laredo, Texas, 1900-1930. 4th CDPG Report, Center for Demographic and Population Genetics, University of Texas Graduate School of Biomedical Sciences, Houston, TX (also, MS thesis, University of Texas School of Public Health).

Buchanan AV, Weiss, KM Mortality Patterns in Texas Mexican-Americans 1969-72. (In preparation).

Creagan ET, Fraumeni JF Jr (1972). Cancer mortality among American Indians, 1950-1967. J Nat Cancer Inst 49:959.

Devor EJ (1982). Ethnogeographic patterns in gallbladder cancer. In Correa P, Haenszel W (eds): "Epidemiology of Cancer of the Digestive Tract," The Hague: M Nijhoff, p 197.

Devor EJ, Buechley RW (1979). Gallbladder cancer in Hispanic New Mexicans. II. Familial occurrence in two northern New Mexico kindreds. Cancer Gen Cytogen 1:139.

Diehl AK (1980). Epidemiology of gallbladder cancer: A synthesis of recent data. J Nat Cancer Inst 65:1209.

Elandt-Johnson RC, Johnson NL (1980). "Survival Models and Data Analysis." New York: Wiley.

Falconer DS (1981). "Introduction to Quantitative Genetics." 2d Ed. London: Longman.

Gottlieb K, Kimberling WJ (1979). Admixture estimates for the gene pool of Mexican-Americans in Colorado. Am J Phys Anthrop 50:444 (abstract).

Heaton KW (1972). "Bile Salts in Health and Disease." Edinburgh: Churchill Livingston.

Heaton, KW (1981). Gallstones. In Trowell HC, Burkitt DP (eds): "Western Diseases: Their Emergence and Prevention," Cambridge: Harvard University Press, p 47.

Hecht F, Kuban DJ, Berger C, Hecht BK, Sandberg AA (1983). Adenocarcinoma of the gallbladder: Chromosome abnormalities in a genetic form of cancer. Cancer Genet and Cytogenet 8:185.

Henson DE (1983). Conference and workshop on cancer epidemiology in Latin America. Opportunities for collaborative research. J Nat Cancer Inst 70:979.

Mack TM, Menck HR (1982). Epidemiology of cancer of the gallbladder and extra-hepatic biliary passages. In Correa P, Haenszel W (eds): "Epidemiology of Cancer of the Digestive Tract," The Hague: M Nijhoff, p 227.

Moriyama IM, Gustavus SO (1972). Cohort mortality and survivorship: United States death-registration states, 1900-1968. Vital and Health Statistics, Ser 3, No 16. Washington: US Govt Printing Office.

Reed TE (1974). Ethnic classification of Mexican-Americans. Science 285:283.

Relethford JH, Stern MP, Gaskill SP, Hazuda HP (1983). Social class, admixture, and skin color variation in Mexican-Americans and Anglo-Americans living in San Antonio, Texas. Am J Phys Anthrop 61:97.

Rios-Dalenz J, Takabayashi A, Henson DE, Strom BL, Soloway RD (1983). The epidemiology of cancer of the extra-hepatic biliary tract in Bolivia. Int J Epidemiol 12:156.

Sampliner RE, Bennett PH, Comess LJ, Rose FA, Burch TA (1970). Gallbladder disease in Pima Indians: demonstration of high prevalence and early onset by cholecystography. New England J Med 283:1358.

Sperling M (1964). Familial biliary tract carcinoma. J Amer Med Assoc 190:944.

Stern MP, Gaskill SP, Allen CR, Garza V, Gonzales JL, Waldrop RH (1981). Cardiovascular risk factors in Mexican Americans in Laredo, Texas. I. Prevalence of overweight and diabetes and distributions of serum lipids. Am J Epidemiol 113:546.

Waterhouse J, Shanmugarantam KC, Muir C, Powell J (1982). "Cancer Incidence in Five Continents," Vol 4, Lyon: International Agency for Research on Cancer.

Weiss KM, Ferrell RE, Hanis CL, Styne P (1984a). Aspects of the epidemiology and genetics of gallbladder disease in New World native peoples. Am J Human Genet 36:1259.

Weiss KM, Ferrell RE, Hanis CL (1984b). New World Syndrome of metabolic diseases with a genetic and evolutionary basis. Yearbook of Physical Anthropology 27:153.

Diseases of Complex Etiology in Small Populations:
Ethnic Differences and Research Approaches, pages 199–225

Chapter 9

THE SEARCH FOR GENETIC FACTORS CONTROLLING PLASMA GLUCOSE LEVELS IN DOGRIB INDIANS

E.J.E. Szathmary

Department of Anthropology, McMaster University, Hamilton, Ontario, Canada

INTRODUCTION

Current opinion holds that genetic and environmental factors are involved in the onset of non-insulin dependent diabetes mellitus (NIDDM) (Friedman and Fialkow, 1980). The exact etiological mechanisms of this disease in Caucasians continue to be debated. Some studies report the existence of a strong within-generation effect that influences glucose tolerance, this effect being due to dominant genes, or within-sibship shared environmental factors, or a combination of these (Beaty et al., 1982). Others argue that NIDDM is "predominantly, almost entirely due to a genetic cause" (Pyke, 1979).

Published studies on North American Indians also indicate familial aggregation of NIDDM, at least in those populations with high prevalence of the disease. However, in the two unrelated tribes subjected to detailed inquiry, the Pima Indians of Arizona (Steinberg et al., 1970) and the Seminole Indians of Oklahoma (Elston et al., 1974), homozygosity for a major gene, transmitted as an autosomal recessive, rather than the combined effect of additive genes, is considered the most likely genetic factor involved in the susceptibility to NIDDM. Among the environmental agents considered to influence the disease, the duration of obesity is known to be an important risk factor in the Pima (Knowler et al., 1981), with maternal diabetes during pregnancy contributing significantly to obesity in the offspring (Pettitt et al., 1983).

Whether the findings in the Pima and Seminole apply generally to other North American Indian populations is open to dispute. While there is little doubt that increasing acculturation to non-Indian lifestyles has contributed to the epidemic-like increase in NIDDM in Indians (West, 1974, 1978), the reliability of the proposed genetic mechanisms (by Steinberg et al., 1970; Elston et al., 1974) has been questioned. Indeed, Neel (1976) has suggested that to elucidate the issue, studies of the familial patterns of glucose tolerance before and after a major cultural transition are desirable.

This paper examines data obtained from a North American Indian population whose current distribution and history approximates the experimental scenario proposed by Neel. The association of impaired glucose tolerance with upper trunk adiposity (but not overall fatness) and village of residence has already been described in this group (Szathmary and Holt, 1983). The focus here is on possible genetic factors influencing plasma glucose levels. Evidence will be sought by (1) examining the population distribution of plasma glucose, (2) assessing the clustering of hyperglycemic individuals within pedigrees, (3) estimating the correlations in plasma glucose levels between spouses, between parents and offspring and among siblings, (4) examining the association between elevated plasma glucose level (hr 2 $\geq$ 200 mg/dl) and a series of genetic markers.

THE POPULATION AND THE SAMPLE

Dogrib Indians are an Athapaskan-speaking Indian population that resides between Great Slave and Great Bear Lakes in Canada's Northwest Territories. The Dogrib are the largest Indian group in the Northwest Territories. Approximately, 1600 persons (in 1979), that is over 75% of the Dogrib in existence, are registered to the Rae Band (Helm, 1981).

Members of the Rae Band are currently dispersed

over four communities: the principal village of Rae and three more northerly settlements, Lac La Martre, Rae Lakes and Snare Lake. Such regional differentiation was a feature of Dogrib existence before the advent of Europeans in their area. Regional bands -- groups of people linked by ties of blood or marriage--tended to occupy and exploit different parts of the Dogrib territory for much of the year. None lived in permanent settlements. Movement into and out of regional bands was always possible, and often necessary dependent on the exigencies of seasonal subsistence. Several times during the year bands coalesced to take part in religious celebrations, for spring and fall caribou hunts, and from 1852 onwards, to trade at Fort Rae, the first trading center established within the Dogrib region (Helm, 1981).

Forty years ago, Dogrib life was much as it had ever been: formal schooling, even in the primary grades was rare, medical services consisted of an annual physician's visit to Rae, and cash income was completely dependent on fur trapping. However, after the Second World War, permanent Euro-Canadian facilities began to be established at Rae. In the early 1950s the majority of the Dogrib still pursued traditional subsistence activities and lived "in the bush", away from these installations (Helm, 1981). The drop in fur prices in that decade, in combination with vigorous expansion of government programs in housing, schooling, and health and welfare services both forced and enticed people into a more sedentary lifestyle at Euro-Canadian points-of-service, indeed, to tie all Indians of the Northwest Territories to a "micro-urban life-way" (Helm, 1980).

Lac La Martre and Rae Lakes are two northern Dogrib settlements that were surveyed for adult glucose intolerance in 1979. Each settlement is located within areas exploited and occupied aboriginally by different socio-territorial groups. Consanguineal and affinal ties link many of the residents in these settlements to people living in the "south", at Rae. The latter community was also surveyed for glucose intolerance in 1979. Rae is the largest Indian village in the Northwest Territories. In 1979 its total population size was approximately five times as great as found in either of the northern settlements. Rae is more cosmopolitan (8.7% of the population in 1979 were non-Dogrib), has a greater number of stores, cafes, and is connected by a permanent road to Yellowknife, the territorial capital. Lac La Martre and Rae Lakes, however, are semi-isolated with no year-round road access available. Each has only one cooperative store, and in 1979 the only non-Indians resident year round were two Euro-Canadian teachers in each community. A far greater proportion of adults in these northern settlements than in Rae trap, hunt, and fish regularly. Within the Dogrib region, then, it is possible to contrast residents of different villages by lifestyle, the Dogrib version of the "rural-urban" contrasts documented in indigenous people in other parts of the world. However, because the populations of all Dogrib communities are genetically related (Szathmary, 1983a), and many residents of different settlements are linked by ties of close kinship and marriage, the entire group can be examined for familial aggregation of glucose levels.

The 157 individuals in this study, 97 females and 60 males, constitute a voluntary sample of adults aged 21 years and older. The mean age of men in the sample is 46.7 ± 15.6 years, of women, 43.5 ± 16.2 years. The sample represents 22.1% of the adults of the Rae Band. Because no Dogrib was known to be diabetic, and because the majority had not heard of the disease at the time of survey, voluntary sampling should not have introduced a bias favoring participation of those with impaired glucose tolerance. Comparison of the sample age-structure with that of the target group found no significant differences (Szathmary, 1983b).

FIELD TEST PROCEDURES

The National Diabetes Data Group's (NDDG, 1979) recommendations concerning oral glucose tolerance (OGT) testing and criteria for judgement of diabetes and impaired glucose tolerance had not been published at the time of fieldwork. The methodology employed in the Dogrib study is described in Szathmary and Holt (1983). Departures in the test procedure from currently recommended methods are two: the use of a 100 gm challenge dose, and absence of dietary preparation. The 100 gm dose was originally selected to allow comparability of the Dogrib findings with Alaskan Indians (Mouratoff et al., 1969) who had also been tested with a 100 gm glucose load. The 75 gm dose, although recommended by the NDDG, is known to produce no significant differences in the plasma glucose levels from those elicited by a 100 gm glucose challenge, at least in normals (Castro et al., 1970). On the other hand, the larger test dose (100 gm) is more likely to detect a diabetic insulin response pattern (de Nobel et al., 1978), including maximal insulin response (Castro et al., 1970) and yields more reproducible glucose tolerance test results (Toeller and Knussmann, 1973).

Dietary preparation of Dogrib participants was not possible. To date, no dietary studies have been carried out on the Dogrib, hence it is not known whether a minimum of 150 gm of carbohydrate is consumed daily. However, the Regional Nutritionist at Yellowknife (Picard, 1983) notes that the "traditional diet" in Rae includes a substantial carbohydrate portion. This deduction is based on informants' reports of standard fare: bannock, made with white flour, lard and water may contain fish eggs, berries, cheese, peanut butter or raisins. Caribou and fish, consumed year-round, are often served as soups containing noodles, rice, or oatmeal, or all three added to potatoes and onions. Canned soups and vegetables are frequently added to the broth, and fish soups contain flour and milk in addition. Tea is consumed daily with evaporated milk and white sugar.

It is worth noting that the first case of clinical diabetes diagnosed in the Rae Dogrib did not occur until November, 1981 (Burke, 1981).

STUDY DEFINITION OF HYPERGLYCEMIA

An earlier report of Dogrib glucose intolerance (Szathmary and Holt, 1983) used a value of 160 mg/dl two hours after the glucose load as the boundary between normals and abnormals. Here, "hyperglycemia" is defined as individuals showing either fasting plasma glucose values >140 mg/dl, or a 2-hour glucose level ≥200 mg/dl. Table 1 gives the % intolerant to glucose by sex and age, using several different diagnostic criteria. The definition adopted here approximates that recommended by the NDDG (1979). In fact 14 of the 15 persons considered abnormal here also have 1-hour glucose values ≥200 mg/dl.

Contrary to expectations, the prevalence of hyperglycemia does not differ significantly between the more acculturated village of Rae and the two semi-isolated villages (Szathmary, 1983b). However, that the Dogrib have a high frequency of abnormal responses compared to other subarctic Athapaskan-speaking Indians is indicated by comparisons with a voluntary sample of Alaskans (Mouratoff et al., 1969). Application to the Dogrib of the diagnostic criteria used in the Alaskan study to identify persons with possible impaired tolerance yields approximately four times the number of candidates for retest than had been found in Alaska. This difference is not due to the different sex-specific age distributions in the Alaskan sample (Szathmary, 1983b). What explanations account for it are unknown.

PRELIMINARY STATISTICAL PROCEDURES

For all calculations, the significance level used in this paper is 0.01. Statistical analysis was done with the SPSS (Nie et al., 1975) program package.

The 2-hour plasma glucose level, shown to be the best measure of glucose tolerance (Unger, 1957; Rushforth et al., 1975) was selected for statistical analysis. Normalization of the within-sex distributions of glucose, to reduce observed significant skewness and kurtosis, was accomplished with the log transformation (Szathmary and Holt, 1983).

Within each sex the regression of log hr-2 glucose on age was significant (Szathmary and Holt, 1983). Stepwise regression showed that the addition to the equation of independent variables reflecting

Table 1. Hyperglycemia in the Dogrib by sex and age, under different criteria of impairment.

		Age in years						
		21-29	30-39	40-49	50-59	60-69	70+	Total
M[1]		8	14	13	12	8	5	60
F		25	13	19	21	10	7	95[2]
2-hour plasma glucose >160mg/dl:								
M	No.	0	1	3	5	2	5	16
	%	0.0	7.1	23.1	47.7	25.0	100.0	26.7
F	No.	0	3	4	6	2	4	19
	%	0.0	23.1	21.1	28.6	20.0	57.1	20.0
NDDG[3] "Impaired Glucose Tolerance":								
M	No.	0	0	1	1	0	3	5
	%	0.0	0.0	7.7	8.3	0.0	60.0	8.3
F	No.	1	2	2	5	3	1	14
	%	4.0	15.4	10.5	23.8	30.0	14.3	14.7
NDDG[4] "Diabetic" plasma glucose levels, single OGT:								
M	No.	0	1	1	3[5]	2	1	8
	%	0.0	7.1	7.7	25.0	25.0	20.0	13.3
F	No.	0	1	2[5]	2	0	1	6
	%	0.0	7.7	10.5	9.5	0.0	14.3	6.3
Hyperglycemia[6] by study criteria:								
M	No.	0	1	1	3	2	1	8
	%	0.0	7.1	7.7	25.0	25.0	20.0	13.3
F	No.	0	1	2	2	0	2	7
	%	0.0	7.7	10.5	9.5	0.0	28.6	7.4

[1]M=males, F=females

[2]Two additional women claiming to be 21 yrs. old (one 19, the other 20) were tested. Both had normal OGTs.

[3]Fasting plasma glucose (FPG) <140, 1-Hr ≥200, 2-Hr 140-200 mg/dl.

[4]FPG ≥140 or; FPG <140, 1-Hr ≥200, 2-Hr ≥200 mg/dl.

[5]Includes one person with FPG >140 mg/dl.

[6]FPG>140 or 2-Hr ≥200 mg/dl.

"fatness" or patterning of body fat [i.e. the first and second principal components obtained from principal component analysis of skinfolds (Szathmary and Holt, 1983)] did not significantly improve the percent variance in plasma glucose already explained by age. Age explains 15.9% of the variation in men, but only 8.0% of the variation in log glucose in women.

To maximize sample size, male and female subsamples were combined, a step permissible (Pedhazur, 1982) because analysis of covariance showed there were (1) no significant differences between the slopes of the within sex regressions on age, and (2) the y-intercepts in the sex-specific regression equations did not differ significantly.

Examination of the combined sample also showed that the addition of "fatness" to the regression equation did not significantly improve upon the variability in log glucose already explained by age. The combined samples were subsequently adjusted for age by adding the residuals arising from the regression of log plasma glucose on age in the whole sample (N=157) to the glucose level expected for a man of average age (46.7 years) in the sample. All subsequent analyses were carried out on these age-adjusted data.

POPULATION DISTRIBUTION OF PLASMA GLUCOSE

Bimodality in the distribution of a quantitative trait may be indicative of the existence of a major gene that controls the trait. Under the model of a two allele autosomal locus with dominance, each mode in the observed distribution would represent mean values of the trait associated with the dominant (AA + Aa) and recessive (aa) genotypes.

Elston (1980) has detailed the assumptions and procedures involved in pedigree analysis under different models of genetic causation. Under a monogenic model for NIDDM as given above, the age-corrected log glucose measure of each person in the population is assumed to derive from one of two normal distribution with common variance. The distributions correspond to the genotypes AA + Aa and aa. Within a pedigree the probability of each parent belonging to a particular genotype can be specified, with the probabilities summing to one. The distribution to which each offspring in a pedigree belongs depends on the transmission probabilities of the parental genotypes: for example, the probability that aa transmits a to an offspring, that AA transmits A, and that Aa transmits A, as well as their complementary probabilities (Elston and Stewart, 1971).

The starting point for the application of this approach to the Dogrib glucose values was testing the hypothesis that the age-corrected log glucose measures of each person in the population derives from one of two distributions. Kaplan and Elston's (1972) maximum likelihood estimation program was used in the attempt to fit two log normal distributions to the data. Log normal distributions were attempted because other studies on Indians (Pima: Steinberg et al., 1970; Seminole: Elston et al., 1974) have shown that derived distributions using log-transformed glucose values fit the observed data better than derived curves formed from the raw data. Furthermore, when the cumulative age-unadjusted, within sex Dogrib glucose values were plotted on log probability paper, two different straight line segments were present in each sex, suggesting a mixture of two log normal distributions (Szathmary, 1983b). The parameters to be estimated initially by maximum likelihood were two means, a common variance and two admixture proportions. The likelihood of this set of data was also to be obtained by maximization.

Contrary to expectations, whatever starting values were provided as parameter estimates, one of the admixture proportions converged to a bound and was fixed. In effect, only one distribution could be fitted to the age-adjusted log glucose data, this having a mean of 2.09 and a variance of .019. The joint log likelihood was 87.14. There is, therefore, no support for the hypothesis that the distribution of age-adjusted log plasma glucose in the Dogrib represents a mixture of two underlying distributions, each of which depends upon different genotypes.

It is worth noting, that when sex-specific age-unadjusted data were used in the initial step, similar conclusions were reached, but for different reasons. For example, one, two and three distributions were each fitted to the female log plasma glucose data. Whether the two or three distribution models are each a significant improvement over the unimodal model can be tested. In the case of the bimodal model, twice the difference in log likelihood between the best fitting single distribution and a mixture of two normal distributions is distributed asymptotically as X^2 with 2 d.f.(Elston et al., 1975). Twice the difference amounted to 1.08, which with 2 degrees of freedom is not significant. A non-significant result was also obtained when the trimodal model was assessed against the unimodal [twice the difference = 3.60, df = 4, NS], and similar findings obtained in men [twice the difference = 3.25, df = 2, NS; twice the difference = 4.58, df = 4, NS].

Unlike the findings in the Pima and Oklahoman Seminole, the distribution of log glucose in the Dogrib is not bimodal, nor can it be dissected into a mixture of two distributions. There is no evidence here of a major gene controlling plasma glucose levels.

AGGREGATION OF HYPERGLYCEMICS IN PEDIGREES

NIDDM is thought to be a "new" disease among North American Indians, one that results from the interaction of a susceptible genotype with an altered environment. Although the unimodal distribution of log glucose in the Dogrib does not offer support for the existence of a major gene, familial aggregation, especially if it occurs among relatives who have not shared a common household environment for decades, is suggestive of the existence of underlying genetic factors in susceptibility.

The reconstruction of pedigrees is always a difficult task. Among a people with no written record, nor any tradition that requires the oral transmission of genealogical information beyond the depth of three generations, the usual difficulties are compounded.

The pedigrees that have been reconstructed in this study are based on missionary records. The first representative of the Oblates of Mary Immaculate visited Dogrib territory in 1859. The first conversions to Catholicism took place that year, and the Christianization of a whole people was essentially complete by 1869 (Helm, 1981). This fact, however, does not preclude the appearance in the records of new adult converts throughout the latter part of the 19th century. These persons are very probably kinsmen of Dogrib already in the mission records, although neither the degrees of relationship nor type of relationship (affinal or consanguineal) they may have had with others was written down.

Accuracy of the Dogrib lineages from the present extending back 3 or 4 generations is very high. However, problems do exist with the first two recorded generations, where consanguineal linkages among apparently independent individuals (and therefore their descendants) must have existed, but were not noted by the missionaries. The reasons for this are manifold. They include the fact that Dogrib prior to baptism did not use surnames, and that an individual during his lifetime could have several different names. What are surnames today can be shown to be the Indian names of ancestors in use at the time of conversion. Thus, several different families, with distinct family names can be traced back to a single sibship. For example, the individuals Angele Tsezere wife of Witcho, Baptiste Ndekette, Francoise Louwa wife of Tlaadi (or Klaadi), and Lucien Lize were all children of Dekon and Etlaadi. Other such sibships have been identified. However, because the missionaries did not compile family lists until the turn of the century, there is no assurance for the first recorded generations that all sibs that left descendants who participated in this study have been identified. This is particularly so for adult women baptized with their husbands, who may not have given the same name for parents as used by other siblings baptized at other times. Additional complications arise from the pre-Christian practice of polygamy--for example, is Dekon husband of Etlaadi, the same as

Dekon, husband of Niklene. Lastly, the most obvious source of error centers on the transliteration of Dogrib names in the first recorded generations. Dogrib was and is not a written language, hence the missionaries had to invent an orthography to transcribe sounds with which they were unfamiliar. The linguistic capabilities of the priests varied. There are examples in the records of very different spellings of the name of one individual. However, not all such confusions can be identified. Hence there is a possibility that some persons treated as different may in fact be the same, and apparently unlinked pedigrees, were the details known, would coalesce in the same ancestors.

Participants in this study were traced as far back as possible without allowing any ambiguity of identification. Many pedigrees are 6 generations deep, a few are 7. The founders of at least 37 different genealogies into which the 157 study participants can be fitted have been identified. There are numerous cross-linkages among the pedigrees, and all include "unrelated" individuals who married into the groups.

Table 2 shows the consanguineal relationships identified among the 15 Dogrib hyperglycemics, and places these individuals into 8 genealogies headed by apparently unrelated individuals. There are clear clusters within genealogies, there is also overlap among some of these 8 genealogies. For example, 40% (6/15) of the hyperglycemics occur in Pedigree I, in which there is striking occurrence of hyperglycemia in 4 first cousins. Pedigree I also includes one of 2 sets of hyperglycemic spouses. Three of the people in this pedigree, however, including a pair of sibs are also linked by descent to Pedigree II and hence to still another hyperglycemic. An even more striking cluster of relatives is represented by Pedigrees V and VI, these including a consanguineally unrelated husband and wife and two of their adult offspring.

In these aggregations, only two occur between unrelated individuals (spouses) sharing the same household. Thus, while a common household environment may be a factor in the onset of hyperglycemia, the

Table 2. Familial relationships among 15 Dogrib hyperglycemics and clustering of hyperglycemics in pedigrees.

Individuals ID:ID	Total in pedigree	r[1]	Kin category
Pedigree I:	6		
13:115		1/2	siblings
46:116:49:59		1/8	1st cousins
13,115[2]:46, 116[2],49,59		1/64	2nd cousins once removed (2½)
Pedigree II:	4		
13:115		1/2	siblings
13,115:46		1/32	half 1st cousins once removed (half 1½)
13,115:238		1/16	1st cousins once removed (1½); half 2nd cousins
46:238		1/64	half 2nd cousins
Pedigree III:	2		
238:116		1/32	1st cousins twice rem. (1¼)
Pedigree IV:	2		
238:28		1/256	3rd cousins once rem. (3½)
Pedigree V:	4		
210:215		1/2	siblings
209[2]:210,215		1/2	parent-child
209:67		1/16	1st cousin once rem. (1½)
67:210,215		1/32	2nd cousins
Pedigree VI:	3		
210:215		1/2	siblings
204[2]:210,215		1/2	parent-child
Pedigree VII:	1		
99[3]		-	-
Pedigree VIII:	1		
88			

[1]r=coefficient of relationship
[2]Husband-wife pairs: 115-116, 204-209
[3]Has Caucasian ancestors

impression left by the clustering of hyperglycemics in particular pedigrees is that of an underlying genetic base to the impairment of glucose tolerance. This is reinforced by the finding that the one case of Dogrib NIDDM diagnosed in 1981 by medical personnel occurs in a first cousin of ID's 115 and 13, hyperglycemics in Pedigree II (Table 2). This diabetic was unaware of any illness in 1979 and had not participated in the 1979 survey.

The last observation worthy of note here is that the pedigrees indicate that if genes are involved in the onset of glucose intolerance, then the genes responsible are indigenous to the Dogrib and cannot be ascribed to European sources. While maximum European admixture in the Dogrib sample is 8.5% (Szathmary, 1983b; Szathmary et al., 1983), only one of the hyperglycemics (Table 2) has European ancestors through his Métis antecedents. This individual may well have inherited his predisposing "glucose intolerant genes" from his Dogrib ancestors.

CORRELATION OF GLUCOSE LEVELS AMONG DIFFERING SETS OF FIRST DEGREE RELATIVES AND SETS OF SPOUSES

When genetic factors and environmental factors are thought to bear influence on the manifestation of a quantitative trait, the total phenotypic variance of the trait can be partitioned as

$$V_P = V_G + V_E + V_R,$$

where V_P is the total variance, V_G is the variance due to genes, V_E is the environmental variance, and V_R is a residual variance. Falconer (1960) has discussed the relationship between these components of variance and correlation. When the latter is obtained from standardized variables, then the correlation between any two persons is the function of covariance only. Given a linear model that specifies a set of variance components due to genes and environment, the covariances can be used in path analysis to estimate path coefficients, the squares of which are estimates of the variance components in the model (Li, 1975). Correlations, then, provide the starting point for the application of methods that seek to assess the relative importance of genetic factors compared to environmental factors in the regulation of a quantitative trait, such as glucose level.

Table 3 shows the number of sets of first degree relatives contained in the Dogrib sample. The "unrelated" group contains persons whose pairwise coefficient of relationship ranges from 0 to less than 1/2.

Table 3. Categories of relatives sampled in Dogribs.

Relationship	Number	
	Families	Individuals
Parents and Offspring[1]:		
Both Parents - 1 Child	4	12
Both Parents - 2 Children	3	12
Both Parents - 4 Children	1	6
One Parent - 1 Child	11	22
One Parent - 2 Children	2	6
One Parent - 3 Children	1	4
Total	22	62
Siblings:		
Pairs of sibs	25	50
3 Sibs	6	18
4 Sibs	1	4
Total	32	72
Unrelated[2]		52
Correction factor[3]		-29
Total sampled		157

[1]Only adult offspring were tested.
[2]"Unrelated" means the coefficient of relationship ranges between 0 and <1/2.
[3]"Correction factor" is the number of persons counted more than once. That is, for example, a person who is a parent and also a sib of study participants.

Prior to the computation of correlations the distributions of age-adjusted log glucose values within each kinship category were checked for normalcy with Kolmogorov-Smirnov tests (Sokal and Rohlf, 1969). All the statistics were non-significant. The age-adjusted glucose values were then standardized within groups: that is, separately for each set of fathers, mothers, father's offspring, mother's offspring, siblings and husbands and wives. The means of the distributions within each of these groups were 0 and the variances 1. The standardized distributions did not deviate significantly from normal.

Four sets of interclass correlations were obtained with the standardized data. The intra-class correlation was obtained from a one-way analysis of variance of standardized glucose levels of sibs within sibships (Sokal and Rohlf, 1969). Because some parent-offspring correlations involved averages (for example, father's glucose level with the standardized value of his children's average glucose level) pairwise parent-child correlations were obtained by multiplying the correlations by K, the correction factor given by Annest et al. (1979). In particular, $K = [1 + r_{OO} (s-1)]/s$, where s is the average sibship size, and r_{OO} is the intra-class correlation among sibs.

Z-transformations of the father-offspring and mother-offspring correlations were corrected for bias as described in Sing and Orr (1978). Methods described by Snedecor and Cochran (1967) were followed to determine whether they differed significantly. The results ($Z = .55$, $P = .21$) indicated that they could be combined into an average parent-offspring correlation.

Lastly, because many of the 52 "unrelated" Dogrib in this study are distantly related, the possibility exists that they too share genes that influence glucose levels. Accordingly, the inter-class correlation was computed between 26 pairs of "unrelated" persons. Assignment of individuals to a pair was random. Procedures detailed above were followed in the derivation of this correlation coefficient.

Table 4 shows the results of these calculations. All correlations involving first degree relatives or people residing in the same household are positive. Only the correlation between unrelated people residing in separate households is negative. The sign of these coefficients suggests, therefore, a positive relationship between glucose level and shared household environment, and glucose level and close genetic relationship. However, it must be stressed that the only correlation that differs significantly from zero is that between siblings ($r = +.507$, $df = 30$, $P < .01$). While the small number of family sets available for analysis is probably the cause of the lack of significance observed in the other correlations, this is an inference from studies in non-Indian populations in which the familial nature of NIDDM is well established (Beaty et al., 1982; Tattersall and Pyke, 1972).

Table 4. Estimates of correlation in plasma glucose level between relatives and between unrelated individuals.

Relatives	N[1]	Correlation	Standard error[2]
Interclass:			
Father-Offspring	9	+.253	±.331
Mother-Offspring	21	+.001	±.224
Parent-Offspring	30	+.062	±.185
Husband-Wife	30	+.185	±.179
Unrelated Pairs	26	-.188	±.193
Intraclass:			
Sib-Sib	32	+.507*	±.12

[1]Number of sets of relatives or unrelated pairs.
[2]The standard error of an intraclass correlation is

$$\sqrt{\frac{2[sN-1]\ [1-r]^2\ [1+(s-1)r]^2}{s^2(s-1)\ (N-1)N}}$$ (Swigler et al., 1964).

Here s=2.215. The standard error of an interclass correlation is $(1-r^2)\ /\ \sqrt{N-1}$ (Fisher, 1958).
*P < 01. Test of Ho: $\rho = 0$, Ha: $\rho \neq 0$.

Two facts argue against attempts to use the data in Table 4 in any subsequent analysis to portion phenotypic variance in glucose level. The most obvious is that, with one exception, all correlation estimates are essentially zero. Secondly, the theoretical approach for using input data from different family sets assumes that the sets are independent (Elston, 1975). Clearly this is not the case here. For example, the parents used in the parent-offspring correlation calculation are identical to 28% of the pairs of husbands and wives. There is also overlap between the offspring and sibling sets.

Can any interpretation be placed on the observed correlation between adult Dogrib siblings? Certainly the finding suggests that a within-generation effect influences plasma glucose levels in the Dogrib. Were the genetic basis of impaired glucose tolerance in Indians multifactorial, this effect could be due to variance of dominant genes, or a within-sibship environmental effect, or both. Because all the sibs are adults (average age 42.1 ± 13.4 yrs.), most of whom have not shared a common household environment for many years, a recent common household effect is not likely. However, a generational effect, such as a relatively rapid and sudden onset of a changed lifestyle could affect a cohort of sibs profoundly, with only marginal effects on their parents. The Dogrib experienced such a cultural transition in the 1950s, hence this is an experience shared at some point in individual life cycles, by 78% of the total sample. Were any genetic susceptibility present in the group, this could manifest itself in specific sibships in the altered environment.

Reinforcement for these notions is provided by the observation that the age-adjusted plasma glucose levels of sibs of hyperglycemics are elevated ($P < .05$) compared to glucose levels of sibs of normoglycemics (Szathmary, 1983b). No such elevations were seen in the comparisons of other first degree relatives of hyperglycemics compared to first degree relatives of controls (Szathmary, 1983b). The scenario outlined above predicts plasma glucose increases in sibs of hyperglycemics, and it is doubtful that the observation found in Dogrib is due to chance. A strong within-generation effect that influenced both test response and risk to diabetes was also found in a study of first degree relatives of Caucasian diabetics (NIDDM) in Michigan (Beaty et al., 1982).

In sum, the Dogrib data suggest that intra-generational environmental influence must not be excluded from any model that seeks to explain variation in plasma glucose levels. More specifically, the most likely model that needs to be explored with better data than available here must include variance components due to additive genes, genes with dominant effects as well as an intra-generational environmental variance component.

GENETIC MARKER PHENOTYPES AND PLASMA GLUCOSE LEVELS

Reports in the literature have noted that significant differences exist between Pima diabetics and normals in the distribution of Phosphoglycolate Phosphatase (PGP) phenotypes (Cadien et al., 1979). Kirk et al. (1983) have found in addition that in Polynesians--a group in which NIDDM has also increased with the onset of Westernization (West, 1974; Zimmet et al., 1981), non-insulin dependent diabetics have a significant excess of $\underline{GLO}^{2}$ (Glyoxalase) and $\underline{Gc}^{1}$ (Group Specific Globulin, or Vitamin-D binding protein). There is great interest in such associations because proof for the existence of a major gene controlling a quantitative trait could be supplied by showing the trait is linked to a qualitative marker (Elston et al., 1974). Although the Dogrib data did not support the major gene model, I thought it would be worthwhile to examine genetic marker data for evidence of association with glucose level. It should be noted that for the 3 systems considered below chi-square analyses showed no significant differences in the distribution of phenotypes between hyperglycemic and normoglycemic persons (Szathmary, 1983b).

Table 5 shows that age-adjusted log glucose levels do not differ significantly among the three Glyoxalase phenotypes, this in spite of the fact that the Glyoxalase locus is linked to the HLA complex on chromosome six, and HLA-2 in the Pima is said to contribute to an earlier age of onset of NIDDM in these Indians (Williams et al., 1981).

Cadien et al.(1979) did not state which PGP phenotype was associated with elevation in plasma glucose in the Pima. The Dogrib data (Table 5) indicate that PGP (1-1) may have this effect.

Table 5. Age-adjusted plasma glucose levels by phenotype.

Phenotype	$\log_{10}$ (Plasma Glucose mg/dl) N	$\bar{X} \pm$ SD	Statistic (with df)
Phosphoglycolate Phosphatase[2]:			
PGP (1-1)	131	2.20±.13	
PGP (2-1)	26	2.04±.16	$t_{155} = 2.03$
Glyoxalase:			
GLO (1-1)	2	2.13±.15	
GLO (2-1)	36	2.10±.14	
GLO (2-2)	119	2.09±.14	$F_{2,156} = 0.18$
Group-Specific Component (Vitamin-D Binding Globulin):			
Gc 1S-1S	51	2.12±.16	
Gc 1F-1F	23	2.08±.12	
Gc 1F-1S	61	2.08±.14	
Gc 2-1S	11	2.13±.09	
Gc 2-1F	11	2.05±.09	$F_{4,156} = 1.22$
Gc(1S-1S)+(2-1S)	62	2.12±.15	
Gc(1F-1F)+(2-1F)+(1S-1F)	95	2.07±.13	$t_{155} = 2.14$
Gc(1S-1S)+(2-1S)	62	2.12±.15	
Gc(1F-1F)+(2-1F)	34	2.07±.11	$t_{94} = 1.88$

[1]Age-adjustment is to that of a male, aged 46.7 yrs.
[2]Only one person (female) was PGP (2-2) in phenotype. This phenotype is grouped with (2-1). The woman's raw 2-hr glucose level was 157 mg/dl, or 2.19 $\log_{10}$(mg/dl).
[3]Exact probabilities are shown.

Analysis of variance of age-adjusted plasma glucose by Gc phenotype showed no significant differences in the Dogrib (Table 5). However, the data do suggest that $\underline{Gc}^{1S}$ may be linked with elevation of plasma glucose level in all instances except when present with $\underline{Gc}^{1F}$. When data are grouped to reflect this, that is Gc (1S-1S) + Gc (2-1S) versus Gc (1F-1F) + Gc (2-1F) + GC (1F-1S), the difference in mean glucose levels between these groups is again not significant by the criteria used in this paper, but a marked difference is evident. This is also seen when the contrast excludes heterozygotes for Gc (1S-1F).

Kirk et al (this volume) did not specify which of the two $\underline{Gc}^{1}$ genes, $\underline{Gc}^{1F}$ or $\underline{Gc}^{1S}$ is significantly associated with NIDDM in Polynesians. The glycoprotein products of these genes bind Vitamin D and its metabolically active derivatives (van Baelen et al., 1978). In turn, 1,25 $(OH)_2D_3$ is known to act directly on the β-cells of the pancreas (Clark et al., 1980b) and serves to increase insulin production. A positive feedback relationship between insulin level and 1,25 $(OH)_2D_3$ by Gc phenotypes could have an effect on insulin production and subsequently on glucose level. The studies that have examined binding differences (e.g. Daiger and Cavalli-Sforza, 1977) reported only slight differences by phenotype in the affinity of the Gc proteins to Vitamin D_3 and its metabolites. No specific mention was made of differences in binding affinity of Gc 1 subtypes (Daiger and Cavalli-Sforza, 1977). The findings in experimental animals suggest that Gc may have a role to play in the transport or release of 1,25 $(OH)_2D_3$ to target cells in the pancreas. If this is also true in humans, then the differences in glucose level by Gc phenotype in the Dogrib may be more than just coincidence. These possibilities, however, require confirmation from other population surveys, from assessment of <u>unrelated</u> individuals, and from laboratory analyses.

DISCUSSION AND CONCLUSIONS

The delineation of the specific genetic and environmental variables involved in the etiology of

NIDDM in Amerindians is of importance, given the epidemic-like increase of the disease in most North American Indian groups (West, 1978). This paper has focused attention on evidence for the existence of genetic factors that influence plasma glucose level in an Indian population in which NIDDM had never been diagnosed nor suspected. While the test methodology used in the 1979 survey of the Dogrib did use a higher glucose challenge dose than currently recommended, the higher test dose should not have had an impact on responses were all Dogrib normal. That some hyperglycemic responses did occur indicates the presence of some abnormality of glucose metabolism in some of these Indians.

The American National Diabetes Data Group (1979), and the WHO Expert Committee on Diabetes Mellitus (1980) agree that standardization of glucose tolerance test procedures and a more uniform interpretation of test responses is necessary if we are to achieve understanding of the etiology of NIDDM. Under the guidelines established by the NDDG (1979) none of the hyperglycemics in this study can be called "diabetic". The question to be resolved is whether these hyperglycemics can be said to display Impaired Glucose Tolerance (IGT), at least for epidemiologic purposes which allow the use of data obtained on a single screening test (NDDG, 1979) as was done here. Medical opinion does not equate IGT with NIDDM. However, the two are linked, for some individuals with IGT do convert to NIDDM at the rate of 1-5% per year (NDDG, 1979). Furthermore, follow up studies have shown that those who do develop NIDDM tend to have some impairment of their responses to glucose challenge some time before the disease appears (Beaty et al., 1982).

The criteria by which hyperglycemia is defined in this study are rigorous. The boundaries were set high deliberately, to offset the possible small increase in plasma glucose (15 mg/dl at hour-2, WHO, 1980) produced by a 100 gm challenge dose. There can be no doubt that at the very least the hyperglycemics in this study fall into the category now labelled "IGT". Accordingly, the model of regulation of plasma glucose level indicated by this study has direct bearing on our understanding of the etiology of NIDDM in Indians.

That there is a genetic basis to dysfunction of carbohydrate metabolism in some Dogrib is shown by the clustering of hyperglycemic Dogrib in pedigrees. One of these pedigrees connects hyperglycemics in the least acculturated and most acculturated settlements, and is also the pedigree that contains the only known case of clinical diabetes in the Dogrib, diagnosed two years after the survey on which this study is based.

In spite of the clustering of hyperglycemics in pedigrees, the distribution of plasma glucose level in the Dogrib is unimodal. This observation affords no support for the notion that a major gene, probably transmitted as an autosomal recessive (Elston et al. 1974; Steinberg et al., 1970) is responsible for the regulation of glucose level in all Indians. This study was also unable to confirm the differential distribution of specific genotypes (systems GLO, PGP and Gc) in hyperglycemics compared to normals. Nevertheless, some elevations of plasma glucose by PGP or Gc phenotype were apparent. Confirmation of these associations needs to be done by studies conducted on unrelated persons.

The major positive and important finding in this study was the highly significant correlation of glucose level observed among siblings, but not among other first degree relatives, or spouses, or among unrelated individuals selected at random. This finding, when coupled with the observation that (1) plasma glucose is elevated in sibs of hyperglycemics compared to sibs of normoglycemics but not in other groups of first degree relatives (Szathmary, 1983b), and that (2) the Dogrib have experienced a major cultural shift to sedentism within the past thirty years, suggests that a within-generation environmental effect is influencing glucose levels in this population. Significant sib-sib covariance for a quantitative trait is also dependent on variance components due to genes with additive effects and genes with dominant effects (Cavalli-Sforza and Bodmer, 1971). Accordingly, the model of plasma glucose regulation that is suggested by the results of this study includes the operation of additive as well as dominant genes and the operation of an intra-generational environmental effect.

ACKNOWLEDGMENTS

To all the Dogrib people who participated in this study: Massi cho! This study was supported by Health and Welfare Canada Grant 6606-1609-46.

LITERATURE CITED

Annest JL, Sing CF, Biron P, Mongeau J-G (1979). Familial aggregation of blood pressure and weight in adoptive families. I. Comparisons of blood pressure and weight statistics among families with adopted, natural, or both natural and adopted children. Am J Epidem 110:479.

Beaty TH, Neel JV, Fajans SS (1982). Identifying risk factors for diabetes in first degree relatives of non-insulin dependent diabetic patients. Am J Epidem 115:380.

Burke E (1981). Personal Communication from the Director of the Rae-Edzo Cottage Hospital. Edzo, Northwest Territories.

Cadien JD, Mamula PW, Hecht F (1979). Phosphoglycolate phosphatase phenotypes and association with Pima Indian diabetes. Am J Hum Genet 31:40A.

Castro A, Scott JP, Grettie DP, Macfarlane D, Bailey RE (1970). Plasma insulin and glucose responses of healthy subjects to varying glucose loads during three-hour oral glucose tolerance tests. Diabetes 19:842.

Cavalli-Sforza LL, Bodmer WF (1971). "The Genetics of Human Populations." San Francisco: W.H. Freeman.

Clark SA, Stumpf WE, Sar M (1980a). Effect of 1,25 Dihydroxy-vitamin D_3 on insulin secretion. Diabetes 30:382.

Clark SA, Stumpf WE, De Luca HF, Tanaka Y (1980b). Target cells for 1,25 Dihydroxyvitamin D_3 in the pancreas. Cell Tissue Res. 209:515.

Daiger SP, Cavalli-Sforza LL (1977). Detection of genetic variation with radioactive ligands. II.Genetic variants of Vitamin D-Labelled Group Specific Component (Gc) proteins. Am J Hum Genet 29:593.

de Nobel E, vaan't Laar A (1978). The size of the loading dose as an important determinant of the results of the oral glucose tolerance test.

Diabetes 27:42.
Elston RC (1975). On the correlation between correlations. Biometrika 62:133.
Elston RC (1980). Segregation analysis. In Mielke JH, Crawford MH (eds): "Current Developments in Anthropological Genetics." Vol. 1, New York: Plenum Press, p 327.
Elston RC, Stewart J (1971). A general model for the analysis of pedigree data. Human Hered 21:523.
Elston RC, Namboodiri KK, Glueck CI, Fallat R, Tsang R, Leuba V (1975). Study of the genetic transmission of hypercholesterolemia and hypertriglyceridemia in a 195 member kindred. Am Hum Genet 39:67.
Elston RC, Namboodiri KK, Nino HV, Pollitzer WS (1974). Studies on blood and urine glucose in Seminole Indians: Indication for segregation of a major gene. Am J Hum Genet 26:13.
Falconer DS (1960). "Introduction to Quantitative Genetics." London: Longman Group.
Friedman JM, Fialkow PJ (1980). The genetics of diabetes mellitus. Prog Med Genet 4:199.
Fisher RA (1958). "Statistical Methods for Research Workers." New York: Hafner.
Helm J (1980). Indian dependency and self determination: Problems and paradoxes in Canada's Northwest Territories. In Schusky EL (ed): "Political Organization of Native North Americans," Washington: University Press of America, p 215.
Helm J (1981). The Dogrib. Helm J (ed): "The Subarctic. Handbook of North American Indians." Vol. VI, Washington: Smithsonian Institution, p 291.
Kaplan EB, Elston RC (1972). A subroutine package for Maximum Likelihood Estimation (MAXLIK). Institute of Statistics Mimeo Series No. 823. Chapel Hill: Department of Biostatistics.
Knowler WC, Pettitt DJ, Savage PJ, Bennett PH (1981). Diabetes incidence in Pima Indians: Contributions of obesity and parental diabetes. Am J Epidem 113:144.
Li CC (1975). "Path Analysis--A Primer." Pacific Grove, CA: The Boxwood Press.
Mouratoff GJ, Carroll NV, Scott EM (1969). Diabetes mellitus in Athabaskan Indians in Alaska. Diabetes 18:29.
National Diabetes Data Group (1979). Classification and diagnosis of diabetes mellitus and other

categories of glucose intolerance. Diabetes 28:1039.
Neel JV (1976). Diabetes mellitus--a geneticist's nightmare. Creutzfeldt W, Köbberling, Neel JV (eds): "The Genetics of Diabetes Mellitus," New York: Springer-Verlag, p 1.
Nie NH, Hull CH, Jenkins JG, Steinbrenner K, Bent DH (1975). "SPSS. Statistical Package for the Social Sciences." Second Ed. New York: McGraw-Hill.
Pedhazur EJ (1982). "Multiple Regression Research." 2nd Ed. New York: Holt, Reinhart, and Winston.
Pettitt DJ, Baird HR, Aleck KA, Bennett PH, Knowler WC (1983). Excessive obesity in offspring of Pima Indian women with diabetes during pregnancy. New Eng J Med 308:242.
Picard L (1983). Personal communication from the Regional Nutritionist, Health and Welfare Canada. Yellowknife, Northwest Territories.
Pyke DA (1979). Diabetes: The genetic connections. Diabetologia 17:333.
Rushforth NB, Bennett PH, Steinberg AG, Burch TA, Miller M (1975). Diabetes in Pima Indians. Evidence of bimodality in glucose tolerance distributions. Diabetes 20:756.
Sing CF, Orr JD (1978). Analysis of genetic and environmental sources of variation in serum cholesterol in Techumseh, Michigan. IV. Separation of polygene from common environmental effects. Am J Hum Genet 30:491.
Snedecor GW, Cochran WG (1967). "Statistical Methods." 6th Ed. Ames: The Iowa State University Press.
Sokal RR, Rohlf FJ (1969). "Biometry." San Francisco: W.H. Freeman.
Steinberg AG, Rushforth NB, Bennett PH, Burch TA, Miller M (1970). On the genetics of diabetes mellitus. In Cerasi E, Luft R (eds): "The Pathogenesis of Diabetes Mellitus," New York: John Wiley & Sons, p 237.
Swigler LA, Harvey WR, Everson DO, Gregory KE (1964). The variance of intraclass correlation involving groups with one observation. Biometrics 20:818.
Szathmary EJE (1983a). Dogrib Indians of the Northwest Territories, Canada: Genetic diversity and genetic relationship among subarctic Indians. Annals of Human Biology 10:147.
Szathmary EJE (1983b). Athapaskan speakers: Glucose

Intolerance, Genes and Obesity. Final Report to Research Directorate, Health and Welfare, Canada.

Szathmary EJE, Holt N (1983). Hyperglycemia in Dogrib Indians of the Northwest Territories, Canada. Association with age and a centripetal distribution of of body fat. Hum Biol 55:493.

Tattersall RB, Pyke DA (1972). Diabetes in identical twins. Lancet ii:1120.

Toeller M, Knussmann R (1973). Reproducibility of oral glucose tolerance tests with three different loads. Diabetologia 9:102.

Unger RH (1957). The standard two-hour oral glucose tolerance test in the diagnosis of diabetes mellitus in subjects without fasting hyperglycemia. Ann Int Med 47:1138.

Van Baelen H, Bouillon R, De Moor P (1978). The heterogeneity of human Gc-globulin. J of Biol Chem 25:6344.

West KM (1974). Diabetes in American Indians and other native populations of the New World. Diabetes 23:841.

West KM (1978). Diabetes in American Indians. Adv Metab Disord 9:29.

WHO Expert Committee on Diabetes Mellitus (1980). WHO Tech Rep Series 646. Geneva: WHO.

Williams RC, Knowler WC, Butler WJ, Pettitt DJ, Lisse JR, Bennett PH, Mann DL, Johnston AH, Terasaki PI (1981). HLA-A2 and Type 2 (insulin independent) diabetes mellitus in Pima Indians: An association of allele frequency with age. Diabetologia 21:460.

Zimmet P, Faaiuso S, Ainuu J, Whitehouse S, Milne B, De Boer W (1981). The prevalence of diabetes in the rural and urban Polynesian population of Western Samoa. Diabetes 30:45.

Diseases of Complex Etiology in Small Populations:
Ethnic Differences and Research Approaches, pages 227–244

Chapter 10

GENEALOGICAL APPROACH TO THE GENETIC STUDY OF HYPOACUSIA IN A CARIBBEAN ISOLATE

F.M. Mayer[1], C. Bonaïti[2], J. Benoist[3]

[1]Centre de recherches caraïbes, Université de Montréal, Montréal, Quebéc, Canada; [2]Groupe de recherches de génétique épidémiologique, Institut national de la santé et de la recherche médicale, Paris, France and [3]Laboratoire d'écologie humaine de l'Université de Droit, d'Economie et des Sciences d'Aix-Marseille, Pavillon de Lenfant, Aix-en-Provence, France

INTRODUCTION

The population of the island of St.Barthélemy in the French West Indies presents a high rate of hypoacusia. Clinically detected but not yet studied, this pathology has been the object of a request for aid from the local authorities. The Centre de recherches caraïbes (Université de Montréal) and the Groupe de recherches de génétique épidémiologique (Institut national de la santé et de la recherche médicale, U. 155, Paris) had put together in 1977 a joint research project to study deafness in St.Barthélemy in the context of the social and the genetic structure of the population. Four years later, they were joined by the Laboratoire d'ecologie humaine (Université d'Aix-Marseille III).

The purpose of the present article is to present the first results of the genealogical approach followed by these teams in their effort to elucidate the hereditary nature and the mode of transmission of this pathology. A segregation analysis is concurrently being carried on by C. Bonaïti (INSERM). Through the search for common ancestors of the individuals suffering from deafness, this study allowed us, as well, to go further in the identification of the population structure.

The study of hypoacusia runs into many difficulties. Some are tied up with the characteristics of the pathology as it presents itself on the island. The audiological examinations were performed with a Philips portable audiometer mainly at schools and at numerous organized meetings, or at people's homes when they did not come spontaneously to those meetings. To date 1450 individuals have been tested, and more than 1900 examinations executed, for numerous persons have been examined twice. This was done to estimate the "repeatability" of the measures or to control doubtful audiograms. This study cannot be exhaustive (60% of the population was tested) for many reasons: refusals, adolescents studying in Guadeloupe or in France, persons too young or too old. A particular effort has been made to reconstitute nuclear families (father, mother and children) in order to obtain the most complete information for the genetic analysis. One hundred seventy-three families have been so examined.

The results obtained thus far allow one to characterize hypoacusia in the following ways:

(1) It is a sickness that affects adults essentially and which develops in a progressive way. It initially affects high frequencies. We found numerous young people who have no functional constraint but whose threshold on frequency 8000 has broken down.

(2) It seems that onset is precipitated by aggravating factors. Many observations show revealed or aggravated hypoacusia after a medical or a surgical stress, particularly after a small number of ototoxic antibiotic injections.

(3) It is very often difficult to differentiate the "normal" from the "pathological" subject using the usual criteria of normality. This is due on the one hand to the less than ideal examination conditions; on the other hand to the fact that deafness is not total. Presbyacusia (hypoacusia related with senescence) which is particularly frequent (almost no individual

over 60 years of age has a normal audiogram according to the habitual criteria) is also a confounding factor. In addition, about 20% of the subjects have an audiogram on the borderline, that is, near the threshold of normality.

(4) Hearing troubles are particularly frequent since 30% of the subjects show clear pathological audiograms.

(5) A certain number of severely impaired individuals are closely related by kinship, but this is not the case for all the affected subjects.

Other difficulties of this research are related to the complexity of the genealogical network. Even if the population of St. Barthélemy is divided into geographical and sociological endogamous subunits (Benoist, 1964; 1966) the pathology is present in all these groups. Accordingly the study cannot be limited to the examination of a few pedigrees but shall explore the nature of the genetic exchange between all the units.

The genealogical approach has been carried on through the use of a population register built by the Montreal team from archival sources. The quality and richness of the data rendered this task possible. The population file is principally based on the exploitation of the civil records (birth, marriage, death); secondly on nominative census lists; and finally on other sources, mainly notarial papers (e.g. inheritance records, mortgages). The civil records are found chiefly in the parish registers of St. Barthélemy at the Archives départementales de la Guadeloupe and the Evêché de Basse-Terre (Guadeloupe); census lists and other auxiliary sources are located at the Archives d'Outre-mer (Aix-en-Provence), Fonds St. Barthélemy.

The data are computerized and linked in order to produce a demographic corpus which will permit a genetic and demographic analysis. The population file, still in the process of being completed, is now mainly built on civil records from 1977 back to 1820. The data prior to this period (civil records and notarial papers) are in the process of being inventoried, computerized or linked. The census lists are also computerized but not yet linked with the population file.

The Population of St. Barthélemy

The population of St. Barthélemy numbers roughly 2500 people and is mainly white, essentially rural, Catholic and of French tradition. The black community of 200 individuals, English speaking and Anglican, is located in the town of Gustavia. Most of its members are from the neighboring English islands.

The first settlement dates to 1659 when a small group of settlers, originating from the western provinces of France, established themselves on the island. However, subsequent frequent wars led to deportations followed by returns. For these reasons the first lasting settlement dates to the mid-eighteenth century. There has been no major contribution added to the original settlement (Benoist, 1964). This is clearly shown by the fact that the majority of the population shares only ten major surnames which are found again and again in the old parish registers. Immigration into the white population has been continuous but in small numbers until 1830 when the island was almost closed to all exterior contact. The Swedish possession of the island from 1784 to 1878 (when it was retroceded to France) and the presence of slaves engaged in domestic and agricultural work on small familial holdings did not leave marks on the socio-cultural and biological characteristics of the population.

A 1961 study conducted by J. Benoist (1964, 1966) through a survey of the origins of the couples in the three major districts of the island, as well as an examination of the marriages registered on the island since 1862, showed a very high rate of endogamy. Of 717 marriages only eight included a partner of colored origin and one, an immigrant from France. According to Benoist, the descendants of the marriages between the whites and colored ceased to reside in the white community, and the only foreigner having married a white woman from St. Barthélemy had gone back to France. This produced an exceptionally high rate of endogamy of almost 100% for those one hundred years. Moreover, the sociological study and the examination of the marriage structure since 1862 revealed that the isolate of St. Barthélemy was also divided into two highly endogamous units which correspond, sociologically, to the two parishes of the island and, geographically, to its two halves, the windward and the leeward. The parish of Lorient which groups the rural windward districts showed a rate of endogamy of 96% while the parish of Gustavia, regrouping the rural leeward districts had an endogamous rate of 89.5% over one hundred years. The districts themselves also showed a relatively high endogamous rate.

The biological study carried on at the same time by Benoist and dealing particularly with the blood groups ABO, showed that the population of St. Barthélemy is significantly different from the French population. It also showed that the subisolates are different from one another.

MATERIALS AND METHODS

Of the 1450 individuals who took the audiometric test, 37 left no doubt concerning the severity of their deafness. Only 32 of the latter individuals (20 women and 12 men from 17 to 78 years of age) have been selected for this study. One sibling of each of the six pairs of siblings present in the group has been set aside. Also, three subjects who could not be found in the recent genealogies were replaced by a brother or sister and in one case by both his parents. Siblings and parents were identified through the medical questionnaire. The birthplace in all 32 cases was St. Barthélemy, 11 districts being represented of the 15. In 23 cases, the place of residence was the same as the birthplace. Two pairs are composed of closely related individuals (father and son and mother and daughter). There is also one pair of aunt and niece, one pair of aunt and nephew, one pair of uncle and niece and one pair of grandmother and grand daughter. There are two pairs of great aunt and great niece, nine pairs of first degree cousins and eleven pairs of second degree cousins once removed.

This study consists of three components: (1) The reconstruction of the 32 genealogies using the records covering the period from 1977 to 1820. (2) The examination of the interferences between the genealogies in order to identify the common ancestors. (3) The analysis of the exchanges between the genealogies through the successive generations in order to compare their eventual pattern with the actual population structure. The results represent a first step toward identifying the hereditary mode of transmission of this pathology and the investigation of the population dynamics which favor this mechanisms.

In the reconstruction of the genealogies these procedures were followed: (1) All the ancestral pairs in the genealogies were identified as were all the 32 genealogies in which these pairs were cited with the frequency with which they appear. (2) For each genealogy all the pairs mentioned were again identified, this time taking into account the generation depth where these pairs were found. It was also noted whether the pair was cited for itself or as the parent or ancestor of a pair appearing elsewhere in the genealogies. Note should be taken that a pair could appear more than once in the same genealogy.

RESULTS AND DISCUSSION

Study of the Common Ancestors

Through the genealogies, each pair mentioned last in the lines of ascent was identified. These ancestral pairs are called "founding" pairs and total 124. For each "founding" pair, the number of different genealogies in which the pair appears, as well as the frequency with which it occurs was indicated. This appears in the form of a ratio (Table 1). Those "founding" pairs cited only once were classified by approximate date of marriage, from the earliest to the more recent. It was also indicated in which genealogy and at which generation they appeared (Table 2).

Table 1. Ratio for each "founding" pair between the number of different genealogies in which it appears more than once and the total number of times it appears.

Pair No.	Year[1] Marr	Ratio	Pair No.	Year Marr	Ratio	Pair No.	Year Marr	Ratio
1	1802	16/28	31	1822	7/8	60	1803	3/5
2	1786	12/18	32	1806	7/7	61	1811	3/5
3	1786	12/18	33	1808	6/17	62	1789	3/4
4	1806	12/16	34	1800	6/8	63	1802	3/4
5	1802	11/18	35	1800	6/6	64	1889	3/4
6	1745	10/25	36	1810	5/7	65	1759	3/3
7	1745	10/25	37	1787	5/6	66	1759	3/3
8	1801	10/25	38	1787	5/6	67	1796	3/3
9	1776	10/22	39	1807	5/6	68	1802	3/3
10	1801	10/17	40	1819	5/6	69	1823	3/3
11	1811	10/16	41	1843	5/6	70	1829	3/3
12	1790	10/10	42	1793	5/5	71	1827	2/4
13	1776	9/16	43	1814	5/5	72	1829	2/3
14	1793	9/14	44	1819	5/5	73	1829	2/3
15	1788	9/12	45	1802	4/7	74	1795	2/2
16	1816	8/13	46	1798	4/6	75	1800	2/2
17	1807	8/12	47	1793	4/5	76	1800	2/2
18	1740	8/10	48	1801	4/5	77	1802	2/2
19	1793	8/9	49	1806	4/5	78	1803	2/2
20	1794	8/8	50	1811	4/5	79	1815	2/2
21	1790	7/13	51	1787	4/4	80	1815	2/2
22	1790	7/11	52	1793	4/4	81	1818	2/2
23	1804	7/11	53	1793	4/4	82	1818	2/2
24	1800	7/10	54	1793	4/4	83	1820	2/2
25	1749	7/9	55	1815	4/4	84	1823	2/2
26	1794	7/9	56	1829	4/4	85	1834	2/2
27	1812	7/9	57	1838	4/4	86	1834	2/2
28	1799	7/8	58	1798	3/5	87	1845	2/2
29	1810	7/8	59	1803	3/5	88	1865	2/2
30	1819	7/8						

[1]The approximate year of marriage has been calculated by subtracting 28 years from the marriage date of the offspring. This figure, representing one generation span, corresponds to an estimated mean age of the mothers at delivery.

Table 2. Distribution of "founding" pairs present in only one genealogy according to the approximate year of marriage[1].

Pair No.	Year Marr	Genealogy No.	Generation No.	Pair No.	Year Marr	Genealogy No.	Generation No
89	1759	3	7	107	1822	17	5
90	1759	3	7	108	1822	17	5
91	1788	3	6	109	1823	11	5
92	1790	6	7	110	1824	11	5
93	1795	8	7	111	1824	6	6
94	1795	11	6	112	1831	2	6
95	1808	7	5	113	1832	14	6-6
96	1810	8	6	114	1832	4	5
97	1812	13	7-7	115	1834	32	6
98	1813	13	7-7	116	1836	32	6
99	1816	6	6	117	1838	17	5
100	1817	25	6	118	1839	14	6-6
101	1818	25	6	119	1839	9	6
102	1820	8	5	120	1840	12	6
103	1820	14	6-7	121	1848	12	5
104	1820	17	5	122	1860	4	4
105	1821	7	5	123	1889	16	4
106	1821	25	6	124[2]	1894	23	4

[1]The approximate year of marriage has been calculated by subtracting 28 years from the marriage date of the offspring. This figure, representing one generation span, corresponds to an estimated mean age of the mothers at delivery.
[2]Unwed mother.

The high number of "founding" pairs mentioned only once cannot be explained entirely by deficiencies in the sources, because they occur in 15 different genealogies, and are identified in the 4th to the 7th ascending generations. Furthermore, most of the approximate dates of marriage of these once cited "founding" pairs are similar to those of the pairs which are found in more than one genealogy.

An arbitrary choice could have been made to end the observations at the sixth generation but the fact that the 32 deaf individuals have an age span of 40 years would have made this choice fictitious. Moreover, it was interesting to find out how the furthest known ancestors were distributed in the 32 genealogies. The distribution of all 124 "founding" pairs, according to the frequency of their presence in the genealogies, is negative exponential (Figure 1). The fewer number of "founding" pairs present in several different genealogies are in most cases mentioned more than once in a single genealogy. This indicates a strong lineage endogamy.

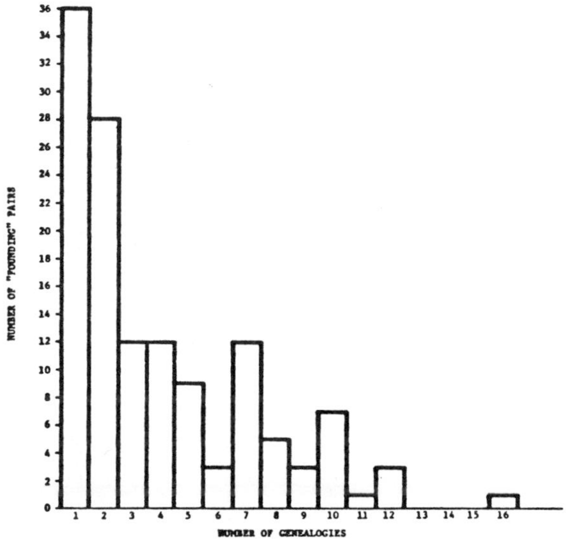

Figure 1. Distribution of "founding" pairs according to the number of different genealogies in which they are present.

Seventy "founding" pairs were found to be present in three or more genealogies and were then classified according to each genealogy in which they are cited. The distribution of these pairs in the genealogies follows a definite pattern that did not develop by accident. The pairs present in a certain number of

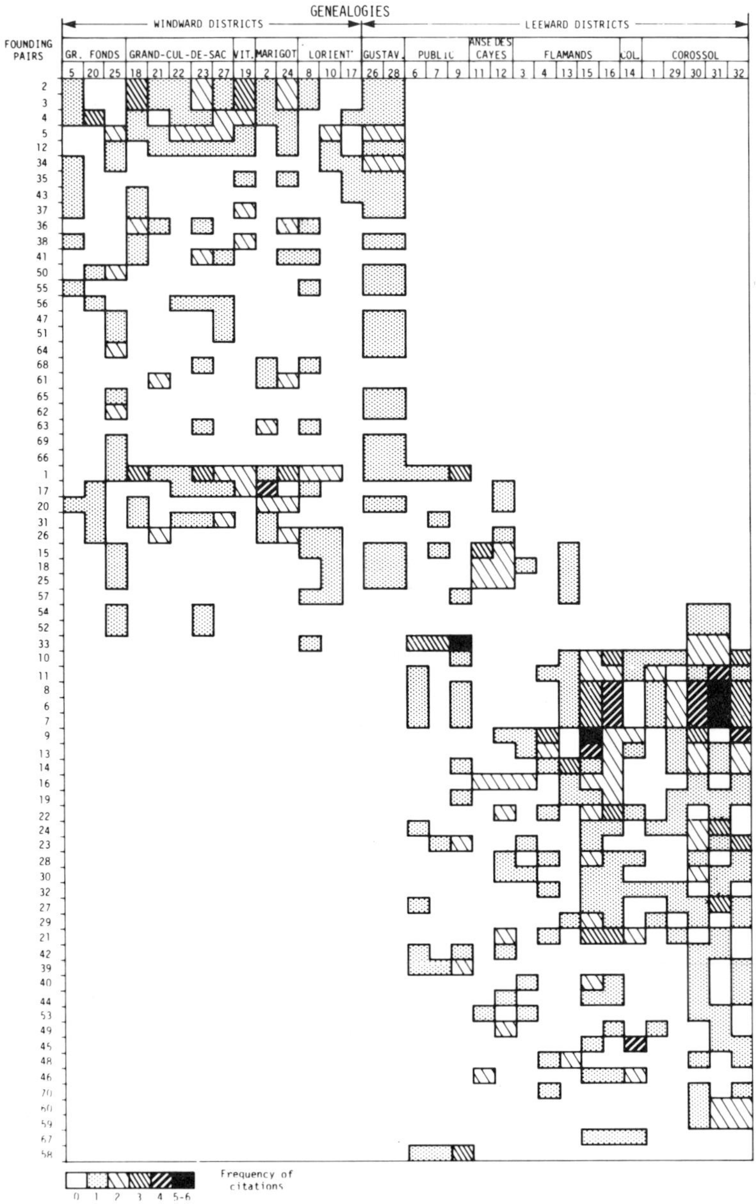

Figure 2. Distribution of "founding" pairs present in three or more genealogies according to those genealogies in which they appear.

genealogies are systematically absent from the others and conversely. This means that the majority of the "founding" pairs divide themselves into two groups of ancestors according to their preferential links with one of the two sets of genealogies. There are only a few exceptions to this observation.

In order to illustrate more clearly the two patterns of presence of the "founding" pairs, the classification of the genealogies was purposely reorganized (Figure 2). Classification was done by the birthplace of the 32 individuals, covering the windward districts of the island and then leeward ones, rather than by numerical order from 1 to 32 (corresponding to the alphabetical order of the 32 cases). This latter method did present the same pattern, but in a far more disparate and therefore less effective manner. Secondly, the consecutive order of presentation of the "founding" pairs was altered to further emphasize the two patterns.

The two groups thus delineated correspond to the two endogamous isolates first identified by Benoist (1964). The present research, however, goes 50 years beyond that study. The two isolates are in fact the social and geographical subunits of the Lorient and Gustavia parishes. More precisely, these are the leeward and the windward sections of the island. Figure 3, sections A and B shows with two examples the two patterns of presence.

The identification of the common ancestors for the 32 individuals suffering from severe deafness necessitated further analysis. Because the sources presently available do not allow one to go further back in the genealogies to pinpoint these ancestors, the study required an indirect approach in order to identify at least one group of potential founders. In so doing, we tried to identify the minimum number of "founding" pairs who, through their lines of descent would be included in all the 32 genealogies. Each time, at least five pairs were needed to attain full coverage. If only three were taken, four genealogies were systematically left out, and two more pairs were always needed to fill the void. The most effective combination of pairs of ancestors are shown in Table

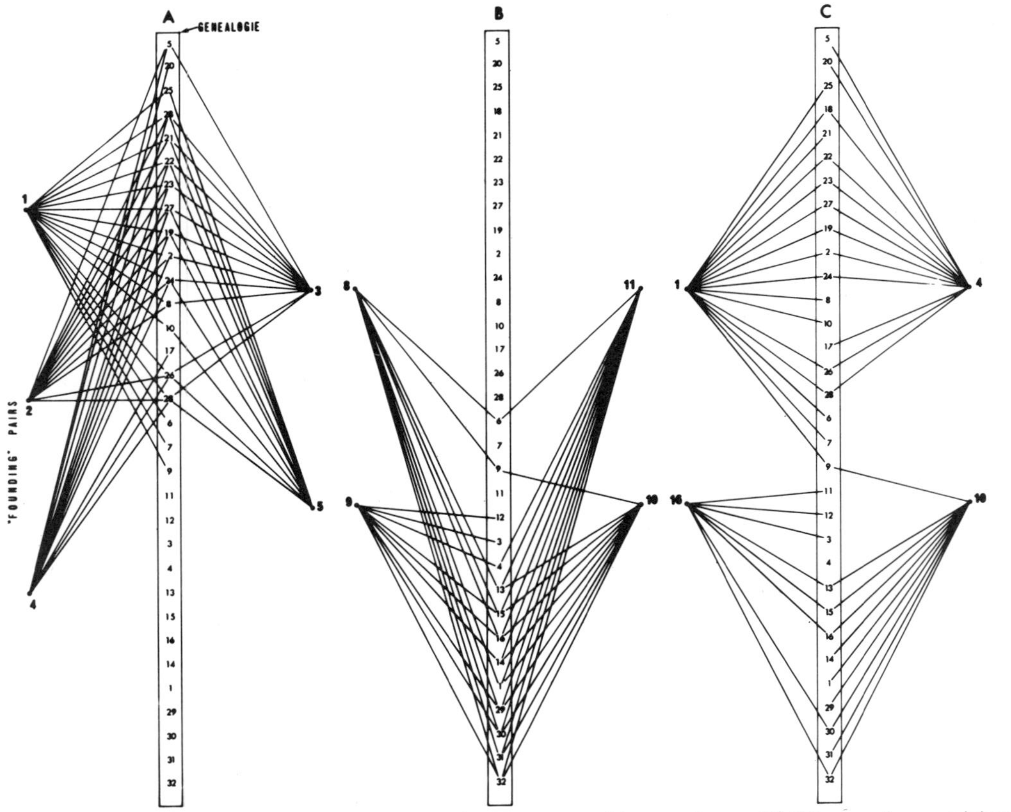

Figure 3. Distribution of "founding" pairs according to different patterns of presence in the genealogies.

3. The combinations in Table 3 show that there are eight pairs whose presence was essential to attain full coverage: 1, 4, 10, 11, 9, 16, 2 and 3. More particularly, Figure 3 section C gives an example of near total coverage of the 32 genealogies with four pairs of ancestors. Only genealogy number 4 is left uncovered.

Table 3. Most effective combinations of "founding" pairs: covering as many of the 32 genealogies as possible.

Number of Genealogies Covered			
29	28		27
1-9-4	1-10- 4	1- 9-43	(2 or 3)-10-(18 or 15)
	1-20-20	1- 9- 6	(2 or 3)-11-(18 or 15)
	1-10- 9	1- 9- 7	(2 or 3)- 8-(18 or 15)
	1-10-16	1- 9-16	(2 or 3)- 6-(18 or 15)
	1-10-18	1- 9-29	(2 or 3)- 7-(18 or 15)
	1-11- 4	1- 9-15	(2 or 3)- 9-(18 or 15)
	1-11-20	1- 9-18	
	1-11-31	1- 9-25	
	1-11-18	1-13-15	
	1- 9-20	1-13-18	
	1- 9-34	1-14-15	
	1- 9-35	1-14-18	
		4- 9-15	

So far, two concluding points may be derived from this analysis. First, a potential founder who could have introduced the pathology to the island will have to be found in a period prior to the one studied here (1977 to 1820). The introduction of this pathology into the population is therefore very old, and it is necessary to pursue the reconstruction of the genealogies with a population register covering the entire eighteenth century. If sources permit, reconstruction should extend into the latter half of the seventeenth century. Secondly, it is clear that the pathology has been transmitted into both of the subunits of the total population of the island. Defined through the pairs of ancestors to which they are linked, these two subpopulations will have to be compared qualitatively and quantitatively in their manifestation of hypoacusia. It may be possible that differences will appear similar to those found for the genetic markers between the two endogamous isolates.

Study of the Exchanges Between the Genealogies

In order to study the interrelations between the 32 genealogies a triangular matrix was built that indicates the exchanges and their frequencies for each genealogy in relation to all the others. In order to make the representation clearer, the matrix was made symmetrical and the genealogies were classified by the birthplace of the 32 individuals, going from the windward to the leeward part of the island (Figure 4). Figure 5, A, B and C illustrates with three examples the intensity and the duration of the exchanges through the generations. From these figures emerge two very distinct patterns of exchange between the genealogies (Figure 4). It is worth noting that the exchange between preferential genealogies is continuous through several generations (Figures 5, A and B). The mode of exchange for the genealogies that do not fit exclusively in one of the two patterns is hazy, each acting differently as to the generation when the exchanges took place as well as to their duration. For example, genealogy number 9 (Figure 5, C) exchanges with almost all the genealogies, but only at the seventh generation.

This preferential pattern of exchange corresponds to the structure drawn from the study above on common ancestors, and, in addition, gives it more accuracy. The two subpopulations remained permanent on a historical continuum of over a century and a half. Over this period of time, the two endogamous subunits had a few interactions that are reflected through a certain number of genealogies for which ancestors are related to both groups. The vast majority of the genealogies, however, coalesce into one or the other of the two distinct groups.

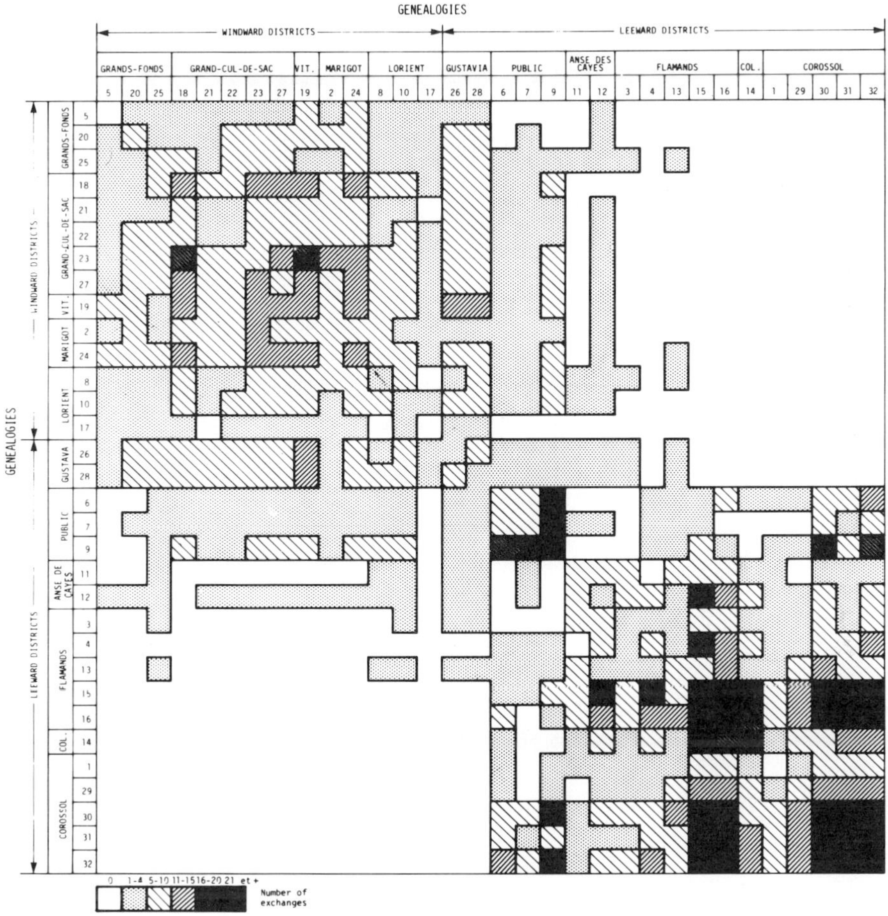

Figure 4. Matrix showing exchanges and intensity of exchanges between the genealogies.

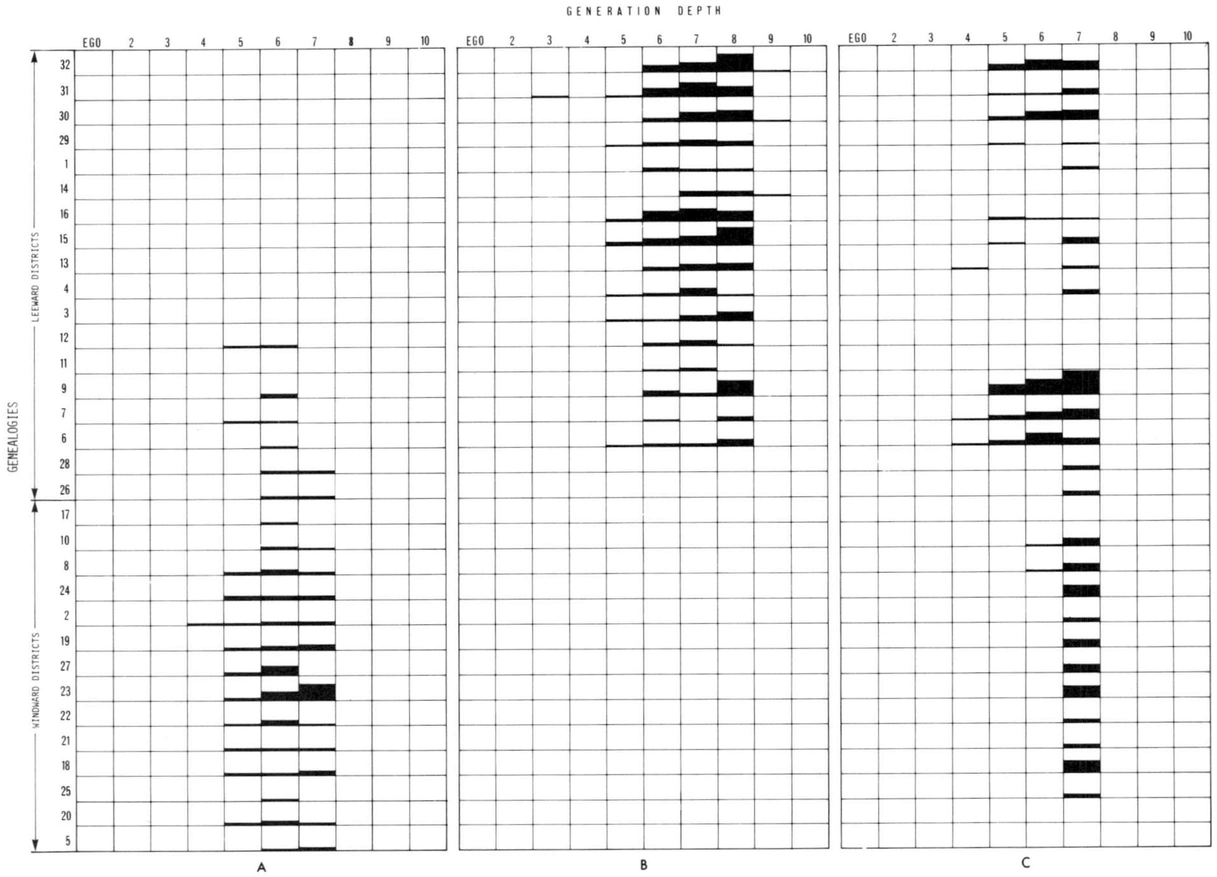

Figure 5 A, B, C. Exchanges between genealogies 2, 30 and 9 respectively and the 31 others according to generation depth.

CONCLUSION

The investigation into the nature of these exchanges, be it concerning the connections between the genealogies or the variations of the exchanges from generation to generation show certain regularities. A more sophisticated study of the matrix is presently underway to gain further insight into the nature of these exchanges. The interpretation of our results, however, will have to await the findings of the historical and demographic studies currently being done. Through the examination of the old census lists and the archival sources (mainly inheritance papers), it will be possible to identify the sociological component of the endogamy, as well as the nature of the exchanges which sometimes may reduce this endogamy.

It would be premature here to do more than underscore this level of articulation between the social organization of the St. Barthélemy community and the genetic structure of the population.

ACKNOWLEDGEMENTS

These analyses have been made possible with the assistance of the St. Barthélemy research team in Montréal (Centre de recherches caraïbes): M.T. Duquette, F. Nault, L. Roy, and S. St. Germain, and with the collaboration of Lise Hamel-Robillard of the Centre de calcul de l'Université de Montréal.

The English text was reviewed by Carolyn Fick of the Centre de recherches caraïbes. The treatment of the data was done on a Cyber-855 computer (Control Data Corporation, Canada). The drawings were made by Lucien Goupil, Département d'anthropologie, Université de Montréal.

The research at the Centre de recherches caraïbes has been made possible through two grants from the Social Sciences and Humanities Research Council of Canada, nos: 410-78-0067 and 410-80-0292 and a grant from CAFIR (Comité d'attribution de fonds internes de recherche de l'Université de Montréal). The research at the Groupe de recherches de génétique épidémiologique has been financed by two grants from DGRST (Délégation générale à la recherche scientifique et technique), nos: 80-704-06 and 81-L0529 and by a grant from INSERM (Institut national de la santé et de la recherche médicale), no :CRL 79-5-009-1. Finally, the work at the Laboratoire d'écologie humaine has received funds from the Ministère de la recherche, Paris, CORDET, Sciences humaines.

LITERATURE CITED

Benoist J (1964). St.Barthélemy: Physical anthropology of an isolate. Am J Phy Anth 22:473.

Benoist J (1966). Du social au biologique:étude de quelques interactions. L'Homme 6:5.

SECTION III
ENVIRONMENTAL AND/OR CULTURAL FACTORS AND RISK TO DISEASE

Diseases of Complex Etiology in Small Populations:
Ethnic Differences and Research Approaches, pages 247–254

SECTION III. INTRODUCTORY REMARKS

E.J.E. Szathmary and R. Chakraborty

It is a truism that populations differ in their responses to environmental stress such as heat, cold, aridity, humidity and altitude. Human populations also display a range in levels of social organization and sociocultural complexity. The interaction of the latter phenomena with a variety of habitats likely gave rise to different adaptive strategies that influenced and may still influence food acquisition, resource utilization and levels of physical activity within human populations.

It is also a truism that few if any peoples remain untouched by the intense post World War II cultural changes often referred to as "Westernization". Nutritional shifts, improvements in sanitation and health care and amelioration of the stresses of physical climate occur together with population size increases and increases in average longevity. The altered conditions, however, are not entirely beneficial, for the diseases of "civilization" (Damon, 1975; Wadsworth, 1984), the chronic diseases that afflict the middle aged and the elderly also make their appearance and increase in frequency in societies undergoing Westernization.

This section examines some of the environmental and cultural factors that may constitute risks for the alteration of health status and therefore perhaps for diseases of complex etiology. Two of the chapters deal with phenomena that undergo major changes during the process of Westernization: Haas and Greksa discuss the role of nutrition on biological fitness and Adams and Smouse describe some consequences of demographic changes in human groups. The remaining four chapters examine patterns of morbidity and mortality in different parts of the world. While the latter chapters do not encompass all geographic regions of the globe, nor all ethnic groups, they all show that generalizations about health status and the roles played by ethnicity and physical habitat are poor substitutes for observations obtained from field investigations. Indeed, some of the chapters question conventional wisdom about the effects of physical habitat on mortality and morbidity, as have a few studies in the literature (e.g. Baker, 1978; Goldstein et al., 1983).

The role of nutrition on biological fitness is complex, for nutritional status is both an index of fitness, as well as a determinant of fitness. Haas and Greksa are careful to note that their definition of biological fitness is not synonymous with Darwinian fitness. Rather, they define biological fitness as a measure of individual well-being in a particular environment at a particular point in time. In addition to having a direct impact on biological fitness, nutrition also has indirect impact because it affects so many other parameters that also impinge on fitness. For example, mortality, morbidity, reproduction and physical working capacity all have complex interrelationships with nutriture. Haas and Greksa focus their attention on the influence nutritional variability exerts on energy reserves. They suggest that energy imbalance may best serve as a risk factor for the reduction of biological fitness in populations. Because energy imbalance can be measured by several different approaches, valuable information about the degree of nutritional stress within a group can be obtained. This information is worth having in epidemiological studies, for alteration of energy balance through changes in the pattern of food intake and changes in the relative proportions of major nutrients have different consequences dependent on the age at which the shifts occurred (Greene, 1980). Duration of acute nutritional stress and resultant energy imbalance may also have a role in the onset of some chronic diseases.

Adams and Smouse discuss the genetic consequences

of demographic change, that is, shift from high birth and death rates typical of pre-industrial societies, to low birth and death rates typical of modern, highly industrialized (i.e. "Western") societies. By using data obtained from Sweden for the period 1780 to 1965, a period during which the Swedish population was in demographic transition, they are able to show decreases in the intensities of selection against three hypothetical disorders: a trait (1) with early and minimally variable age of onset; (2) one with medium and a more variable age of onset; (3) one with late and highly variable age of onset. Pattern (3) in particular is typical for several chronic diseases. The diminished selection against all three varieties of disease classes was due to two factors: a continual lowering of mortality rates during the given 185 years, and a reduction of generation times because of altered age-specific fertility rates. Large increases in selection coefficients also occurred, but were transient and dependent on a short period of demographic instability. Adams and Smouse also show that differences in most published values for the index of opportunity for selection can be explained on the basis of differences in the age structure of the populations and do not imply genetic differences in fitness. These observations suggest that accumulation of "disease susceptibility" genes in populations undergoing demographic transition may be rapid and substantial. Furthermore, increase in the number of such genes may have bearing on the increase in the incidence of chronic diseases that is so marked in recently Westernized societies.

Salzano describes succinctly what is entailed in the process of "Westernization" by South American Indians. In addition, he reviews briefly the epidemiology of tuberculosis, the prevalence of pyoderma, HLA distribution and catecholamine excretion rates among Brazilian Indians. Salzano notes the considerable problems entailed in the investigations of these phenomena in indigenous Brazilians, but he also indicates that further studies are warranted. For example, he wonders whether the course of tuberculosis in Brazilian Indians, which was quite unlike that expected in groups without previous history of the disease, occurred because infection was with a new strain of *M. tuberculosis*. The pattern of skin infections in response to *Staphylococcus* species suggests the existence and possible action of some naturally occurring antibiotic substances. Of greater ramification for the onset of chronic diseases is the observation that some Brazilian Indians have higher average catecholamine levels than do Englishmen. High adrenaline output is certainly an indicator of stress, yet no such evidence for stress was expected in the recently accultured Indian group that was sampled. Although the finding appears unusual, it is worth noting that intragroup stress has been convincingly argued for some northern North American native groups pursuing *traditional* lifestyles (e.g. Savishinsky, 1974; Chance, 1968), although these assessments were not based on catecholamine levels. If these assessments are correct, there may be disease consequences in the longer-living, post-acculturation populations. Catecholamine response to stress has been shown to influence the occurrence of hypertension in white Americans (Sterling and Eyer, 1981) and Samoans (Scheder, 1983), and to be involved in the onset of Type II diabetes in migrant Mexican Americans (Scheder, 1981).

Whether variations in infant and adolescent mortality rates are associated with altitudinal variation is the subject considered by Basu, Gupta, Bharati, Mukhopadhay and Roy. The study focuses on populations residing in central Nepal (upper Khumbu area), east central Sikkim (Lachen, Lachung areas), the Kalimpong area of northern West Bengal (just south of the Sikkim-India border) and two lowland areas of southern West Bengal. The experimental design of the study allowed several within and between group comparisons to assess the roles played by altitude, by concomitant sociocultural factors, and by sociocultural and ethnic factors independent of altitude. The results did not show any effects of altitude on mortality rates. However, sociocultural factors and ethnicity do have effects. These findings challenge prevailing views that regard altitude (e.g. hypoxia, cold, terrain) as an environment that consistently provokes a uniform set of physiological and physical responses from humans. While it is possible that the altitudinal differences within the mountain zone of this study may not have been sufficient to produce enough hypoxia related stress factors that affected mortality, it is fact that within the mountain zone at the same altitude socio-cultural differences did affect mortality. This suggests at minimum that socio-cultural factors must not be overlooked when mortality patterns of high altitude populations are assessed. Furthermore, it should not be assumed a priori that high altitude peoples are subject to greater selection pressures during development than are other populations. To make such a judgement one must be assured that socio-cultural differences have been controlled.

In the next chapter, Rothhammer, Castillo and Schull continue to focus on the effects of high altitude on human populations. They are particularly concerned with altitudinal effects on cardiovascular pathology in Amerindian populations residing in five different altitudinal regions (from 125 m to over 6,000 m) of Chile and Bolivia. Contrasts were also possible within country, for certain regions (e.g. the altiplano differs by altitude, humidity, settlement pattern and access to medical care). The findings show two distinctions in patterns of morbidity, at least for Indians of Chile: populations residing at elevations greater than 2,500 m had higher prevalences of infectious, respiratory and sense organ disorders, but a lower prevalence of borderline hypertension and other circulatory disorders. On the other hand, no differences were seen in the frequency of acute hypertension among Aymara Indians from the altiplano, sierra and coast. The latter observation and three others suggest that altitude related hypoxia does not have a "protective" effect against cardiovascular disease: (1) systolic and diastolic blood pressures varied directly with the Body Mass Index [(weight)/(stature)^2] in Chilean Indians living at all altitudes; (2) non-Aymara residents of the same altitudinal regions displayed the same pattern of morbidity as did the Aymara; (3) compared to Chilean Caucasians, Aymara Indians did not have unusually low rates of cardiovascular disease. Rothhammer et al. suggest that the patterns of cardiovascular pathology they observed are more likely secondary consequences of altitude, the more direct effects being those involved with nutrition, subsistence patterns and lifestyles. It is worth noting that although this study focused on evidence for a claimed protective effect of high altitude against a chronic disease while Basu et al. concentrated on evidence for a detrimental effect on high altitude on health, neither study could show direct altitudinal effects separate from sociocultural and/or ethnic effects. Both studies dispute the "truism" that for humans, altitude represents a specialized environment.

The last chapter in this section by Lefèvre-Witier focuses on the epidemiology of diseases associated with single gene defects in the northern half of the African continent. The geographic region is vast; in it arid and subarid climatic zones are defined by latitude, and populations in these zones are widely dispersed. The difficulties of obtaining reliable epidemiological data in these regions should not be underestimated. Nevertheless Lefèvre-Witier has gathered an impressive amount of information on the distribution of hemoglobin defects and glucose-6-dehydrogenase deficiencies (G-6PD) that show a variety of pathological forms.

One of the more interesting findings in this study concerns the role aridity has had in influencing the fitness of Hb AS heterozygotes. Increasing dessication of North Africa since the epipaleolithic led to the formation of two very different biotopes in which different balanced polymorphisms occur. A very severe malaria, for example, is present in the humid equatorial forest, and its spread is associated with a rise in the frequency of $\underline{Hb}^S$. However, the extent of the dry season in the equatorial steppe has modified the epidemiology of malaria. Accordingly, there is less advantage conferred by the Hb AS phenotype on populations residing in the steppe and savanna than elsewhere, and in the former areas other hemoglobinopathies tend to prevail.

Lefèvre-Witier explains the current distribution of hemoglobin defects and G-6PD deficiencies in North Africa through a complex interplay of aridity-influenced selective vectors, population migrations and population-specific mating patterns. Enhancing the effects of selection are the effects of chronic malnutrition, as well as the consumption of certain foods and more recently, medicines. Lefèvre-Witier sees the old patterns changing but not necessarily ameliorating under the process of urbanization. Emigration from rural communities to the cities has enhanced genetic exchanges between groups, and has also led to founder effects, both of which could reduce the risks for hemoglobinopathy. However, in the humid tropical forest endemic malaria has maintained a reservoir of heterozygous individuals with steady concomitant risks of lethal hemoglobin disease.

The papers in this section testify that environmental risk to disease is not a single-factor phenomenon. Even in the single instance in which habitat did have an extremely strong role in disease occurrence (the North African hemoglobinopathies) sociocultural effects (e.g. inbreeding) and their own specific risks could not be ignored. On the other hand, the other specialized environment examined in this section, namely altitude, did not constitute a direct risk factor for morbidity or mortality of populations. Certain disease occurrences in recently contacted South American Indians also do not follow expectations. The role that environment plays in the onset of diseases, chronic, infectious and genetic, clearly is a complex one. Unequivocally albeit implicitly the population based studies in this section and the two concerned with demographic change and nutrition proclaim the need for more concentration on sociocultural variables in any genetic-epidemiologic investigation. Sociocultural variables may constitute direct population specific risk factors for disease. Accordingly, less emphasis on identification and assessment of physical environmental factors may be warranted, for these appear to have only secondary consequences for human health. The best approach is likely synthetic, combining biomedical and biocultural investigative techniques in the search to understand the onset of disease and disease responses of human groups (Johnston and Low, 1984).

LITERATURE CITED

Baker PT (ed) (1978). "The Biology of High-Altitude Peoples." Cambridge: Cambridge University Press.
Chance HA (1968). Implications of stress: Strategies of developmental change in the north. Arch Enviro Hlth 17:571.
Damon A (ed) (1975). "Physiological Anthropology." New York: Oxford University Press.
Goldstein MC, Tsarong P, Beall CM (1983). High altitude hypoxia, culture and human fecundity/ fertility: A comparative study. Am Anthropologist 85:28.
Greene LS (1980). Factors affecting nutritional status, physical growth, and neurological development: Final comments. In Greene LS, Johnston FE (eds): "Social and Biological Predictors of Nutritional Status, Physical Growth, and Neurological Development." New York: Academic Press, p 311.
Johnston SE, Low SM (1984). Biomedical anthropology: An emerging synthesis in anthropology. Yearbook of Phys Anthrop 25:215.
Savishinsky JS (1974). "The Trail of the Hare. Life and Stress in an Artic Community." New York: Gordon Branch, Science Publishers.
Scheder JC (1983). Chronic disease and disorders of adaptation in migrant and modernizing populations. Am J Phys Anthrop 60:250.
Scheder JC (1981). Diabetes and Stress among Mexican-American Migrants. Ph.D. Thesis, University of Wisconsin-Madison.
Sterling P, Eyer J (1981). Biological basis of stress-related mortality. Soc. Sci. Med. 15E:3.
Wadsworth G (1984). "The Diet and Health of Isolated Populations." Boca Raton: CRC Press.

Diseases of Complex Etiology in Small Populations:
Ethnic Differences and Research Approaches, pages 255–281

Chapter 11

NUTRITION AND BIOLOGICAL FITNESS

J.D. Haas[1] and L.P. Greksa[2]

[1]Division of Nutritional Sciences, Cornell University, Ithaca, New York and [2]Department of Anthropology, Case Western Reserve University, Cleveland, Ohio

INTRODUCTION

This paper examines the relationship between nutrition and biological fitness and demonstrates the importance of considering nutrition in all studies of human populations, including epidemiological ones. Our discussion of nutrition will focus primarily, although not exclusively, on energy reserves as reflected in body composition. The term biological fitness is often used in human population adaptation studies but is frequently used in subtly different ways and may not be a familiar concept to everyone. Therefore, we will first describe what we mean by biological fitness.

We conceive of biological fitness as a multifactorial measure of individual adaptation within a specific environment and at one point in time. Biological fitness thus provides a measure of biological well-being within a specific environmental context or, in a sense, a measure of the biological "quality" of life. Such assessments are, of course, often central to epidemiological investigations. It should be noted that biological fitness, as defined here, can be considered indicative of future evolutionary success only if one assumes a constant environment, an unlikely event in the groups currently studied by anthropologists.

Biological fitness may be assessed through

evaluation of a number of interrelated parameters, or domains, including physical fitness, mortality, fertility, health, growth and development and nutrition (Mazess 1975). In fact, biological fitness is ideally assessed by measurements of as many domains as possible, with the only limitation being that individual variation within that domain has functional consequences. Only such variation will have an impact on overall biological well-being. The reason for multiple measures is, of course, because humans live in multi-stress environments and evaluation of overall well-being, or the ability to cope with the total environment, requires consideration of numerous domains. It is these various domains as they relate to health that makes them relevant to epidemiological investigations. An anthropological approach to the effects of nutritional variation on functional performance may provide insights to disease causality and environmental health that has heretofore been lacking (Haas and Harrison, 1977).

The rationale for focusing on nutrition and biological fitness is that nutrition, besides being an indicator of biological fitness, is also an environmental factor which affects individual variation in functional capacity in most domains of biological fitness. Nutritional variation can thus have broad consequences for the biological fitness of individuals. In this sense, nutrition can be viewed as a risk factor which affects biological fitness both directly and indirectly through other domains. The indirect consequences may be very complex, although our ability to comprehend them is limited. For example, protein-energy malnutrition (PEM) can cause a decrease in physical working capacity, which may result in a decreased capacity to produce nutrient resources, which may affect nutritional status, health, and so on. Nutrition is especially interesting as a determinant of biological fitness because, in many cases, functional capacity is affected, although in different ways, by both an excess and deficit in nutrient consumption. Thus, the total spectrum of nutritional variability can have consequences for biological fitness.

Because of its wide ranging biological impact,

nutritional variability is likely to be an important factor in all epidemiological investigations. Even if nutrition is not a direct intervening variable it may very well have an indirect effect through another domain. This paper will review the effects of nutritional variability, particularly in energy reserves, on biological fitness, focusing on the better documented and more relevant cases.

NUTRITION, NUTRITIONAL STATUS AND BODY COMPOSITION

Nutrition

The concept of nutritional risk factors associated with illness, biological fitness and general dysfunction is not new. The health effects of acute food shortages due to famine have been documented for centuries (Keys et al., 1950). Specific nutrient deficiency diseases have been recognized as such for hundreds of years even if the specific causal sequences were not understood until recently. Current confusion over the role of nutritional variation on health and biological function relates to the definition of malnutrition one uses and methods used to diagnose malnutrition in individuals and groups.

Malnutrition, in its most general sense, refers to deviation from meeting the nutrient demands for optimal physiological function. This includes both over and under consumption of many nutrients. There are over 40 nutrients and their multiple combinations that make up one's definition of nutrition. Thus, there is a tremendous number of potential situations in which malnutrition could be defined. It is not the purpose of this review to cover all of these potential nutritional deficiencies and excesses as they affect biological fitness. Rather, we will focus on several indicators of nutritional status that relate to one aspect of nutrition, food energy. This is not to suggest that other nutrients are unimportant. However, since energy intake reflects the overall quantity of food ingested, it also often reflects the quantity of specific nutrients as well. This is especially true for cases of specific nutrient deficiencies, such as those related to an insufficient consumption of protein or of the B-vitamins, which generally occur under conditions of insufficient food intake. Hence, many specific types of malnutrition occur under generalized conditions of negative energy balance. Likewise, the condition of positive energy balance due to overconsumption is often related to ingestion of energy-dense foods, usually associated with a high proportion of fats and refined carbohydrates.

While monitoring energy intake may not result in the specificity one desires for certain epidemiological investigations of diet and disease, it does provide a relatively good proxy for many macronutrients such as fats and protein that have been implicated in the etiology of certain broad classes of diseases. In addition, the extremes of energy balance alone have been shown to be related to reduced biological fitness in populations living under many different environmental situations. It is clear, however, that such a general measure of dietary quality as energy intake provides only crude information about the role of diet and nutrition on biological fitness. Nevertheless it is a good starting point for epidemiological studies given the relative ease with which energy intake can be estimated and disturbed energy balance can be assessed.

Nutritional Status

As McLaren (1976) and Habicht et al. (1979) point out, there is a need to distinguish between nutrition, nutriture and nutritional status. McLaren states that nutrition is "the process by which the organism uses food, or anything normally ingested through digestion, absorption, transport, storage, metabolism and elimination for purposes of maintenance of life, growth, normal functioning of organs and the production of energy." Thus nutrition is essential for the maintenance of all of the individual adaptive domains described by Mazess (1975). McLaren further notes that nutriture is "the state resulting from the balance between supply of nutrition on one hand and the expenditure of the organism on the other." The direct measurement of this balance is difficult if not impossible and we must rely on the measurement of specific indicators of nutritional status to evaluate the nutriture of an individual. Indicators of nutritional status vary widely depending on the specific aspect of nutrition to be assessed and the level of technological sophistication available for measurement. There are numerous methods employed by clinicians, researchers and laymen to evaluate one of several aspects of energy balance in humans. All of these indicators of energy nutritional status rely on an evaluation of one or more of the 3 components of the energy balance equation:

Energy ingested = Energy expended + Energy stored.

Energy ingested can be estimated through the application of various methods designed to quantify food intake. These include the 24 hour dietary recall, food record or diary, food weighing and diet history. All methods have inherent sources of systematic and random measurement error which detract from their use in research on individual energy balance (Sanjur, 1982). For example, the most widely used method is the 24 hour dietary recall which is estimated to have an interindividual interdaily reliability, as indicated by test-retest correlations, that varies around 0.60 (Lechtig et al., 1976). Other more time consuming methods do not fare much better.

In addition to the random error inherent in the 24 hour recall, it is also subject to systematic bias. In the U.S. there is a tendency for individuals whose energy intakes fall at the upper end of the distribution to underreport the quantity of food ingested, while those at the lower end of the distribution tend to overestimate intake (Gersovitz et al., 1978; Linusson et al., 1974). Since it is the extremes of the distribution of food consumption, and by inference body weight, that are of the most interest to the epidemiology of many chronic diseases, this type of bias renders the dietary recall virtually useless for those studies which propose to examine the link between diet and disease. Finally, if there is a degree of variation in metabolic efficiency in the utilization of food energy, and this variation is greatest at the extremes of under and over consumption

(Sukhatme and Margen, 1982), then food consumption, even when accurately measured, may be inappropriate for epidemiological and clinical studies.

Energy expenditure has been estimated by many different methods. These range from the pioneering direct calorimetry of Atwater and Benedict (1903) and its recent modifications (Webb et al., 1980), through indirect calorimetry (Durnin and Passmore, 1967), and through heart rate monitoring and time motion studies (Bradfield, 1971). While the direct and indirect calorimetry are more reliable than dietary intake, these methods are too invasive and time consuming to be used in large scale epidemiology surveys.

Body Composition

Due to the limitations in estimating intake and expenditure, estimates of energy storage are by far the most practical and commonly used methods for inferring energy balance in humans. The rationale for this class of nutritional status indicators is that interindividual imbalance between energy intake and expenditure is reflected in morphological variation for those body components that reflect stored energy. Energy stores can be broadly defined as any tissue component of the body. Therefore, caloric deficit during growth will result in reduced size of a child, and the degree of undernutrition among children can be inferred by the relative size rankings of these children in terms of stature and weight. These indicators, however, are not specific to energy deficiency and should be used with some caution when direct effects of energy deficiency are being studied.

Energy intake above expenditure is best reflected by changes in the body mass and more specifically in the fat component of the total body composition. Also, growing children and adults who are undernourished with respect to energy show marked changes in body composition that can be used as indicators of nutritional status. Therefore, the preferred indicators of deficient or excessive energy intake (relative to expenditure) seem to be measurements of body mass and body composition. They include such nonspecific anthropometric indicators as body weight and circumferences to more sophisticated indicators of the dimensions of specific body components such as fat and lean tissue.

Body weight as a composite indicator of total body mass is the most widely used anthropometric indicator of nutritional status. Its application to all age groups and throughout the range of undernutrition to overnutrition have been well documented. Weight is usually expressed relative to standards for healthy individuals of the same age as is the case with children, or for individuals of the same height as is the case throughout the life cycle.

Weight relative to height has been shown to be the most acceptable expression of weight for most situations in epidemiological surveys (Flegal, 1982). Hence overweight or underweight is expressed by deviation from a normal pattern for such indices as:

height/weight
weight/height^2 (body mass or Quetelet index)
weight/height$^{1/3}$ (ponderal index)
weight^n/height (Benn index) and
Metropoliton Life Insurance standard weight.

Deviation can be expressed as a percent of a specific population mean, as a percentile placement, or as a standardized Z-score. In addition, the reference standard could be the mean or median value for the population being studied, or for another population of known health and demographic parameters. While all of these indices of weight corrected for height have similar properties, several studies suggest that the body mass index and the Metropolitan Life standard weight may be the most appropriate for epidemiological surveys that focus on obesity as a risk factor (Flegal, 1982; Keys et al., 1972; Khosla and Lowe, 1967; Florey, 1970; Billewicz et al., 1962). However, it is important to note that the best indicator for males may not be the best one for females and that racial factors may also affect the choice of the best index for epidemiological studies of obesity and overweight (Flegal, 1982).

For underweight there is relatively little information available to validate the different indices. Several studies in developing countries have demonstrated the efficiency of reduced body weight relative to other anthropometric measures to predict prospective risk of death in children (Chen et al., 1980; Cogill, 1982; Jahari, 1982; Gomez et al., 1956; Kielman and McCord, 1978). For children, standards of weight for a given height or age in the U.S. population (NCHS, 1977) are widely used around the world to identify acute malnutrition which results in weight loss. Likewise these reference standards have been used to identify obese children with excess weight for given height, either when age is considered as a conditional factor or the weight-for-height references are used independent of age (Neumann, 1979).

Measurements of body girth at specific locations have been used as an alternative to body weight in epidemiological and clinical studies. The relationship between weight and certain circumferences is fairly strong when they both serve as indicators of body mass. The most commonly used measure of girth is the circumference of the upper arm. This measurement reflects the dynamic relationship between brachial muscle and fat which is presumed to be indicative of the general status of these two soft tissue components in the total body. Mid upper arm circumference has become a very popular screening device for protein-energy malnutrition in young children, especially under conditions where the measurement of body weight is impractical (Delgado et al., 1983; McDowell and King, 1982; Sommer and Lowenstein, 1975; Trowbridge and Staehling, 1980; Jelliffe, 1966). Other circumferences that have been used for identifying the malnourished have included the calf and thigh measurements, which have similar properties to the mid upper arm, and the waist and chest measurements which are primarily used as indicators of overweight. Bray et al. (1978) have shown that changes in weight, and presumably fat, are better reflected by changes in waist circumference than by more direct measures of adiposity such as skinfold.

More direct measures of energy excess have employed techniques which measure the fat component of the soft tissue, and by subtraction the muscle or lean component can be estimated. Measurements of the thickness of the subcutaneous fat layer, as reflected in the skinfold or fatfold thickness are the most practical methods by which body fat can be estimated. Skinfolds have been used to quantify the amount of body fat at specific sites around the body as well as to provide inference to the distribution of fat across the body. The utility of skinfolds is widely accepted but often used without recognition of some major problems in its determination and interpretation (Himes, 1980; Haas and Flegal, 1981). The triceps skinfold combined with measurement of mid upper arm circumference has been used to compute the fat and lean components of the arm and thus provide a more specific indication of energy stores in the body (Jelliffe, 1966; Frisancho, 1981).

More sophisticated, time consuming and invasive methods of determining body fat have been widely used in clinical and human biology research. These include estimates of total body fat by densitometry, and lean body mass by measuring body water and body potassium (Grande and Keys, 1980; Malina, 1980). These techniques have served as a means of validating the less invasive methods described above. However, their utility in epidemiological research is limited to work on relatively small samples of individuals who have access to the sophisticated laboratory facilities needed for these assessments.

It should be noted that all measures of body composition which reflect energy deficit or excess are indirect methods with varying degrees of reliability and accuracy in indicating the true composition of the body. A major problem arises in using most of the anthropometric indicators in that they do not permit a very accurate distinction between obesity tissue and overweight or between the components of tissue wasting or growth failure associated with underweight. A judicious use of multiple indicators might prove to be a more satisfactory application of nutritional anthropometry to distinguish between the various components of body composition.

NUTRITIONAL STATUS AND ITS RELATION TO INDICATORS OF BIOLOGICAL FITNESS

While considerable evidence exists in the literature to relate nutritional stutus to performance in many of the functional domains described by Mazess (1975), this review will deal only briefly with some of these domains. The domains of mortality, morbidity and fertility will be presented to demonstrate some efforts to validate specific indicators of nutritional status as well as to point out the role that nutrition may have played in some of the more commonly used definitions of biological fitness. However, if we expand the definition of fitness to areas other than health and recognize that the consequences of protein-energy malnutrition may be reflected in functional domains other than those related directly to reproduction and survival, the research on the effects of malnutrition on physical performance becomes an important area to review. Therefore, more attention will be given to the relationship between nutritional status and physical work capacity as an example of potentially important topics for future research.

Mortality

Population mortality statistics reflect the overall severity of disease load, as well as providing an indication of the evolutionary forces which may operate in that population. The general fitness of a population can be reflected in various aspects of mortality. The role that nutritional variation plays in mortality risk has served as a basis for evaluating various indicators of undernutrition and overnutrition with respect to maintaining energy balance. Childhood malnutrition, due primarily to protein and energy deficiencies, are reflected in reduced growth. Indicators of these growth parameters have been related to prospective risk of death at various phases of the life cycle. The most common example of this research is the analysis of birth weight specific mortality during the neonatal period, which has been analyzed for many populations around the world (Goldstein and Peckham, 1976; Jayant, 1966; Lubchenco et al., 1972; Sansing and Chinnici, 1976; VanValen and

Mellin, 1967). Birth weight is often used as a sensitive but nonspecific indicator of maternal nutritional status during pregnancy (Habicht et al., 1974). The relationship of birth weight to mortality is well known to represent a reversed J-shape curve. Mortality risk is lowest in the birth weight categories between 3,000 and 3,500 grams. The risk progressively increases as weights fall below this level to the point where very small infants at birth have an extremely high risk of dying in the next 28 days. Risk of death also increases at higher birth weights but for reasons that may not necessarily be related to fetal malnutrition.

Studies in preschool children of weight, height and upper arm circumference in relation to prospective risk of death over a one-two year period have been the basis for the validation of anthropometric indicators of nutritional status. Studies in Bangladesh suggest that weight-for-age and height-for-age criteria provide good discrimination between children who survive versus those who die over a 2 year period of demograhic surveillance (Cogill, 1982; Chen et al., 1980). Moreover, these measures proved to be better indicators than weight-for-height or arm circumference. However, slightly different results were observed for a population of preschool children living in Western Java (Jahari, 1982). In this case, height-for-age proved to be less useful than weight-for-age and arm circumference. Population differences in the sensitivity of various indicators of nutritional status to predict mortality risk may be associated with differences in causes of death and age groupings, even within a fairly narrow five year preschool age period.

Analysis of prospective risk of death in adults was the basis for the popular Metropolitan Life Insurance Company (1959) tables of ideal weight commonly used to evaluate obesity and underweight. These tables were developed from actuarial statistics of insured individuals in the United States whose weight and height were available at the time they purchased their insurance policies. Mortality risk clearly increased with weight within specific height categories. Thus, it was possible to identify an optimal range of weight for a given height based on their association with the lowest mortality risk. While the relationship between overweight and high mortality appears logical, the precise reason why overweight or obesity should lead to increased risk of death is not so clear (Mann, 1974; Andres, 1980). The increased risk of death at lower weight is an unexpected phenomenon which has been shown in the Framingham Heart Study to be related to a higher prevalence of smoking related deaths among lighter compared to average weight subjects (Garrison et al., 1983).

Morbidity

Morbidity has been analyzed in a similar fashion as mortality as it relates to underweight, overweight and obesity. The relationship between PEM, as measured by anthropometry, and infection in preschool children is an often stated characteristic of the etiology of disease in developing countries. The general consensus is that malnourished children who are small or light have an increased risk of contracting gastrointestinal and respiratory illness, presumably because of a reduced resistance to disease. Moreover, children who are sick generally have reduced appetites and increased energy requirements which may precipitate malnutrition (Scrimshaw et al., 1968; Martorell, 1980). However, there is some debate regarding the causal relationship between malnutrition and infection given the evidence from Bangladesh that suggest that reduced weights and heights do not increase risk of infection in rural preschool children (Chen et al., 1981).

Overweight in children has been associated with hypertension, especially during adolescence. Moreover, fat patterning as well as thickness of the adipose tissue seems to be important in the identification of children at risk of hypertension (Stallones et al., 1982) and various chronic diseases in adults (Vague, 1956; Damon et al., 1969). In adults obesity and overweight and the pattern of fat distribution have been related to a large number of diseases such as coronary heart disease, hypertension, non-insulin-dependent diabetes mellitus, breast cancer, gout and arthritis (Vague, 1956; Salans, 1979; Rimm and White,

1979). However, many of these relationships are weak and do not suggest any specific causal mechanisms. A recent study of obesity and blood pressure from the Health Examination Survey of the United States (Flegal, 1982) sheds some important light on the use of various indicators of obesity in epidemiological surveys. Flegal found that weight-for-height is a better indicator of body fatness for use in population research than either triceps or subscapular skinfolds, and triceps skinfold is a particularly poor indicator. Also, while weight adjusted for height is a preferred method of expressing overweight, there is very little difference between the various indices described above in regard to their ability to identify hypertensive individuals.

Reproduction

The relationship between nutrition, body composition and fertility is a very complex one. It involves, among other things, the independent effects of malnutrition on fecundity, fetal growth and survival, lactation performance, and postpartum amenorrhea. This topic has been reviewed extensively by Butz and Habicht (1976) and Huss-Ashmore (1980) and will only be discussed briefly here. Much interest in this area has been generated since the provocative work of Frisch and colleagues (Frisch and Revelle, 1970; Frisch, 1975 a,b) which attempts to link body fatness with menstrual dysfunction, menarche, and fecundity. Huss-Ashmore finds little evidence for direct effects of fatness on fecundity. Also, while both overnutrition and undernutrition interfere with reproductive function, it is only at the extremes of body fat that this relationship is reasonably strong.

There is good evidence of effects of maternal malnutrition during pregnancy on fetal growth and survivorship (Stein and Susser, 1975; 1976; Stein et al., 1978). However, much of the literature on nutritional effects on fecundity and fertility are confounded by lactation. Maternal malnutrition may affect lactation performance following a birth, but maternal malnutrition is also influenced by the duration and extent of lactation. What is clear from much of this research is that, as in the case of the research on mortality and morbidity, very few causal links have been established between overnutrition or undernutrition and reduced reproductive performance. It appears more logical that the indicators of nutritional status commonly employed in these studies reflect a general state of dysfunction which is not specific to malnutrition.

Work Capacity

The final functional area to be discussed is work capacity, as evaluated by cardiorespiratory endurance. The best overall index of cardiorespiratory endurance is generally considered to be aerobic power, or $\dot{V}O_2$ max, the maximum amount of oxygen which can be utilized by the body's muscles during maximal exercise involving large muscle groups (Buskirk and Taylor, 1957). $\dot{V}O_2max$ is most often expressed in ml/kg/min in order to standardize for differences in body size.

Measurements of cardiorespiratory endurance provide particularly useful indices of biological fitness since the cardiorespiratory system is an important determinant of both overall health and an individual's ability to perform work (Astrand and Rodahl, 1977). An additional practical advantage is that biological fitness at one point in time and within a specific environmental context can be accurately quantified by measurement of $\dot{V}O_2max$. In addition, $\dot{V}O_2max$ tends to be reasonably responsive to environmental change and therefore alterations in biological fitness over time or due to a change in environmental context can be quantified. In fact, of all the available indices of biological fitness, $\dot{V}O_2max$ and related measures probably provide the greatest potential for evaluating the effect of environmental stress on the biological fitness of individuals. For example, the effect of altitude on $\dot{V}O_2max$ can be evaluated by testing the same person at various altitudes while the effect of altitude on an index such as fertility must be evaluated by comparing different groups of women residing at various altitudes.

There are, of course, also disadvantages to the use of measures of cardiorespiratory endurance as indices of biological fitness. The same characteristic which makes the cardiorespiratory system a useful index of biological fitness, its central importance to optimal body functioning, also limits its usefulness. This is because, not unexpectedly, such an important biological system is affected by a number of diverse behavioral, environmental and biological factors (Astrand and Rodahl, 1977). The focus of this discussion, nutritional status and body composition, is only one of these factors. The practical consequence is that it is often difficult to determine the effect of variation in one specific parameter on biological fitness, except under extreme conditions.

As noted earlier, our discussion of the effect of nutritional variation on biological fitness, as measured by $\dot{V}O_2$max, will focus on energy reserves. Also, given the epidemiological focus of this volume our examples are drawn primarily from studies with a population approach, rather than from the numerous purely laboratory studies of various aspects of the effect of nutritional variability on work capacity (e.g. Buskirk and Taylor, 1957; Keys et al., 1950; Welch et al, 1958). Also, for the reasons just described, the effect of variation in energy reserves will be reviewed by focusing on the extremes of energy balance, obesity and protein-energy malnutrition (PEM).

We will begin by reviewing the effect of positive energy balance, or obesity, on $\dot{V}O_2$max (ml/kg/min). The negative effect of obesity on $\dot{V}O_2$max (ml/kg/min) is well documented (Dempsey, 1974). Body fat is equivalent to an excess load which must be transported during any activity requiring body movement. Increased body fatness, therefore, produces a decrease in $\dot{V}O_2$max (ml/kg/min) and an increase in the energetic cost of many types of submaximal work. Due to both of these trends, increased body fatness also results in an increase during submaximal work in relative work intensity, or the ratio of submaximal to maximal $\dot{V}O_2$. This relationship is extremely important since the physiological strain associated with submaximal work is positively related to its relative work intensity.

Thus, obese individuals undergo greater physiological strain than lean individuals during the performance of equivalent tasks (Buskirk, 1974).

The relationship between obesity and work capacity will be illustrated with exercise data collected on American Samoan males residing on Tutuila, the principal island of American Samoa. These data were collected as part of a Pennsylvania State University project designed to evaluate the biological effects of modernization in Samoans. American Samoans are ideal for our purposes since they are currently among the fattest peoples in the world (Bindon, 1981). For example, adult American Samoans are approximately the same stature as U.S. adults but their median triceps skinfolds are two or more times greater than in U.S. adults (Greksa, n.d.). This comparison is especially striking when it is remembered that the U.S. population is itself noted for a high prevalence of obesity.

The data to be considered here consist of the physiological responses to submaximal and maximal exercise of 34 Samoan males between the ages of 18 and 30 years (Greska and Baker, 1982). Body fatness was evaluated with the sum of 6 skinfolds: triceps, subscapular, midaxillary, suprailiac, forearm and medial calf. Skinfold frequency distributions tend to be right skewed and therefore must be normalized prior to statistical analysis (Edwards et al., 1955). Normally a logarithmic transformation is appropriate. The excessive fatness of American Samoans, however, results in a skinfold frequency distribution which is less skewed than in most populations. As a result, the most appropriate transformation, and the one which will be used in the following analyses, is a square root (Greksa, n.d.).

Mean aerobic power ($\dot{V}O_2max$) in this sample was, not unexpectedly, very low, or only 38.9 ml/kg/min. The low levels of physical fitness in this sample can be emphasized by noting that mean $\dot{V}O_2max$ in American Samoans is even less than found among Easter Islanders (Ekblom and Gjessing, 1968), a Polynesian population cited for its extremely low level of physical fitness.

The relationship between $\dot{V}O_2max$ (ml/kg/min) and the transformed sum of 6 skinfolds is shown in Figure 1. There is a highly significant ($p<.001$) negative relationship between these variables, with a correlation coefficient of -0.70. In other words, almost 50% of the variation in $\dot{V}O_2max$ in this sample is associated with variation in body fatness. The relationship between body fatness and relative work intensity was also evaluated. This relationship is weaker than that between $\dot{V}O_2max$ and body fatness but is nevertheless statistically significant ($r = 0.40$; $p<.05$). Thus, as expected, increasing fatness is associated with a decrease in $\dot{V}O_2max$ and an increase in the physiological strain of submaximal work, both of which decrease biological fitness.

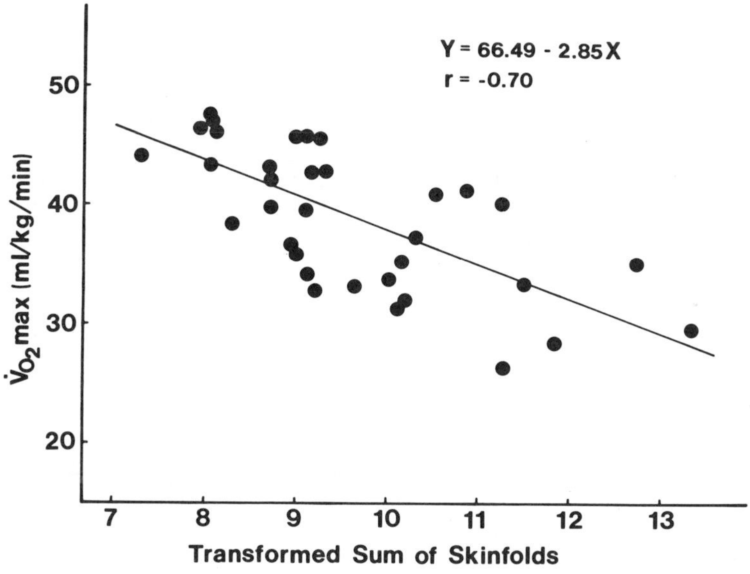

Figure 1. Relationship between $\dot{V}O_2max$ (ml/kg/min) and body fatness in Samoan males.

The opposite end of the energy balance spectrum, or PEM, is also associated with a decrease in work capacity (Consolazio et al., 1967; Keys et al., 1950). For example, in a series of classic experiments with human volunteers. Keys and colleagues (1950) found a rapid decrease in $\dot{V}O_2max$ following weight losses of 10 to 16% of normal body weight. The biosocial implications of this relationship may be extremely important. Undernutrition tends to be widespread in those parts of the world where human power plays a significant role in the performance of essential tasks, including the acquisition of food resources. In such cases, a decrease in work capacity may result in a decrease in productivity (FAO, 1962). Such a relationship obviously has the potential of developing into a positive feedback system affecting entire families, with the level of malnutrition becoming increasingly severe.

The available data on the relationships between nutrition, work capacity and productivity are extensively summarized by Spurr (1983). We will illustrate these relationships with selected findings from a series of elegant studies conducted by Spurr and colleagues in a rural Colombian population. The first study from this project demonstrates the relationship between varying levels of protein-energy malnutrition and work capacity (Barac-Nieto et al., 1978). Adult males were classified as being severely (N=18), intermediately (N=20), or mildly (N=11) malnourished on the basis of weight-for-height, serum albumin and the creatine/height index. Data on a group of nutritionally normal laborers (N=99) from the same area of Colombia were also presented. Mean $\dot{V}O_2max$ for each nutritional category is presented in Figure 2. As can be seen, there is a rapid and highly significant ($p<.001$) decrease in $\dot{V}O_2max$ as nutritional status decreases from mild to severe PEM, with the greatest difference being between severely and intermediately malnourished men. In addition, $\dot{V}O_2max$ in the normal control group is significantly greater than in the mildly malnourished group (1-tail t-test; $p<.01$). There were other differences between these latter two groups, such as activity level, which also affect work capacity. Nevertheless, this finding suggests that even mild malnutrition may result in a decreased $\dot{V}O_2max$.

Additional comparisons between these groups indicated that submaximal work performance was also related to energy reserves (Spurr et al., 1979). For example, predicted heart rate at a constant work load consistently increased with decreasing nutritional status. Heart rate did not differ significantly between the normal controls and the mildly malnourished group but did differ significantly

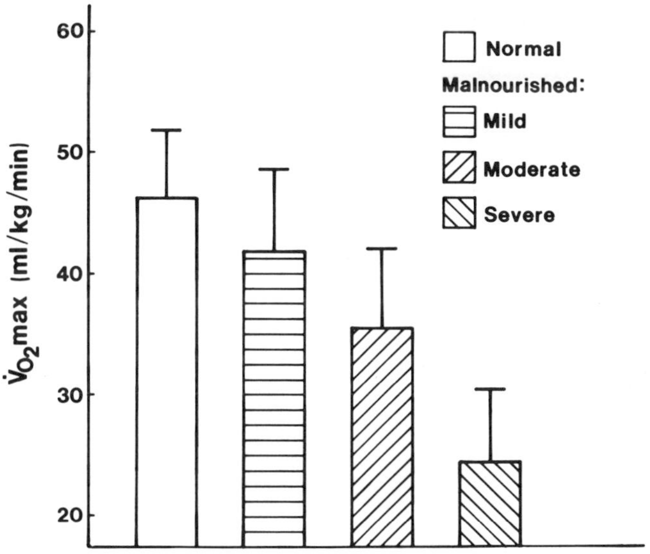

Figure 2. Relationship between $\dot{V}O_2$max (ml/kg/min) and nutritional status in Colombian males (adapted from Barac-Nieto et al., 1978).

between the three malnourished groups ($p<.001$). This finding was due primarily, of course, to the positive relationship between energy reserves and $\dot{V}O_2$max, so that relative work intensity increased with decreasing nutritional status. However, it was also partially due to differences in the relationship between heart rate and work load in the severely malnourished group. Thus, when heart rate was predicted at a constant relative work intensity, it was significantly higher in the severely malnourished group ($p<.01$) than in the remaining groups.

These studies indicate a decrease in both submaximal and maximal work capacity, and thus biological fitness, with decreasing energy reserves. Spurr and colleagues investigated the possible effect of this relationship on productivity by studying men working in the sugar cane industry. The first study involved 46 sugar cane cutters (Spurr et al., 1977a). Sugar cane cutting is continuous and strenuous work. Productivity in the cutters was significantly related to several anthropometric measures of nutritional status, including stature, weight, and fat-free body weight ($p<.01$). In addition, productivity was moderately correlated ($r=0.34$; $p<.05$) to $\dot{V}O_2max$ (ml/kg/min). A second study of sugar cane loaders provided somewhat less consistent results (Spurr et al., 1977b). Loading is intermittent work, since men must await the availability of wagons, and is less strenuous than cutting. In this case, productivity was significantly related to body fatness ($r=-0.38$; $p<.05$) but was unrelated to body size and to $\dot{V}O_2max$, although the relationship approached significance in the latter case.

Studies such as these indicate that variation in productivity is to some extent related to variation in physical fitness and nutritional status. Much more research is needed in this important field, however. For example, are these relationships valid for a wide range of occupations or do they only apply to specialized occupations, such as cane cutting? The weaker relationship between $\dot{V}O_2max$ and productivity in cane loaders, whose occupation is less strenuous and less dependent on aerobic mechanisms than cane cutting, tends to support the latter hypothesis. Also, even if a wide range of occupations are affected, does the variation in productivity which is related to variation in $\dot{V}O_2max$ result in real interfamilial differences in resource acquisition? Finally, what effect would energy supplementation have on $\dot{V}O_2max$ and thus productivity? Studies to-date have been largely inconclusive, finding no increase in productivity with supplementation (Wolgemuth et al., 1983). However, by all indications, the workers in these studies were not greatly, if at all malnourished. Supplementation in malnourished individuals, given the relationships noted earlier, might have a significant positive impact on work capacity and, thus, biological fitness. Whether this would also result in an increase in productivity would, however, depend on the strength of the relationship between work capacity and productivity in their respective occupations.

CONCLUSIONS

This review of the relationship between nutrition and biological fitness is limited by our definitions of nutrition and fitness. Nutrition is defined primarily in terms of food energy intake and nutritional status is defined in terms of indicators of energy balance. Biological fitness is defined in terms of functional categories associated with a specific time in the individuals life cycle and specific environmental conditions. Due to the lack of specificity of various indicators of energy nutritional status employed in the studies reviewed here, it is impossible to identify causal relationships between nutrition and fitness.

The majority of the evidence suggest that reduced biological fitness is best observed at the extremes of energy imbalance. The evaluation of the relationship between nutrition and function among those in the normal range of energy balance is hampered by reduced specificity of indicators of nutritional status as well as possibility for a different set of causal mechanisms that link nutrition to function in this segment of the population.

Many of the relationships between the state of energy balance and specific functional domains used to define fitness must be viewed with caution. It would be dangerous to generalize these relationships to populations whose dietary quality may vary with energy intake and whose evaluation of function or dysfunction may be affected by nonnutritional factors specific to the environment of that population. However, the consistent trend of a statistical link between nutritional status and biological function suggests that indicators of energy imbalance may serve as significant risk factors for reduced biological fitness in many human populations.

LITERATURE CITED

Astrand PO, Rodahl K (1977). "Textbook of Work Physiology." 2nd ed. New York:McGraw-Hill.
Andres R (1980). Effect of obesity on total mortality. Int J Obesity 4:381.
Atwater WO, Benedict FG (1903). Experiments on the metabolism of matter and energy in the human body. U.S.D.A., Office of Experimental Station, Bulletin No. 136.
Barac-Nieto M, Spurr GB, Maksud MG, Lotero H (1978). Aerobic work capacity in chronically undernourished adult males. J Appl Physiol 44:209.
Billewicz WZ, Kemsley WFF, Thomson AM (1962). Indices of adiposity. Brit J Prev Soc Med 16:183.
Bindon J (1981). Genetic and environmental influences on the morphology of Samoan adults. Ph.D. Dissertation, Penn. State Univ., Univ. Park, Pa.
Bradfield RB (1971). A technique for determination of usual daily energy expenditure in the field. Am J Clin Nutr 24:1148.
Bray G, Greenway FL, Molitch ME, Dahms WT, Atkinson RL, Hamilton K (1978). Use of anthropometric measures to assess weight loss. Am J Clin Nutr 31:769.
Buskirk ER (1974). Obesity: A brief overview with emphasis on exercise. Fed Proc 33:1948.
Buskirk ER, Taylor HL (1957). Maximal oxygen uptake and its relation to body composition, with special reference to chronic physical activity and obesity. J Appl Physiol 11:72.
Butz WP, Habicht JP (1976). The effects of nutrition and health on fertility: Hypotheses, evidence, and interventions. In Ridker RG (ed): "Population and Development: The Search for Selective Intervention," Baltimore: John Hopkins Univ. Press, p 210.
Chen LC, Chowhurry AKMA, Huffman SL (1980). Anthropometric assessment of energy-protein malnutrition and subsequent risk of mortality among preschool age children. Am J Clin Nutr 33:1836.
Chen LC, Hug E, Huffman SL (1981). A prospective study of the risk of diarrheal diseases according to the nutritional status of children. Am J Epidem 114:284.
Cogill B (1982). Ranking anthropometric indicators using mortality in rural Bangledesh children. M.S.

Thesis, Cornell University, Ithaca, New York.
Consolazio CF, Nelson RA, Johnson HL, Matousch LO, Krzywicki HJ, Issac GJ (1967). Metabolic aspects of acute starvation in normal humans: performance and cardiovascular evaluation. Am J Clin Nutr 20:684.
Damon A, Damon ST, Harpending HD, Kannel WB (1969). Predicting coronary heart disease from body measurement of Framingham males. J Chronic Dis 21: 781.
Delgado HL, Valverde V, Klein RE (1983). Analysis critico de la validez del brazo como indicador del estado nutricional proteineco-energetico en ninos preescolares. Arch Latinamer Nutr 33:170.
Dempsey JA (1974). Exercise and obesity. In Ryan AJ, Allman PL (eds): "Sports Medicine," New York: Academic Press, p 557.
Durnin JVGA, Passmore R (1967). "Energy, Work and Leisure." London: Williams Heineman.
Edwards DAW, Hammond WH, Tanner JM, Whitehouse RH (1955). Design and accuracy of calipers for measuring subcutaneous fat thickness. Br J Nutr 9:133.
Ekblom B, Gjessing E (1968). Maximal oxygen uptake of the Easter Island population. J Appl Physiol 25:124.
FOA (1962). Relation between diet and working capacity. In "Nutrition and Working Efficiency," FFHC Basic Study No. 5, Rome.
Flegal KM (1982). Anthropometric evaluation of obesity in epidemiologic research on risk factors: Blood Pressure and Obesity in the Health Examination Survey. Ph.D. Dissertation, Cornell University, Ithaca, New York.
Florey C (1970). The use and interpretation of ponderal index and other weight-height ratios in epidemiological studies. J Chronic Dis 23:93.
Frisancho AR (1981). New norms of upper limb fat and muscle areas for assessment of nutritional status. Amer J Clin Nutr 34:2540.
Frisch RE (1975a). Demographic implications of the biological determinants of female fecundity. Soc Biol 22:17.
Frisch RE (1975b). Critical weights, a critical body composition, menarche, and the maintenance of menstrual cycles. In Watts ES, Johnson FE, Lasker FW (eds): "Biological Interrelations in Population

Adaptation," The Hague: Mouton, p 319.
Frisch RE, Revelle R (1970). Height and weight at menarche and a hypothesis of critical body weights and adolescent events. Science 169:397.
Garrison RJ, Feinleib M, Castelli WP, McNamara PM (1983). Cigarette smoking as a confounder of the relationship between relative weight and long term mortality in the Framingham heart study. JAMA 249:2199.
Gersovitz M, Madden JP, Smiciklas-Wright H (1978). Validity of the 24-hour dietary recall and seven day record for group comparisons. J Amer Diet Assoc 73:48.
Goldstein H, Peckham C (1976). Birthweight, gestation, neonatal mortality and child development. In Roberts DF, Thomson AM (eds): "The Biology of Human Fetal Growth," London: Taylor & Francis, p 81.
Gomez F, Ramos-Galvin R, Frank S, Cravioto J, Chavez R, Vazquez J (1956). Mortality in second and the third degree malnutrition. J Trop Paediat 2:77.
Grande R, Keys A (1980). Body weight, body composition and calorie status. In Goodhart RS, ME Shils (eds): "Modern Nutrition in Health and Disease," 6th Ed. Philadelphia: Lea and Febiger, p 3.
Greksa LP (n.d.). Some aspects of the triceps skinfold frequency distribution in an obese population. Manuscript.
Greska LP, Baker PT (1982). Aerobic capacity of modernizing Samoan men. Hum Biol 54:777.
Haas JD, Flegal KM (1980). Anthropometric measurements. In Newell GR, Ellison NM (eds): "Nutrition and Cancer: Etiology and Treatment," New York: Raven Press, p 123.
Haas JD, Harrison GG (1977). Nutritional anthropology and biological adaptation. Ann Rev Anthrop 6:69.
Habicht JP, Lechtig A, Yarbrough C, Klein RE (1974). Maternal nutrition, birthweight and infant mortality. In Elliot K, Knight J (eds): "Size of Birth," Ciba Foundation Symposium 27. Amsterdam: Elsevier, p 353.
Habicht JP, Yarbrough C, Martorell R (1979). Anthropometric field methods: Criteria for selection. In Jelliffe DB, Jelliffe EFD (eds): "Nutrition and Growth," New York: Plenum Press, p 365.
Himes JH (1980) Subcutaneous fat thickness as an

indicator of nutritional status. In Greene LS, Johnston FE (eds): "Social and Biological Predictors of Nutritional Status, Physical Growth, and Neurological Development," New York: Academic Press, p 9.

Huss-Ashmore R (1980). Fat and fertility: Demographic implications of differential fat storage. Yearbook Phys Anthrop 23:65.

Jahari AB (1982). Anthropometric measures for use in monitoring risk of death in under five years of age for the nutritional surveillance system in Indonesia. M.S. Thesis, Cornell University, Ithaca, New York.

Jayant K (1966). Birthweight and survival: A hospital survey repeated after 15 years. Ann Hum Genet 29:367.

Jelliffe DB (1966). The assessment of the nutritional status of the Community. Geneva: World Health Organization Monograph No. 53.

Keys A, Fedanza F, Karvonen MJ, Kimura N, Taylor HL (1972). Indices of relative weight and obesity. J Chronic Dis 25:329.

Keys A, Brozek J, Henschel A, Mickelsen O, Taylor HL (1950). "The Biology of Human Starvation." Minneapolis: Univ. of Minn. Press.

Khosla T, Lowe CR (1967). Indices of obesity derived from body weight and height. Brit J Prev Soc Med 21:122.

Kielman AA, McCord C (1978). Weight-for-age as an index of risk of death in children. Lancet ii:1247.

Lechtig A, Yarbrough C, Martorell R, Delgado H, Klein RE (1976). The one-day recall dietary survey: A review of its usefullness to estimate protein and calorie intake. Arch Latinamer Nutr 26:243.

Linusson EEI, Sanjur D, Erickson EC (1974). Validating the 24-hour recall as a dietary survey tool. Diet Latinamer Nutr 24:277.

Lubchenco LO, Searls DT, Brazie JV (1972). Neonatal mortality rate: Relationship to birthweight and gestational age. J Pediat 81:814.

Malina RM (1980) The measurement of body composition. In Johnston FE, Roche AF, Susanne C (eds): "Human Physical Growth and Maturation: Methodologies and Factors," New York: Plenum Press, p 35.

Mann GV (1974). The influence of obesity on health. New Eng J Med 291:178.

Martorell R (1980). Interrelationships between diet, infectious disease, and nutritional status. In Greene LS, Johnston FE (eds): "Social and Biological Predictors of Nutritional Status, Physical Growth, and Neurological Development," New York: Academic Press, p 81.
Mazess RB (1975). Biological adaptation: Aptitudes and acclimatization. In Watts ES, Johnston FE, Lasker GW (eds): "Biosocial Interrelations in Population Adaptation," Hague:Mouton, p 9.
McDowell I, King FS (1982). Interpretation of arm circumference as an indicator of nutritional status. Arch Dis Child 57:292.
McLaren DS (1976). "Nutrition in the Community." New York: Wiley.
Metropolitan Life Insurance Company (1959).Statistical Bulletin 40:1.
Neumann CG (1970). Reference data. In Jelliffe DB, Jelliffe EFP (eds): "Nutrition and Growth," New York: Plenum Press, p 299.
NCHS (1977). NCHS growth curves for children: Birth - 18 years. Vital and Health Statistics, Series 11, No. 165. Hyattsville, Md: U. S. Dept. Health, Education, and Welfare.
Rimm AA, White PL (1979). Obesity: Its risks and hazards. In Bray G (ed): "Obesity in America," Washington: DHEW Publ. (NIH) No. 79-359, p 103.
Salans LB (1979). Natural history of obesity. In Bray G (ed): "Obesity in America," Washington: DHEW Publ. (NIH) No. 79-359, p 69.
Sanjur D (1982). "Social and Cultural Perspectives in Nutrition." Englewoods Cliffs, NJ: Prentice-Hall.
Sansing RC, Chinnici JP (1976). Optimal and discriminating birthweights in human populations. Ann Hum Genet 40:123.
Scrimshaw NS, Taylor CE, Gordon JE (1968). Interactions of nutrition and infection. Geneva: World Health Organization Monograph Series 57.
Sommer A, Lowenstein MS (1975). Nutritional status and mortality: A prospective validation of the QUAC stick. Am J Clin Nutr 28:287.
Spurr GB (1983). Nutritional status and physical work capacity. Yearbook Phys Anthropol 26:1.
Spurr GB, Barac-Nieto M, Maksud MG (1977a). Productivity and maximal oxygen consumption in sugar can cutters. Am J Clin Nutr 30:316.

Spurr GB, Maksud MB, Barac-Nieto M (1977b). Energy expenditure, productivity, and physical work capacity of sugar cane loaders. Am J Clin Nutr 30:1740.

Spurr GB, Barac-Nieto M, Maksud MG (1979). Functional assessment of nutritional status: Heart rate response to submaximal work. Am J Clin Nutr 32:767.

Stallones L, Mueller WH, Christiansen BL (1982). Blood pressure, fatness and fat patterning among USA adolescents from two ethnic groups. Hypertension 4:483.

Stein Z, Susser M (1975). Fertility, fecundity, famine: Food rations in the Dutch famine 1944/5 have a causal relation to fertility and probably to fecundity. Hum Biol 47:131.

Stein Z, Susser M (1976). "Famine and Human Development: The Dutch Hunger Winter of 1944/45." New York: Oxford University Press.

Stein Z, Susser M, Rush Z (1978). Prenatal nutrition and birthweight: Experiments and quasi-experiments in the past decade. J Reprod Med 21:287.

Sukhatme PV, Margen S (1982). Autoregulatory homeostatic nature of energy balance. Am J Clin Nutr 35:355.

Trowbridge FL, Staehling N (1980). Sensitivity and specificity of arm circumference indicators in identifying malnourished children. Am J Clin Nutr 33:687.

Vague J (1956). The degree of masculine differentiation of obesities: A factor determining predisposition to diabetes, atherosclerosis, gout and uric calculous disease. Am J Clin Nutr 4:20.

VanValen L, Mellin G (1967). Selection in natural populations. 7. New York babies (Fetal Life Study). Ann Hum Gen 31:109.

Webb P, Annis JF, Troutman SJ (1980). Energy balance in man measured by direct and indirect calorimetry. Am J Clin Nutr 33:1287.

Welch BE, Reindeau RP, Crisp CE, Isenstein RS (1958). Relationship of maximal oxygen consumption to various components of body composition. J Appl Physio 12:395.

Wolgemuth JC, Latham MC, Hall A, Chester A, Crompton DWT (1983). Worker productivity and the nutritional status of Kenyan road construction laborers. Am J Clin Nut 36:68.

Diseases of Complex Etiology in Small Populations:
Ethnic Differences and Research Approaches, pages 283–299

Chapter 12

GENETIC CONSEQUENCES OF DEMOGRAPHIC CHANGES IN HUMAN POPULATIONS

J. Adams[1] and P.E. Smouse[2]

[1]Division of Biological Sciences, [2]Department of Human Genetics, University of Michigan, Ann Arbor, Michigan

INTRODUCTION

The importance of stable unacculturated populations to studies of human population genetics has long been recognized, but the number of such populations available for further study is dwindling rapidly. Many of the unacculturated populations of 20 years ago have been 'discovered' and can now be considered to be in a state of transition towards the modern world. As this trend continues, attention is beginning to shift toward transitional populations. The changes experienced by such populations are demographic, cultural and environmental. In this paper, we will focus on demographic changes, and will show how changing vital rates may influence the genetic structure of a population, particularly as it relates to genetically mediated disease.

Keyfitz and Flieger (1971) classify present day human populations into three broad categories, on the basis of demographic vital rates. The first category is characterized by high birth and death rates. A consequence of both high birth and death rates is that the intrinsic rate of natural increase (r) is low, with a doubling time on the order of 35 years. These populations are typified by a strongly tapering age pyramid, having a high percentage of individuals in the lower age categories. The second category is characterized by high birth rates but low death rates. As might be expected, these populations experience elevated growth rates, and faster doubling times, on the order of 20 years. The third category is characterized by low birth and death rates. This category includes most Western European and North American populations, as well as those of Japan and Australia, populations for which the industrial revolution has already occurred. The lower birth rates in these populations can often be ascribed to parity-specific fertility limitation (Henry, 1961). The age distribution of modern Sweden, a category III population, shows a much higher proportion of individuals in the older age categories than do populations in either category I or category II.

Keyfitz and Fleiger (1968) have suggested, on the basis of studies in western European populations, that these three categories represent successive stages in the demographic evolution of a population. While the appropriateness of this particular model for non-European populations has been questioned (eg. Teitelbaum, 1975), recent empirical studies have largely supported its wider applicability (cf. Knodel, 1977; Coale, 1983). To investigate the role of demographic evolution on the genetic structure of a population, we consider the demographic changes experienced by the population of Sweden between 1780 and 1965. We present in Figure 1 the birth and death rates and a measure of demographic stability over this period. It can be seen that both birth rates and death rates drop steadily, indicating the transition from a category (stage) I population to a category (stage) III population. During the initial period, 1800 to 1860, birth rates remain high and approximately constant, while mortality rates drop continuously, representing a transition to stage II. From 1860 to the present, mortality rates have continued to drop steadily and birth rates have declined precipitously, indicating a transition to stage III. We also plot the index of demographic stability (Δ), which is the sum of the absolute differences between observed and the predicted stable age-distribution values, expressed as percentages. Note that between 1910 and 1940, this index first rises rapidly and then falls. We will have occasion to refer to this demographic pulse later.

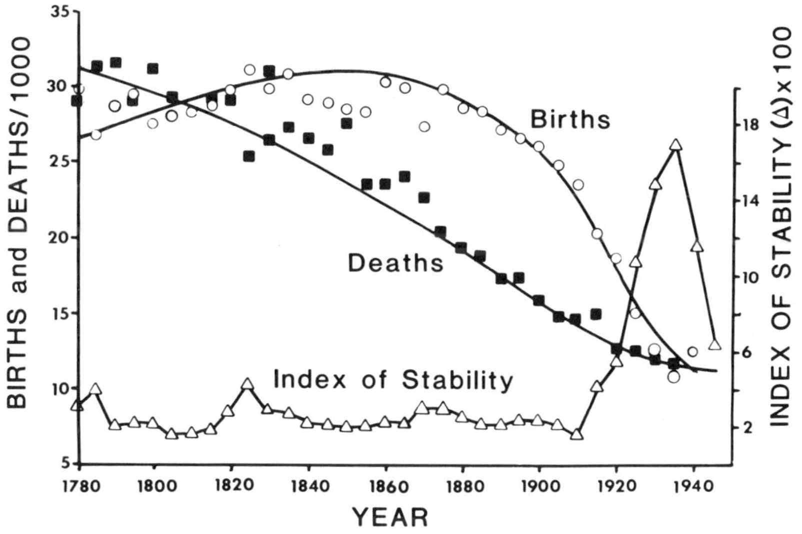

Figure 1. Birth rates, death rates, and the index of demographic stability (Δ) for the population of Sweden from 1780 to 1965. Birth and death rates are standardized on the 1960 U.S. population.

SELECTION IN AGE-STRUCTURED POPULATIONS

It is clear that any measure of relative fitness in human populations must take into account age-specific mortality and fertility rates. A number of procedures for fitness estimation have been proposed in the past, but probably the most widely used and most satisfactory approach utilizes differences in the net rates of reproduction for different genotypes (Charlesworth and Charlesworth, 1973; Charlesworth, 1980). The following approach is modified from Bodmer (1968).

The net reproductive rate of a population (R) is defined as

$$R = \sum_x \ell_x m_x = e^{rT} \qquad (1)$$

where ℓ_x is the probability of survival from birth to age x, m_x is the age-specific birth rate, r is the intrinsic rate of natural increase, and T is the generation interval (Keyfitz, 1968). The fitness (w_i) of genotype i, relative to that (w_j) of genotype j, is conceptually easy to define as

$$w_i / w_j = e^{(r_i T_i - r_j T_j)} \qquad (2)$$

where the subscripts (i) and (j) index the i-th and j-th genotypes, respectively. A satisfactory approximation for small differences in (r) and (T) is given by

$$w_i / w_j \approx 1 + r_i T_i - r_j T_j \approx 1 - R_i - R_j \qquad (3)$$

The selective differential (s_{ij}) is given by

$$s_{ij} = R_i - R_j \qquad (4)$$

Although relative fitness is easy to define and understand in these terms, it is nevertheless very difficult to estimate in practice. A major problem is that accurate age-specific fertility and mortality measures are difficult to calculate for genetic traits with variable age of onset, since individuals who have not yet developed the abnormal phenotype are necessarily included among the 'normal' part of the population. In addition, age-specific fertility rates are almost always defined in terms of female-dominant fertility models, because male-dominant fertility schedules are not readily available. To illustrate, Keyfitz and Flieger (1968) were able to find male-dominant period fertility figures for only seven countries, whereas equivalent female-dominant figures are available from over 400 countries.

Therefore, to calculate relative fitnesses in human populations, a number of simplifying assumptions are necessary. (1) First, we must assume that susceptible individuals have normal vital rates until the abnormal phenotype is manifested. Manifestation may be defined operationally as onset of the disease, hospitalization, or even death, depending on the situation. (2) Second, we assume that the age-specific fertility and mortality rates of individuals who already express the trait are independent of the age of onset. The utility of this assumption is that the net reproductive rate for susceptible individuals (R_S) can be written as

$$R_S = \sum_x \ell_x m_x \psi_x \tag{5}$$

where ℓ_x and m_x are the age-specific vital rates for the normal population and ψ_x is the probability of remaining disease-free until age x. Thus, age-specific fertility and mortality rates from the general population can be used. These vital rates are often available from standard sources such as the 'U.N. Demographic Yearbook' and 'Vital Statistics of the United States', published by the National Center for Health Statistics. (3) Third, we calculate selective coefficients for females only. Selective coefficients for males may be calculated by estimating male-dominant fertility schedules from the average difference in ages between the spouses (cf. Bodmer, 1968). Unfortunately, even this age-differential between spouses is unavailable from the majority of demographic surveys.

CHANGING AGE STRUCTURE AND SELECTIVE COEFFICIENTS

We illustrate the genetic effect of changing age structure with the Swedish demographic data alluded to above. It will be remembered that during the period from 1780 to 1965, the population of Sweden evolved from a stage I population (high birth and death rates) to a stage III population (low birth and death rates). We have calculated selective coefficients, as described above, for three hypothetical disease traits. These disorders were chosen as examples of traits with different age of onset patterns. Trait A is an example of a disorder with an early and minimally variable age of onset; Trait B is an example of a disorder with a medium and more variable age of onset; Trait C is a disorder with a late and highly variable age of onset. The age-specific patterns of onset for the three disorders are presented in Figure 2 as the probabilities of remaining disease-free by age x. In fact, these survival data were taken from the literature on actual diseases. The curve for

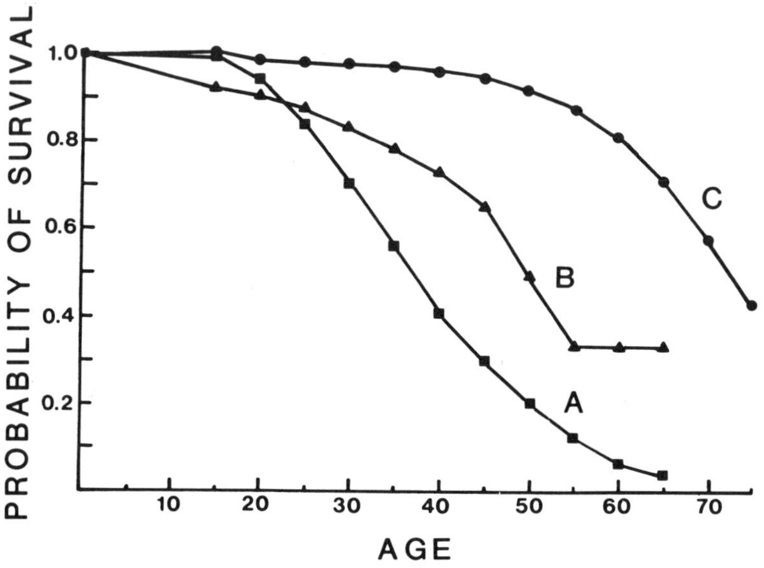

Figure 2. Probability of (disease-free) survival (ψ_x) for three hypothetical disease traits.

trait A is 1 minus the probability of being admitted to a mental institution for schizophrenia by a certain age, and the data are taken from Rosenthal (1966). The curve for trait B is the probability of survival of U.S. females with Marfan's syndrome, and the data are taken from Murdoch et al. (1972). The curve for trait C is the probability of survival of U.S. males and females with maturity-onset diabetes mellitus, and the data are taken from Table 1-26 of the 1978 edition of 'Vital Statistics of the United States' (Anonymous, 1978).

In view of the obvious difficulties in applying contemporary U.S. data to Sweden over this extended period, and in view of the numerous assumptions required, no attempt should be made to extrapolate from the results in Figure 2 to actual selective coefficients for schizophrenia, Marfan's syndrome, and diabetes mellitus. Traits A, B and C should be regarded as hypothetical; our purpose is merely that of illustration. We are concerned here with changing patterns of selective coefficients in general, rather

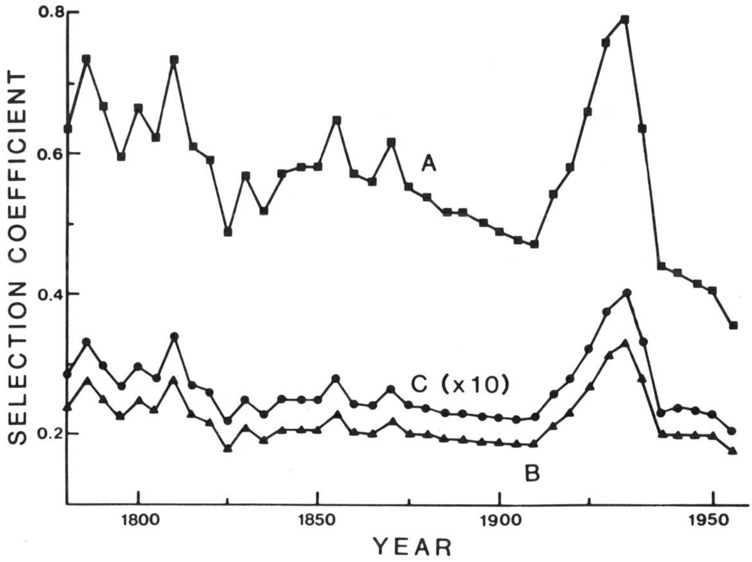

Figure 3. Reconstructed female selective coefficients for the same disease traits as shown in Figure 3 for the population of Sweden between 1780 and 1965. The rates for trait C are multiplied by 10.

than with absolute magnitudes for particular diseases. Figure 3 shows the selective coefficients against Traits A, B, and C that would have obtained over the 1780-1965 period in Sweden.

Between 1780 and 1910, selective coefficients declined steadily for all three traits. This is particularly notable for Trait A, but is also true to a lesser degree for Traits B and C. During that same period, the population evolved demographically from stage I to stage II. The effect of the transition from stage I to stage II on selective coefficients is greatest for traits with an early age of onset, and becomes progressively smaller as age of onset is shifted upwards.

Pre-reproductive mortality rates are decreasing throughout this period, resulting in an increase in the mean age of the population. Reduction in prereproductive mortality, without a concomitant change in fertility rates, would be expected to increase selection intensity for diseases of delayed onset. In actual fact, the intensity of selection is reduced over the period, rather than increased (Figure 3). This decrease is achieved as a result of concomitantly changing patterns of age- specific fertility, manifested as a steady decrease in generation time. The result is that a greater proportion of child-bearing is accomplished at earlier ages, before onset of the disease can take its toll. This result, which is typical of most western European populations, may not apply to other populations. For example, in many Asian and North African populations, there has been an increase in the average age at marriage over the last 30 years (Coale, 1983). Such changes would be expected to alter fertility rates in such a way that selective coefficients would increase over that period, rather than decrease, as in the Swedish example.

Surprisingly, selective coefficients for all these traits show a large but transient increase during the period 1910-1940. The absolute magnitude of this increase is largest for diseases with an earlier age of onset. It should be recalled that it is during this same period that the age-structure of the population becomes unstable (see Figure 1), due to a rapid decline in birth rates. This effect can create serious complications for the human geneticist or epidemiologist who attempts to measure selective coefficients in populations at this stage of demographic evolution. Rapidly rising or rapidly declining selective coefficients, which in another context may say something profound about changing environment, in this context are merely manifestations of a temporary demographic instability.

INDEX OF OPPORTUNITY FOR SELECTION

In the preceding section, we examined the consequences of demographic change on the genetic structure of a population by examining the changes in selective coefficients for three specific phenotypes. An alternative approach is to examine the change in a more general measure, the 'index of opportunity for selection', first defined by Crow (1958). This measure is defined as the square of the coefficient of variation in offspring number

$$I_t = V(w) / w^2 \tag{6}$$

where V(w) is the variance in offspring number and w is the mean number of offspring born during the lifetime of an individual. It can easily be shown that this index is equivalent to the rate of change of mean population fitness, under the assumption that all variation in offspring number is genetically determined (cf. Li, 1955; Crow, 1958).

The total index (I_t) is routinely partitioned into mortality (I_m) and fertility (I_f) components

$$I_t = I_m + (I_f / \ell_a) \tag{7}$$

where ℓ_a is the probability of survival to reproductive age, usually taken to be 15. The mortality index I_m, equal to $(1-\ell_a)/\ell_a$, is that portion of the variance in offspring number attributable to variation in mortality. The fertility index I_f is the square of the coefficient of variation in offspring number for those individuals who have survived to reproductive age, and is defined as

$$I_f = V(w_a) / w_a^2 \tag{8}$$

where the subscript 'a' denotes that fraction of the population surviving to age x=a. This partition is not completely satisfactory, as the fertility index has imbedded within it all of the mortality between the onset of reproduction and its cessation. If mortality during this period is substantial, as it is in many unacculturated populations, then much of I_f may actually be due to mortality variation (Neel and Weiss, 1975). It is possible to continue partitioning I_t by age of mortality, and thereby improve the separation of fertility and mortality components (Kobayashi, 1969; Neel and Weiss, 1975), but that is an option we shall not explore further here. Alternatively, one may calculate the fertility variance from those who survive to the end of the reproductive period only, and this is common practice (eg. Cavalli-Sforza and Bodmer, 1971; Pressat, 1972; Jacquard, 1974). This latter strategy ignores all those who live to reproductive age but who die before the end of it. We would suggest that it is generally best to compute the variance in progeny output in a fashion that includes all of the normal demographic components. We will nevertheless find it useful to examine I_f computed only from those who survive to the end of the reproductive period for comparison with published results.

Although I_t defines the maximum rate at which fitness of the population can change, it is widely recognized (eg. Cavalli-Sforza and Bodmer, 1971; Spuhler, 1976) that the actual genetic variation in fitness represented may, at least in principle, be very small. Unfortunately, if the genetic variation in fitness is zero, it does not follow that the index I_t is also zero, as purely demographic factors may create an I_t significantly greater than zero. Changes in vital rates will therefore change estimates of I_t (cf. Spuhler, 1976). These purely demographic changes reflect alterations in the overall environment which may convey no information about changing selective differentials among genotypes. To the extent that evolution of demographic vital rates for the population does not imply changes in selective differentials, reductions in I_t during demographic transition have no evolutionary consequences. As far as we know, no one has attempted to remove these purely demographic effects from I_t, in an effort to obtain a genetically relevant residual.

In order to assess the magnitude of the purely demographic component, we have estimated the indices of opportunity for selection for the same population of Sweden between 1780 and 1965. We have assumed that all individuals have the same life-table parameters, ie. that there is no genetic variation in fitness. Under this assumption, the variation in offspring number is due solely to sampling considerations. We present in Figure 4 the index of opportunity for selection, partitioned according to Eq. (7), so that the I_f component contains the mortality variation during the fertile period. For each five-year

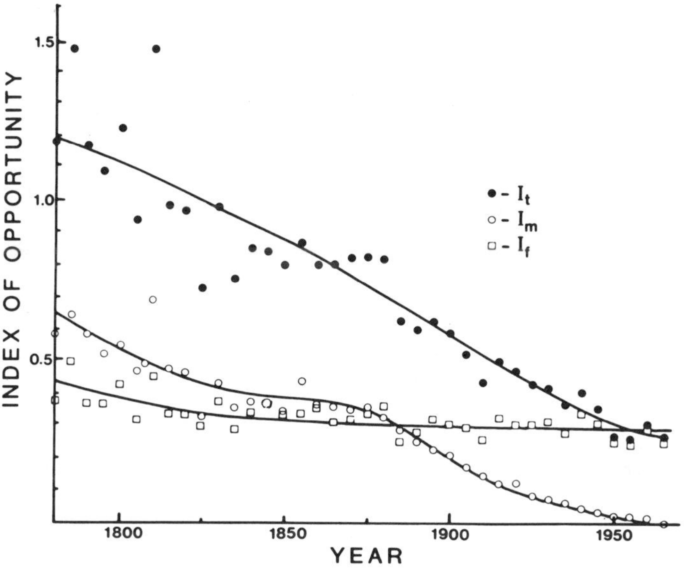

Figure 4. Index of opportunity for selection (I_t) and its components, the index of mortality selection (I_m) and the index of fertility selection (I_f), for the Swedish population (1780-1965).

interval, the mean and variance of offspring born to a female were estimated, using Monte-Carlo simulation. We assume that the probability distributions of the random events which determine the mean and variance are given by the age-specific vital rates for the period in question. For each period, the mean and variance of offspring number were determined from 400 replicates. It is important to note here that with this treatment the offspring number will invariably exhibit a contagious distribution, with the variance exceeding the mean, because different individuals survive to different ages and thus have different expectations for progeny number. It is frequently assumed that such contagious distributions are evidence for genetic differences in fertility, but this need not be the case.

Figure 5 shows the same index of opportunity for selection, but this time computed with the fertility component (I_f) determined only from those who survive

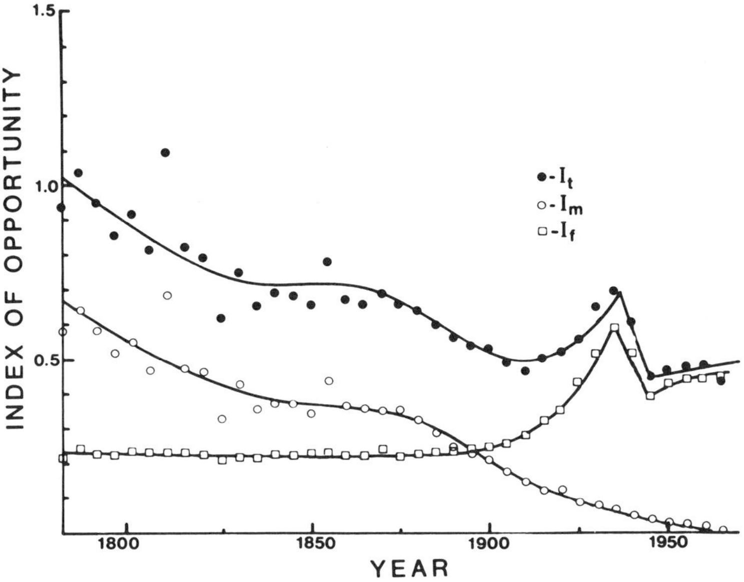

Figure 5. Index of opportunity for selection (I_t) and its components, the index of mortality selection (I_m) and the index of fertility selection (I_f), for the Swedish population (1780-1965). The index (I_f) is calculated from those who survive to the age of 45.

to the end of the fertile period, as is not uncommonly done in practice. Under our assumption that completed family size is determined solely by the age-specific fertility rates, we would expect that the distribution would be Poisson. The expected value of I_f will therefore simply be the reciprocal of the completed family size. It can be seen that the mortality index (I_m), computed as for Figure 4, shows a steady decline throughout the entire period, as the population progresses through its demographic transition. This index is measured as the standardized average prereproductive mortality. Although it would clearly be preferable to know the variance in prereproductive mortality, that information is not available. The assumption implicit in the I_m component is that the larger the mean, the larger the variance. In this respect, we must interpret I_m in a different way from I_f, as described below. The steady decline in I_t over time in both Figures reflects the trend in I_m. The fertility component, I_f, shows a different pattern, depending on the approach used to calculate it. For the first method, I_f remains relatively constant over the whole period. For the second method, I_f is constant for most of the period, but shows an increase in more recent times, and furthermore shows a transient increase and then a decrease during the 1910-1940 period. This brief pulse can again be attributed to the lack of demographic stability during this period. The important point here is that the purely demographic component of fertility variation is relatively unaffected by demographic transition, except perhaps during the unstable period.

Whatever the approach used to calculate these indices, the most striking aspect of the situation is that they are large, on the order of the I-values published for many populations (see review in Spuhler, 1976). It therefore seems necessary to reevaluate the significance of many of the values presented in the literature. The assumption implicit in the use of this index, in particular the use of the fertility index, is that the larger the variance, relative to the square of the mean, the greater may be the fertility differences among genotypes. If our calculations for the Swedish population are typical, they suggest that values of I_f between 0.2 and 0.4, depending on the exact method used to calculate them, would be expected under the null hypothesis of no genetic variation in fertility.

It is easily shown that I_f can be subdivided into a purely demographic sampling component (I_{fd}) and a residual component (I_{fr})

$$I_f = I_{fd} + I_{fr} \tag{9}$$

The latter component (I_{fr}) may contain the genetic variation. In view of this fact, we suggest that the I_f values reported, by way of example, for the Cayapo, Caingang, and Ticuna of 0.34, 0.35, and 0.15, respectively (Salzano, 1961, 1963, 1964, 1971; Salzano et al., 1980) show no real evidence for genetic differences in fertility. On the other hand, values of I_f published by the same workers (Salzano et al., 1980) for the Ayoreo (1.49, 1.56) are undoubtedly significantly different from zero, even after subtracting the demographic component (I_{fd}). The interpretation of these large values is, of course, subject to the usual proviso that I_f (or equally I_{fr}) represents the maximum 'opportunity' for selection. Interestingly, values of I_f reported for acculturated populations in early stage III tend to be fairly high. Values of I_f = 0.84 and 1.14 have been reported for the French cohort of 1900 (Jacquard, 1974) and for the U.S. cohort of 1910 (Cavalli-Sforza and Bodmer, 1971), respectively, and these too may be significantly different from zero after correction for I_{fd}.

DISCUSSION AND CONCLUSIONS

We have shown here that the demographic structure of a population may profoundly influence estimates of the intensity of natural selection. The pattern of change of these coefficients can be complex. Some general trends are nevertheless discernable. Selection due to prereproductive mortality almost always decreases during the demographic transition from stage I to stage III. This point has been made previously by several workers (eg. Cavalli-Sforza and Bodmer, 1971; Jacquard, 1974; Spuhler, 1976; Charlesworth, 1980), but nowhere is this trend more evident than in the reconstructed I_m values for the Swedish population of 1780-1965. In the absence of concomitant changes in fertility rates, a reduced prereproductive mortality rate will result in an increased mean age of the population. However, reductions in the generation interval, T, can lead to a net decrease in the intensity of selection against maturity onset diseases, as shown above.

Trends in fertility selection are more difficult to discern. In a recent review, Spuhler (1976) lists 53 separate estimates of the index of a opportunity for selection (I_t) and its components (I_m and I_f) for a wide range of populations. The average I_f value for these 53 populations is 0.4, and only 7 of the 53 values are greater than 0.5. From the values given in Figures 4 and 5, we suggest that these I_f values provide absolutely no evidence for fertility selection in over 85% of the populations examined. The trend towards higher I_f values in stage III populations is difficult to interpret, although it is consistent with the conclusion of others (eg. Cavalli-Sforza and Bodmer, 1971) that the opportunity for fertility selection is highest in modernized populations. Unfortunately, extensive use of birth control may affect this measure sufficiently to render it of questionable value in modern stage III populations.

We also note that estimators of selection intensity are extremely sensitive to demographic instability. For many populations in the stage II to stage III transition, high I_f values may simply be a consequence of demographic instability, as we have seen from Figure 5. We suggest that the index of demographic stability (Δ) is a statistic worth determining in any future studies of natural selection in human populations.

The pattern of demographic evolution will undoubtedly vary somewhat from population to population; in particular, mortality rates for early agriculturalists may sometimes be higher than for their hunter-gatherer antecedents (Salzano et al., 1980). Moreover, age-specific vital rates can change in a variety of unpredictable ways. On the one hand, juvenile mortality may decrease due to the introduction of antibiotics by missionaries and health personnel. On the other hand, mortality rates may rise among juveniles due to the exposure of acculturating populations to epidemics of newly introduced diseases (Salzano et al., 1967; Neel et al., 1970). Nevertheless, the processes we describe here should serve as a useful guide to the study of the genetic consequences of demographic change in a variety of populations.

We conclude with the often echoed comment that reliable estimates of selection intensity are of paramount importance in understanding human evolution. It is equally often repeated that such estimates in age-structured populations are not easy to obtain. Even though the most reliable demographic data can undoubtedly be obtained from well studied populations in stage III, the most interesting anthropological populations are those currently in the early stages of acculturation, demographically still in the pre-stage I state.

ACKNOWLEDGMENTS

We would like to thank J.C. Long, J.V. Neel, D.F. Roberts and J. W. Wood for helpful criticism. This work was supported by DoE-DE-AC02-82 ER60089.

LITERATURE CITED

Anonymous (1978). Vital Statistics of the United States. Vol. II. Mortality, Part A: Table 1-26. U.S. Dept. Health and Human Services. Natl Cntr Health Statistics.

Bodmer WF (1968). Demographic approaches to the measurement of differential selection in human populations. Proc Nat Acad Sci (US) 59:690.

Cavalli-Sforza LL, Bodmer WF (1971). "The Genetics of Human Populations." San Francisco: W.H. Freeman.

Charlesworth B (1980). "Evolution in Age Structured Populations." Cambridge: Cambridge Univ. Press.

Charlesworth B, Charlesworth D (1973). The measurement of fitness and mutation rate in human populations. Ann Hum Genet 37:175.

Coale AJ (1983). Recent trends in fertility in less developed countries. Science 221:828.

Crow JF (1958). Some possibilities for measuring selection intensities in man. Hum Biol 30:1.

Henry L (1961). Some data on natural fertility. Eugenics Quarterly 8:81.

Jacquard A (1974). "The Genetic Structure of Populations." Berlin: Springer-Verlag.

Keyfitz N (1968). "Introduction to the Mathematics of Population." Reading, Mass.: Addison-Wesley.

Keyfitz N, Flieger W (1968). "World Population: An Analysis of Vital Data." Chicago: Univ. Chicago Press.

Keyfitz N, Flieger W (1971). "Population: Facts and Methods of Demography." San Francisco: W.H. Freeman.

Knodel J (1977). Age patterns of fertility and the

fertility transition: Evidence from Europe and Asia. Population Studies 31:219.
Kobayashi K (1969). Changing patterns of differential fertility in the population of Japan. In "Proc. VIII Intern. Congr. Anthropological and Ethnological Sciences," Tokyo: Science Council of Japan, p 345.
Li CC (1955). "First Course in Population Genetics." Pacific Grove, CA: Boxwood Press.
Murdoch JL, Walker BA, Halpern BI, Kuzma JW, McKusick VA (1972). Life expectancy and causes of death in the Marfan Syndrome. New England J Med 286:804.
Neel JV, Weiss KM (1975). The genetic structure of a tribal population, the Yanomama Indians. XII. Biodemographic studies. Am J Phys Anthropol 42:25.
Neel JV, Centerwall WR, Chagnon NA, Casey HL (1970). Notes on the effect of measles and measles vaccine in a virgin soil population of South American Indians. Am J Epid 91:418.
Pressat R (1972). "Demographic Analysis." Chicago: Aldine-Atherton.
Rosenthal D (1966). The offspring of schizophrenic couples. J Psychiat Res 4:169.
Salzano FM (1961). Studies on the Caingang Indians. I Demography. Hum Biol 33:110.
Salzano F (1963). Selection intensity in Brazilian Caingang Indians. Nature 199:514.
Salzano FM (1964). Demographic studies on Indians from Santa Catarina, Brazil. Acta Genet Med Gemell 13:278.
Salzano FM (1971). Demographic and genetic interrelationships among the Cayapo Indians of Brazil. Soc Biol 18:148.
Salzano FM, Callegari Jacques SM, Neel JV (1980). Genetic demography of the Amazonian Ticuna Indians. J Hum Evol 9:179.
Salzano FM, Neel JV, Maybury-Lewis D (1967). Further studies on the Xavante Indians. I. Demographic data on two additional villages: Genetic structure of the the tribe. Am J Hum Genet 19:463.
Spuhler JN (1976). The maximum opportunity for natural selection in some human populations. In Zubrow EBW (ed): "Demographic Anthropology," Albuquerque, NM: University of New Mexico Press, p 185.
Teitelbaum MS (1975). Relevance of demographic transition theory for developing countries. Science 188:420.

Diseases of Complex Etiology in Small Populations:
Ethnic Differences and Research Approaches, pages 301–323

Chapter 13

CHANGING PATTERNS OF DISEASE AMONG SOUTH AMERICAN INDIANS

F.M. Salzano

Departamento de Genética, Instituto de Biociências, Universidade Federal do Rio Grande do Sul, Porto Alegre, Brazil

THE ROAD TO ACCULTURATION

The course of events that takes place in a South American Indian tribe before and after contact with non-Indians is briefly outlined in Table 1. Before contact they lived in small, isolated nomadic groups, in an intimate relationship with their environment, relying on a subsistence system based on hunting and gathering as well as simple agriculture. Fertility and mortality were moderate, population density low, but population stability high. The types of houses in which they lived were similar, and hygiene practices common. The degree of physical activity was high, with close contacts among individuals in work and play. The diet was diversified and, in terms of disease, epidemics, intestinal parasitic infections, chronic and degenerative illnesses, exposure to toxic substances and introduction of new pathologies were rare. As a result, pre-contact Indians lived in and may still live in a stable ecological and cultural setting.

This way of life changes dramatically after contact with non-Indians. There is a shift of emphasis on elements of the subsistence system, agriculture becoming the dominant activity. Food becomes less varied, with dependence on a major, single crop. Concomitantly, there is aggregation in larger, less isolated, sedentary population units. The lack of adequate sanitation makes individuals from these communities especially vulnerable to sudden, devastating epidemics. Intestinal parasitic infections become universal, exposure to toxic substances increases, and new diseases may occur due to contact with foreigners. Mean ages would increase (since high mortality is coupled with high fertility), and chronic diseases would become more prevalent. There is generally a disruption both in the physical and cultural environment of post-contact Indians.

As a result of these events, there is usually a deterioration of health conditions. Therefore, Indian groups would initially suffer with contact. Recovery

Table 1. Consequences of the acculturation process.

	Degree of contact with non-Indians	
Characteristic	Unacculturated	Acculturated
Population size	Small	Larger
Group mobility	High	Low
Isolation	High	Lower
Fertility	Moderate	High
Mortality	Moderate	High
Population density	Low	Higher
Population stabilty	High	Low
Housing	More similar	Less similar
Hygiene practices	More common	Less common
Physical activity	High	Lower
Physical proximity in work and play	High	Lower
Diet	More diversified	Less diversified
Epidemics	Less common	More common
Intestinal parasitic infections	Less common	More common
Chronic and degenerative disease	Less common	More common
Exposure to toxic substances	Low	Higher
Introduction of new diseases	Uncommon	Common
Ecosystem stability	High	Low
Cultural system	Stable	Unstable

from ill health is gradual, and is dependent on their receiving the benefits of our technological advance.

MEDICAL STUDIES ON SOUTH AMERICAN INDIANS

This situation can be utilized as a tool to answer questions in epidemiology, relating them to genetic and evolutionary aspects of these populations and of our species in general. The philosophy of these investigations, as well as some selected results, can be found in Neel and Salzano (1964), in the proceedings of two subsequent symposia (PAHO, 1968; Ciba Foundation, 1977), and in Garruto (1981). The number of medical studies performed among South American Indians is now very large. Appendix 1 gives a non-exhaustive list. The studies start chronologically with Ranke (1898) and continue to the present. In what follows I will describe some of the studies in which I have been involved, to exemplify some of the possible approaches.

TUBERCULOSIS IN BRAZILIAN INDIANS

During the 1950's and 1960's N. Nutels and coworkers had systematically surveyed many Brazilian Indian populations looking for infections by the tubercle bacillus that was assumed to have been absent from the New World before Columbus. A summary of the tuberculin tests and X-ray investigations conducted among 16 tribes is presented in Table 2. At the time there were still no reactors in many groups, but the situation was changing rapidly. The problem was particularly serious among the Suiá, Txukahamae and Carajá. The high figure observed among the latter must include many non-specific reactions, since it was obtained with a non-standardized solution of tuberculin. However, at least a fraction of the positive responses should represent "real" reactors. The Iawalapti who in 1960 did not have any reactors showed 5 of 37 in 1966.

Nutels (1968) stated that he was surprised at both the clinico-radiological and epidemiological aspects of tuberculosis in "virgin" populations like

Table. 2. Tuberculin tests and X-ray surveys conducted among 16 Brazilian Indian tribes.[1]

	Year of exam	No indiv. examined	% with strong reactions	% with abnormal shadows
Carajá	1952	240	71	3
Gorotire	1957	100	nt	4
7 Xingu tribes	1960	209	0	nt
Same	1966	370	0	nt
Kajabi	1960	63	3	nt
	1966	134	1	nt
Mehinaco	1960	38	5	nt
	1966	34	9	nt
Suiá	1960	42	17	nt
	1966	71	20	nt
Iawalapti	1960	37	0	nt
	1966	37	14	nt
Xavante	1964	84	0	nt
Yanomama	1967	88	0	nt
Txukahamae	1966	114	23	7

[1]Source: Nutels et al. (1967).
nt: not tested

the Suiá and Txukahamae. He would have expected different patterns, such as the so-called infant type in adults and the rapidly evolving acute and miliary forms, similar to those found among the Senegalese soldiers taken to France during the First World War. Instead, he found a disease that in its clinical, radiological, and even epidemiological aspects, could be equated with that of persons with a long experience with the bacillus. The occurrence of previous epidemics among these Indians seems unlikely, due to their isolation. However it is possible that the microorganism responsible for the disease among them is less virulent than that which occurs among whites. Certainly the conclusive identification of pre-Columbian tuberculosis (acid-fast bacilli in rehydrated organs, tubercles in lung, liver and pleura, lumbar kyphosis associated with a psoas abscess) in southern Peru (Allison et al., 1973) lends support to the possibility of a different strain of M.

tuberculosis, at least in some Indian populations. In any case, the current situation in Brazilian Indians is appropriate for planned and controlled research on the response of isolated, previously unexposed populations to the introduction of what may be a new infectious agent.

PYODERMA AND ASSOCIATED PATHOGENS AMONG AMAZONIAN INDIANS

Pyoderma is one of the most common skin diseases among children in the tropics. However, prevalence rates from community-based surveys, as well as bacteriological studies from the material obtained from the lesions, have seldom been reported from remote populations. Such a study was performed by Lawrence et al. (1979), and some of the findings are summarized in Tables 3 to 5. The unadjusted prevalence rates for the four villages surveyed ranged from 7 to 20% (Table 3). The age-adjusted rates, however, did not show significant differences. Children less than 5 years old generally had the greatest frequency of lesions (31%). Prevalence at any age was not affected by sex.

Table 3. Prevalence of pyoderma and bacteriological recovery of pathogens from Amazonian Indians.[1]

Tribe and population	Number studied	% with pyoderma	No. of patients from whom	
			Cultures were taken	A pathogen was isolated
Ticuna				
Umariaçu	389	12	4	4
Vendaval	221	7	12	11
Kashinawa				
Cana Brava	41	20	2	2
Kanamari				
Três Unidos	124	12	11	10

[1]Source: Lawrence et al. (1979).

From 29 of the 87 persons with pyoderma lesions observed in the indicated villages, as well as from 10 others living in communities not surveyed systematically, swabs were taken for bacteriological studies. At least one pathogenic bacterium was recovered from 37 of the 39 persons' cultures, and the results are shown in Table 4. All positive cultures contained Streptococcus pyogenes, and this microorganism was the only pathogen recovered from cultures from 17 (44%) of the 39 individuals tested. All were Lancefield group A. Multiple isolates were recovered from cultures from 20 other subjects (51%) in which S. pyogenes was found with Corynebacterium diphtheriae, Staphylococcus aureus or both. Group G streptococci were isolated once from lesions culture-positive for S. pyogenes and C. diphtheriae, and twice from lesions culture-positive for S. pyogenes, C. diphtheriae, and S. aureus.

Table 4. Pathogenic organisms isolated from Amazonian Indians.[3]

Organisms isolated	Number of patients	% from total
None	2	5
Streptococcus pyogenes	17	44
S. pyogenes[1] + Corynebacterium diphtheriae	6	15
S. pyogenes + Staphylococcus aureus	4	10
S. pyogenes[2] + S. aureus + C. diphtheriae	10	26
Total	39	100

[1]Cultures of 1 of the 6 patients contained Lancefield group G streptococcus as a third pathogenic species.
[2]Cultures of 2 of the 10 patients contained Lancefield group G streptococcus as a fourth pathogenic species.
[3]Source: Lawrence et al. (1979).

While the primary role of the beta-hemolytic streptococcus in causing clinical pyoderma seems well established, additional interest in lesion-associated streptococcal strains derives from the fact that glomerulonephritis can be a fatal non-suppurative complication of pyoderma. Furthermore, it has also been suggested that infection of pyoderma lesions with C. diphtheriae influences the epidemiology of diphtheria.

The 14 pyoderma-associated S. aureus isolates were tested against standard concentration disks containing different antibiotics and sulfa compounds and the results are presented in Table 5. The most interesting result is the presence of resistance to penicillin, erythromycin and tetracycline. Only 3 of the 14 isolates were simultaneously sensitive to all 3 antibiotics.

Table 5. Antibiotic resistance patterns of Staphylococcus aureus isolated from Amazonian Indians.[1]

Antibiotic tested			Number of
Penicillin	Erythromycin	Tetracycline	isolates*
Sensitive	Sensitive	Sensitive	3
Sensitive	Sensitive	Resistant	1
Sensitive	Resistant	Sensitive	1
Resistant	Sensitive	Sensitive	7
Resistant	Sensitive	Resistant	1
Resistant	Resistant	Sensitive	1
Total			14
% resistant 9/14 = 64	% resistant 2/14 = 14	% resistant 2/14 = 14	

[1]Source: Lawrence et al. (1979).
*All isolates were sensitive to 6 other antibiotics and 2 sulfa compounds.

People in the villages reported here have had at least some exposure to pharmaceutical penicillin, but it is doubtful whether eventual treatment programs might have induced the changes in antibiotic susceptibility of the species of interest here. There is a possibility that natural environmental antibiotic substances might have influenced the patterns observed.

HLA DISTRIBUTION AND BALANCING SELECTION

In what way can genetics contribute to the interpretation of the epidemiology of disease in these Indians? Data on the human histocompatibility system may be instructive in this regard. As is shown in Table 6, Black and Salzano (1981) found significantly less HLA haplotype homozygotes (45) than those expected (73) in a total of 459 individuals from eight Amazonian Indian tribes. These results were considered with some diffidence until we discovered a previous paper describing similar findings among Saharan Touaregs (Degos et al., 1974). New, additional evidence for the action of some form of selection favoring the heterozygotes for such haplotypes has now been obtained by Hedrick and Thomson (1983). They examined data from the A and B loci for

Table 6. Expected and observed number of homozygotes in the HLA system in eight tribes of Brazilian Indians.[1]

Population	Number studied	Number of different haplotypes	Expected no.homozygotes	Observed no.homozygotes
Tiriyo	98	18	11	6
Kaxuyana	14	13	2	1
Molokopote	16	6	4	0
Waiãpi	117	21	13	4
Parakanã Novo	31	8	9	6
Parakanã Velho	67	7	19	15
Xikrin	55	14	8	7
Gorotire	30	17	4	2
Mekranoti	31	11	4	4
Total	459	38	73	45

[1]Source: Black and Salzano (1981).

22 populations, which were compared with the expectation of the neutrality theory (for a review see Ewens, 1977). In all cases the observed homozygosity was less than the expected homozygosity assuming neutrality for a given number of alleles and sample size. In addition, the number of alleles represented only once in the sample and the frequency of the most common alleles were lower than those expected with neutrality.

Several explanations can be considered for these findings, and they have been carefully examined by Hedrick and Thomson (1983). They concluded that only symmetrical balancing selection appears to be consistent with these data. A plausible mechanism for such type of selection would be better ability of heterozygotes to cope with infections.

METABOLIC DIFFERENCES

General metabolic regulation is so essential to man that relatively large interpopulation variation in rates are unexpected. However, genetic differences, combined with the varied way in which individuals had grown and lived as adults may condition variability. Why mean blood pressure does not rise with age in several Brazilian Indian tribes, as it does in urban and otherwise "Western" populations has been investigated by Oliver et al. (1975) among the Yanomama, a group that until recently had a "no-salt" culture. They determined Na^+, K^+, Cl^- levels, renin activity and aldosterone excretion. No large differences were observed between the Amerindians and whites submitted to low-salt diets. However, the interpretation of the results is complicated by the high potassium intakes of the Yanomama. J.P.B. Vieira Fº is also performing a series of hormone studies among Brazilian Indians (see the bibliography in the Appendix), but the relative roles of specific genetic factors and the environment in the determination of such levels is far from elucidated.

I have recently participated in an investigation of the relationship of catecholamine excretion rates with lifestyles and environmental influences, and the results obtained are shown in Table 7. A comparison was made between the mean excretion rates of adrenaline and noradrenaline of the Pacaás Novos, a recently acculturated Indian tribe that lives near the Brazilian-Bolivian border, with those of two African and one European population. The noradrenaline averages are not very informative, but for adrenaline the traditional groups showed higher means than the Englishmen. These could have occurred from several causes, but the idea that "primitive people" are happy, unstressed persons may have to be reexamined considering these results. In Oxford, high adrenaline outputs are associated, among other factors, with frustration and general dissatisfaction with life (Harrison et al., 1981; Reynolds et al., 1981).

Table 7. Catecholamine excretion rates in four population groups.[1]

Population	No. individuals studied	Noradrenaline*		Adrenaline*	
		Mean	SE	Mean	SE
Englishmen	41	36.5	2.5	9.7	0.8
Maasai	16	44.9	4.7	12.1	1.8
Mossi	11	27.7	4.1	14.7	3.6
Pacaás Novos	38	37.1	2.0	14.3	1.3

[1]Source: Jenner et al. (1982).
*ng/mg creatinine.

PROBLEMS AND PROSPECTS

The studies reviewed here disclose a series of interesting facts, but do not shed much light on the ways in which hereditary factors interact with the physical and cultural environment to compound the reaction norm of a certain individual to a pathogenic organism or substance. Table 8 focuses on four points: sampling and analytical strategies, study feasibility and definition of problems, when considering questions of health and disease among South American Indians.

Table 8. Problems and prospects for the study of health and disease among South American Indians.

Sampling strategies		
Random samples		
Whole communities:	Cross sectional	
	Longitudinal	
Pooling of data from several tribes		
Study feasibility		
Bureaucratic requirements		
Geographic remoteness		
Language barriers		
Cooperativeness		
Absence of written records		
Definition of problems		
Special foci		
Differential susceptibility to disease		
Effects of:	Physical environment	
	Population structure	
	Culture	
	Genetic factors	
	Physiological factors	
Analytical strategies		
Correlation between:	Antibody levels	
	Genetic markers	
	(isolated or in groups)	
Genetic dissection of the region responsible for the immune process		

In relation to sampling, the generally small sizes of these populations are a problem. This can be partially overcome by the pooling of data from several tribes, when this is feasible. On the other hand, these small sizes make studies of whole communities (or of large parts of it) possible. The problem that remains is the difficulty of unbiased longitudinal investigations, since the sheer presence of the researcher or his (her) group may alter local customs.

As for study feasibility, it is obvious that due

to geographic remoteness these groups are more difficult to study than others, for example, city dwellers. In addition, at least in Brazil, special permission is necessary to reach the tribes. Language barriers and the absence of written records are other problems, but cooperativeness of the subjects is in general good.

In the question of definition of problems, populations showing special foci of specific diseases with high prevalences (while in other places these diseases are rare) merit special attention. Generally, however, differential susceptibility to diseases (especially the infectious ones) involves many factors, that should be duly considered. Some analytical strategies, however, seem promising. Among them I would mention correlations between antibody levels and one or a group of genetic markers, as well as the dissection of the region responsible for the immune process, by the modern techniques of DNA analysis. The possibility of finding differences in remote isolates, as compared to populations from industrialized cities (or racial dissimilarities) should be undoubtedly considered.

ACKNOWLEDGMENTS

Special thanks to Wenner-Gren Foundation for Anthropological Research, which made it possible for me to travel to Canada.

LITERATURE CITED

Allison MJ, Mendoza J, Pezzia A (1973). Documentation of a case of tuberculosis in pre-Columbian America. Amer Rev Resp Dis 107:985.

Black FL, Salzano FM (1981). Evidence for heterosis in the HLA system. Am J Hum Genet 33:894.

Ciba Foundation (1977). "Health and Disease in Tribal Societies". Ciba Foundation Symposium 49. Amsterdam: Elsevier.

Degos L, Colombani J, Chaventre A, Bengston B, Jacquard A (1974). Selective pressure on HLA polymorphism. Nature 249:62.

Ewens WJ (1977). Population genetics theory in

relation to the neutralist-selection controversy. Adv Hum Genet 8:67.
Garruto RM (1981). Disease patterns of isolated groups. In Rothschild HR (ed): "Biocultural Aspects of Disease," New York: Academic Press, p 557.
Harrison GA, Palmer CD, Jenner DA, Reynolds V (1981). Associations between rates of urinary catecholamine excretion and aspects of lifestyle among adult women in some Oxfordshire villages. Hum Biol 53:617.
Hedrick PW, Thomson G (1983). Evidence for balancing selection at HLA. Genetics 104:449.
Jenner DA, Harrison GA, Day JA, Huizinga J, Salzano FM (1982). Interpopulation comparisons of urinary catecholamines: A pilot study. Ann Hum Biol 9:579.
Lawrence DN, Facklam RR, Sottnek FO, Hancock GA, Neel JV, Salzano FM (1979). Epidemiologic studies among Amerindian populations of Amazonia. I. Pyoderma: Prevalence and associated pathogens. Am J Trop Med Hyg 28:548.
Neel JV, Salzano FM (1964). A prospectus for genetic studies of the American Indian. Cold Spring Harbor Symp Quant Biol 29:85.
Nutels N (1968). Medical problems of newly contacted Indian groups. In "Biomedical challenges presented by the American Indian," Washington, D.C.: Pan American Health Organization Scientific Publication No. 165, p 68.
Nutels N, Ayres M, Salzano FM (1967). Tuberculin reactions, X-ray and bacteriological studies in the Cayapo Indians of Brazil. Tubercle 48:195.
Oliver WJ, Cohen EL, Neel JV (1975). Blood pressure, sodium intake, and sodium related hormones in the Yanomama Indians, a "no-salt" culture. Circulation 52:146.
Pan American Health Organization (1968). "Biomedical Challenges Presented by the American Indian." Washington, D.C.: Pan American Health Organization Scientific Publ No 165.
Ranke KE (1898). Beobachtungen über Bevolkerungsstand und Bevölkerungsbewegung bei Indianern Central-Brasiliens. Corresp-Blatt Deutsch Gesellsch Anthropol, Ethnol Urgesch 29:123.
Reynolds V, Jenner DA, Palmer CD, Harrison GA (1981). Catecholamine excretion rates in relation to life-styles in the male population of Otmoor, Oxfordshire. Ann Hum Biol 8:197.

APPENDIX

MEDICAL STUDIES PERFORMED IN SOUTH AMERICAN INDIANS[1]

Alzate H, Gonzáles H, Guzmán J (1969). Lactose intolerance in South American Indians. Am J Clin Nutr 22:122.

Arias S (1976). Etiologia múltiple del enanismo entre los indios Yukpa (Irapa) de la Sierra de Perijá llamados "pigmóides". Bol Indigen Venezol 17:49.

Arias S, Mota M, Pinto-Cisternas J (1976). L'osteochondro-dysplasie spondylo-épiphyso-méta-physaire type Irapa. Nouveau nanisme avec rachis et métatarsiens courts. Nouv Presse Méd 5:319.

Aston DL, Thorley AP (1970). Leishmaniasis in central Brazil: Results of a Montenegro skin test survey among Amerindians in the Xingu National Park. Trans Royal Soc Trop Med Hyg 64:671.

Ayres M, Salzano FM (1972). Health status of Brazilian Cayapo Indians. Trop Geogr Med 24:178.

Barton SA, Lenart V, Palomino H, Murillo F, Weidman W, Schull WJ (1976). High altitude, indigenous origin, and continuous cardiac monitoring. Av Space Environm Med 47:592.

Baruzzi RG (1969/1970). Contribuição para o estudo epidemiológico da toxoplasmose. Levantamento sorológico em índios do Alto Xingu, Brasil Central. Rev Inst Adolfo Lutz 29/30:105.

Baruzzi RG (1970). Contribution to the study of the toxoplasmosis epidemiology. Serological survey among the Indians of the upper Xingu River, Central Brazil. Rev Inst Med Trop São Paulo 12:93.

Baruzzi RG, Abdala N, Black FL (1982). Measles and measles vaccination in isolated Amerindian tribes. II. The 1978/79 Xingu epidemic. Trop Geogr Med 34:7.

Baruzzi RG, Amato Neto V (1966). Inquérito sorológico sumário para toxoplasmose, entre índios do Parque Nacional do Xingu. Rev Inst Med Trop São Paulo 8:277.

Baruzzi RG, Camargo ME, Kameyama I, Hoshino S, Rebonato C, D'Andretta Jr. C (1971). Splenomegalia

[1]This is a non-exhaustive list. Additional references may be found in the papers mentioned. Those included in the bibliography of the present article are not repeated here.

in Brazilian Indians from the "Alto Xingu" (Central Brazil). 1 - Occurrence and results of serological tests for some parasitic diseases. Ann Soc Belge Med Trop 51:205.

Baruzzi RG, Castro RM, D'Andretta Jr. C, Carvalhal S, Ramos OL, Pontes PL (1973). Occurrence of Lobo's blastomycosis among "Caiabi" Brazilian Indians. Int J Dermatology 12:95.

Baruzzi RG, D'Andretta Jr. C, Carvalhal S, Ramos OL, Pontes PL (1967). Ocorrência da blastomicose queloideana entre Indios Caiabi. Rev Inst Med Trop São Paulo 9:135.

Baruzzi RG, Franco LJ, Jardim JR, Masuda A, Naspitz C, Paiva ER, Ferreira-Novo N (1976). The association between splenomegaly and malaria in Indians from the Alto Xingu, Central Brasil. Rev Inst Med Trop São Paulo 18:322.

Baruzzi RG, Iunes M (1970). Levantamento das condições de saúde das tribos indígenas do Alto Xingu. Aplicação de medidas médico-profiláticas para sua prevenção. Parque Nacional do Xingu, Brasil Central. São Paulo: Escola Paulista de Medicina.

Baruzzi RG, Marcopito LF, Iunes M (1978). Programa médico preventivo da Escola Paulista de Medicina no Parque Nacional do Xingu. Rev Anthrop 21:155.

Baruzzi RG, Rodriques MC, Carvalho RP, Dias LCS (1971). Pesquisa de anticorpos neutralizantes contra o vírus do sarampo em índios do Alto Xingu, Brasil Central. Rev Inst Med Trop São Paulo 13:356.

Beaver PC, Neel JV, Orihel TC (1976). Dipetalonema perstans and Mansonella ozzardi in Indians of Southern Venezuela. Am J Trop Med Hyg 25:263.

Bellizzi AM (1960). Alguns dados sobre a incidência nosológica nos índios Karajá. J Bras Med 2:817.

Bellizzi AM (1961). Alguns dados sobre a incidência nosológica nos índios Kayapó. J Bras Med 5:197.

Black FL (1975). Infectious disease in primitive societies. Science 187:515.

Black FL, Woodall JP, Evans AS, Liebhaber H, Henle G (1970). Prevalence of antibody against viruses in the Tiriyo, an isolated Amazon tribe. Am J Epidemiol 91:430.

Black FL, Woodall JP, Pinheiro FP (1969). Measles vaccine reactions in a virgin population. Am J Epidemiol 89:168.

Bloom AD, Neel JV, Tsuchimoto T, Meilinger K (1973). Chromosomal breakage in leukocytes of South American Indians. Cytogenet Cell Genet 12:175.
Bois E, Feingold J (1972). Génétique de l'uricémie: Étude de trois tribus amérindiennes de la Haute-Guyane Française. Ann Génét 15:257.
Brown P, Tsai T, Gajdusek DC (1975). Seroepidemiology of human papovaviruses. Discovery of virgin populations and some unusual patterns of antibody prevalence among remote peoples of the world. Am J Epidemiol 102:331.
Cabannes R, Larrouy G, Ruffié J (1964). Étude clinique et hématologique des indiens du Haut-Oyapock et du Haut-Maroni (Guyane Française) Oyampi, Emerillon et Oayana. Bull Soc Pathol Exot. 57:307.
Campos SS (1960). Estudos sobre cancer nos índios do Brasil. Rev Bras de Canc 17:33.
Candeias JAN, Baruzzi RG, Pripas S, Iunes M (1977). Prevalence of antibodies to the Bk and Jc papovaviruses in isolated populations. Rev Saúde Publ São Paulo 11:510.
Castro RM, Baruzzi RG (1973). Ausgedehnte Keloidblastomykose bei einem Indianer Aus Zentrallbrasilien. Mykosen 16:101.
Coimbra Jr. CEA (1982). Notas para uma análise epidemiológica dos achados de ovos de Capillaria sp. em exames de fezes realizados entre os Suruís do Parque Indígena Aripuanã, Rondônia. Boletim CEPAM 1:5.
Covarrubias E, Barzelatto J, Guiloff R (1969). Genetic questions related to the goiter endemia of Pedregoso (Chile). In Stanbury JP (ed): "Endemic Goiter," Washington, DC: Pan American Health Organization, p 252.
Damianovic J (1948). Realidad sanitaria de la población indígena de la zona austral antártica. Rev Chil Hig Med Prev 10:3.
Degrossi OJ, Altschuler N, Forcher M, Zaninovich AA, Mutchinick OM, Enriori CL (1969). Characteristics of endemic goiter in a Mapuche Indian tribe in Chiquillihuin, El Malleo, Province of Neuquen, Argentine Republic. In Stanbury JP (ed): "Endemic Goiter," Washington, DC: Pan American Health Organizaton, p 149.
Díaz, B, Gallegos D, Murillo F, Covarrubias E, Covarrubias T, Rona R, Weidman W, Rothhammer F,

Schull WJ (1978). The multinational Andean genetic and health program: II. Disease and disability among the Aymara. Bull Pan Am Hlth Organ 12:219.
Dricot JM, Dricot-d'Ans CH (1978). Vision de couleurs, acuité visuelle et sensibilité à la phénylthiocarbamide chez les Indiens Machiguenga de l'Amazonie péruvienne. Bull Soc Roy Belge Anthrop Préhist 89:99.
Dricot-d'Ans CH, Dricot JM (1978). Influence de l'acculturation sur la situation nutritionnelle en Amazonie peruvienne. Ann Soc Belge Méd Trop 58:39.
Dutt JS (1980). Altitude and fertility: The confounding effects of childhood mortality - a Bolivian example. Soc Biol 27:101.
Eichenberger, RW (1966). Una filosofia de salud pública para las tribus indígenas amazónicas. Am Indíg 26:119.
Eveland WC, Oliver WJ, Neel JV (1971). Characteristics of Escherichia coli serotypes in the Yanomama, a primitive Indian tribe of South America. Inf Immun 4:753.
Fagundes Neto U (1977). Avaliação do estado nutricional das crianças índias do Alto Xingu. Ph.D. Thesis. São Paulo: Escola Paulista de Medicina.
Fischman O (1973). Black Piedra among Brazilian Indians. Rev Inst Med Trop São Paulo 15:103.
Freitas Fº AS (1955). Inquérito sanitário entre os índios Xavante. In "SPI", 1954. Rio de Janeiro: Serviço de Proteção aos Indios, p 145.
Freitas Fº AS, Oliveira NB (1955). Estudo sobre o estado nutritivo dos Xavantes. Rev Brasil Med 12:565.
Fribourg-Blanc A, Bois E, Feingold J (1975). Bilan épidémiologique des Amérindiens de Haute-Guyane Française: Sérologie de la toxoplasmose. Med Mal Infect 5:502.
Glanville EV, Geerdink RA (1972). Blood pressure of Amerindians from Surinam. Am J Phys Anthrop 37:251.
Goldsmith RI, Rothhammer F, Schull WJ (1979). The multinational Andean genetic and health program. III.Ophthalmic disease and disability among the Aymara. Bull Pan Am Hlth Organ 13:58.
Guimarães RX (1973). Frequência do antígeno Australia em indivíduos normais índios do Parque do Xingu e portadores de esquistossomose mansônica. Ph. D. Thesis, São Paulo: Escola Paulista de Medicina.

Hecker LH, Allen HE, Dinman BD, Neel JV (1974). Heavy metal levels in acculturated and unacculturated populations. Arch Environm Hlth 29:181.
Hugh-Jones P, Aston DL, Guillebaud J, Jones HI, Mills PH, Rees PH, Thorley AP (1972). Medical studies among Indians of the Upper Xingú. Brit J Hosp Med 7:317.
Kaplan JE, Larrick JW, Yost J, Farrell L, Greenberg HB, Herrmann KL, Sulzer AJ, Walls KW, Pederson L (1980). Infectious disease patterns in the Waorani, an isolated Amerindian population. Am J Trop Med Hyg 29:298.
Kerbauy J, Silva MP (1971). Comportamento em cultura "in vitro" de linfócitos do sangue periférico de índios do Parque Nacional do Xingú sob a ação da fitohemaglutinina (PHA). Rev Bras Pesq Med Biol 4:385.
Kerbauy J (1969). Comportamento em cultura "in vitro" de leucócitos de sangue periférico de índios do Parque Nacional do Xingu. Ph.D. Thesis, São Paulo: Escola Paulista de Medicina.
Lage, HA (1964). Mansonelose em índios do grupo Aruak, do rio Içana. O Hospital 66:557.
Larraya FP (1977). Entre los últimos Sirionó del Oriente de Bolivia. Acta Psiquiat Psicol Am Latina 23:247.
Lawrence DN, Bodmer JG, Bodmer WF (1980). Distribution of HLA antigens in Ticuna Indians of Brazil: Results of typing a leprosy-affected family. Tissue Ant 16: 152.
Lawrence DN, Erdtmann B, Peet JW, Nunes de Mello JA, Healy GR, Neel JV, Salzano FM (1979). Epidemiologic studies among Amerindian populations of Amazônia. II.Prevalence of Mansonella ozzardi. Am J Trop Med Hyg 28:991.
Lawrence DN, Neel JV, Abadie SH, Moore LL, Adams LJ, Healy GR, Kagan IG (1980). Epidemiologic studies among Amerindian populations of Amazônia. III. Intestinal parasitoses in newly contacted and acculturating villages. Am J Trop Med Hyg 29:530.
Layrisse Z, Layrisse M (1968). High incidence cold autoagglutinins of anti-I^T specificity in Yanomama Indians of Venezuela. Vox Sang 14:369.
Layrisse Z, Malavé I (1972). Anticuerpos eritrocitarios y gamma-globulínicos en poblaciones indias venezolanas. Acta Cient Venez 22 (Suppl 3):196.

Lee RV, Black FL, Hierholzer Jr WJ, West BL (1978). A novel pattern of treponemal antibody distribution in isolated South American Indian populations. Am J Epidemiol 107:46.

Leser PG, Camargo ME, Baruzzi RG (1977). Toxoplasmosis serological tests in Brazilian Indians (Kren-Akorore) of recent contact with civilized man. Rev Inst Trop São Paulo 19:232.

Lima PE (1950). Níveis tensionais dos índios Kalapalo e Kamaiurá. Rev Brasil Med 7:787.

Lovelace JK, Moraes MAP, Hagerby E (1978). Toxoplasmosis among the Ticuna Indians in the State of Amazonas, Brazil. Trop Geogr Med 30:295.

Lowenstein FW (1961). Blood-pressure in relation to age and sex in the tropics and subtropics. Lancet i:389.

Madalengoitia J, Ishida N, Umenay T, Miyamoto T, Mejía J, Flores W, Sánchez S, Méndez R (1975). The prevalence of hepatitis B antigen among hepatitis patients and residents of Peru. Bull Pan Am Hlth Organ 9:142.

Makela M, Barton SA, Schull WJ, Weidman W, Rothhammer F (1978). The multinational Andean genetics and health program. IV.Altitude and the blood pressure of the Aymara. J Chron Dis 31:587.

Mattos RB (1958). Acuidade visual para longe e freqüência de discromatopsia em índios brasileiros. Free Dozent Thesis, São Paulo: Escola Paulista de Medicina.

Mattos RB (1970). Estudo oftalmológico dos índios do Médio Xingu. Arq Bras Oftalmologia 31:33.

Mota JL, Motta LS (1955). A epidemia do sarampo no Xingu. In "SPI, 1954." Rio de Janeiro: Serviço de Proteção aos índios, p 131.

Munizaga J, Allison MJ, Aspillaga E (1978). Diaphragmatic hernia associated with strangulation of the small bowel in an Atacamena mummy. Am J Phys Anthrop 48:17.

Munizaga J, Allison MJ Paredes C (1978). Cholelithiasis and cholecystitis in pre-Columbian Chileans. Am J Phys Anthrop 48:209.

Muñoz L, Marconi J, Horwitz J, Naveillan P (1966). Crosscultural definitions applied to the study of functional psychoses in Chilean Mapuches. Brit J Psych 112:1205.

Neel JV (1974). A note on congenital defects in two

unacculturated Indian tribes. In Janerich DT, Skalko RG, Porter IH (eds): "Congenital Defects, New Directions in Research," New York: Academic Press, p 3.
Neel JV, Andrade AHP, Brown GE, Eveland WE, Goobar J, Sodeman Jr. WA, Stollerman GH, Weinstein ED, Wheeler AH (1968). Further studies of the Xavante Indians. IX.Immunologic status with respect to various diseases and organisms. Am J Trop Med Hyg 17:486.
Neel JV, Centerwall WR, Chagnon NA, Casey HL (1970). Notes of the effect of measles and measles vaccine in a virgin-soil population of South American Indians. Am J Epidemiol 91:418.
Neel JV, Layrisse M, Salzano FM (1977). Man in the tropics: The Yanomama Indians. In Harrison GA (ed): "Population Structure and Human Variation," Cambridge: Cambridge University Press, p 109.
Neel JV, Mikkelsen WM, Rucknagel DL, Weinstein ED, Goyer RA, Abadie SH (1968). Further studies of the Xavante Indians. VIII. Some observations on blood, urine, and stool specimens. Am J Trop Med Hyg 17:474.
Neel JV, Salzano FM, Junqueira PC, Keiter F, Maybury-Lewis D (1964). Studies on the Xavante Indians of the Brazilian Mato Grosso. Am J Hum Genet 16:52.
Nutels N, Miranda JAN (1969). Viragem tuberculínica em grupos indígenas vacinados com BCG intradermico. Rev Serv Nac Tuberc 13:79.
Oliveira HC (1952). O estado de saúde dos índios Karajá em 1950. Rev Museu Paul 6:489.
Pazzanese D, Portugal OP, Ramos OL, Finatti AAC, Lanfranchi W, Barreto HPCB, Sustovich DR (1964). Serum-lipid levels in a Brazilian Indian population. Lancet ii:615.
Pereira HG, Baruzzi RG, Carvalho RPS (1971). Estudo dos anticorpos contra o vírus da influenza em índios do Alto Xingu, Brasil Central. Rev Inst Med Trop São Paulo 13:285.
Rassi E, Lacerda N, Guaimaraes JA (1976). Study of the area affected by onchocerciasis in Brazil: Survey of local residents. Bull Pan Am Hlth Organ 10:33.
Ribeiro D (1956). Convívio e contaminação. Efeitos dissociativos da depopulação provocada por epidemias em grupos indígenas. Sociologia 18:3.

Rodrigues MC (1969). Contribuição para o estudo dos entero-vírus em índios do Alto Xingu (Brasil Central) pela pesquisa em anticorpos neutralizantes. Ph.D. Thesis, São Paulo: Universidade de São Paulo.
Rodrigues MC, Carvalho RPS, Baruzzi RG (1973). Pesquisa de anticorpos neutralizantes contra o vírus do herpes simples em índios do Alto Xingu, Brasil Central. Rev Inst Med Trop São Paulo 15:20.
Salzano FM, Neel JV (1976). New data on the vision of South American Indians. Bull Pan Am Hlth Organ 10: 1.
Schaad JDG (1960). Epidemiological observations in Bush Negroes and Amerindians in Surinam. Trop Geogr Med 12:38.
Schwaner TD, Dixon CF (1974). Helminthiasis as a measure of cultural change in the Amazon basin. Biotropica 6:32.
Scolnik R (1955). Observaciones sobre el estado sanitario de algunas tribus indígenas del Brasil Central. Am Indíg 15:89.
Silva MP (1966). Contribuição para o estudo do sangue periférico e da medula óssea em índios do Alto Xingu. Ph.D. Thesis, São Paulo: Escola Paulista de Medicina.
Silva W (1959). Incidência do bócio endêmico sobre índios brasileiros. Bol Indig 19:24.
Soyano A, Layrisse Z, Layrisse M, Neel JV (1979). Hepatitis-Bs antigen in an isolated Indian population of southern Venezuela: A family study. J Med Genet 16:201.
Soyano A, Malavé I, Walder R, Layrisse Z, Layrisse M (1976). Hepatitis-B antigen in an isolated Indian populaton (Yanomama Indians) of Southern Venezuela. Rev Bras Pesq Med Biol 9:247.
Stinson S (1982). The interrelationship of mortality and fertility in rural Bolivia. Hum Biol 54:299.
Sustovich DR, Tucci PJ, Barros Barreto HC, Lima MCC, Ajizen H, Ramos OL (1967). Estudo da hiperlipemia prandial em indivíduos normais, nefróticos, ateroscleróticos e índios. Rev Bras Med. 24:530.
Tato JM, Tato JM (1969). Quelques resultats des examens otologiques et audiologiques des Indiens Sud-Américains. Acta Oto-laryngol 67:277.
Tenbrinck MS (1964). Blood pressure comparisons in tropical Africans and Peruvians. N York State J Med 64:2584.

Van Mazijk J, Pinheiro FP, Black FL (1982). Measles and measles vaccine in isolated Amerindian tribes. I.The 1971 Trio (Tiriyo) epidemic. Trop Geogr Med 34:3.
Vianna MC (1966). Aspectos sócio-econômicos e sanitários dos Fulni-ô de Aguas Belas - Pernambuco. Recife: SUDENE.
Vieira Fº JPB (1970a). Vacinação dos índios Suruí contra o sarampo. Rev Ass Med Bras 16:183.
Vieira Fº JPB (1970b). Vacinação dos índios Xikrin, Suruí e Gaviões contra a varíola. Rev Ass Med Bras 16:357.
Vieira Fº JPB (1972). Considerações a propósito da inexistência de bócio entre os indígenas brasileiros Xikrin. Rev Ass Med Bras 18:345.
Vieira Fº JPB (1974). Considerações acerca da incidência do diabetes mellitus entre os Ameríndios. Rev Ass Med Bras 20:447.
Vieira Fº JPB (1975). Análise das glicemias do índios das aldeias Suruí, Gaviões e Xikrin. Rev Ass Med Bras 21:253.
Vieira Fº JPB (1977). O diabetes mellitus e as glicemias de jejum dos índios Caripuna e Palikur. Rev Ass Med Bras 23:175.
Vieira Fº JPB (1978a). Heredograma e coeficiente de endocruzamento de uma família indígena com pseudo-hermafroditismo masculino e pé torto congênito. Rev Ass Med Bras 24:36.
Vieira Fº JPB (1978b). Indio Paracanã com hipogonadismo hipogonadotrópico idiopático. Rev Ass Med Bras 24:363.
Vieira Fº JPB (1978c). O diabetes mellitus entre os índios dos Estados Unidos e os do Brasil. Rev Antrop 21:53.
Vieira Fº JPB (1978d). Medicina indígena e medicina científica. Rev Antrop 21:171.
Vieira Fº JPB (1979). Médico constata ausência de bócio entre os Xikrin. Rev Atual Indíg 3(15):13.
Vieira Fº JPB (1981a). Deficiência de 17,20-desmolase (lyase) e pseudo-hermafroditismo masculino entre índios do rio Curipi. Rev Assoc Med Bras 27:257.
Vieira Fº JPB (1981b). O bócio entre os índios brasileiros. Rev Ass Med Bras 27:285.
Vieira Fº JPB, Tatit ED, Baruzzi RG (1972). O poder de ligação da triiodotironina radioativa entre índios do Alto Xingu. Rev Ass Med Bras 18:471.

Vieira Fº JPB, Tatit ED, Pinheiro FP (1973). Dosagem da tiroxina no soro dos índios das tribos Menkranoiti e Kuben-Kran-Kegn. Rev Ass Med Bras 19: 193.

Vieira Fº JPB, Vieira JGH, Novo NF (1982a). Níveis séricos de testosterona, sulfato de deidroepiandrosterona, cortisol e prolactina entre os silvícolas Paracategê. Arq Bras Endocr Metab 26:102.

Vieira Fº JPB, Vieira JGH, Novo NF (1982b). Níveis séricos de cortisol dos silvícolas Xikrin. Arq Bras Endocrinol Metabol 26:61.

Vieira Fº JPB, Vieira JGH, Russo EMK (1979). Determinação dos níveis sangüíneos de tiroxina, triiodoirotnina, testosterona e sulfato de deidroepiandrosterona dos silvícolas Xikrin e Suruí. Rev Ass Med Bras 25:208.

Vieira Fº JPB, Vieira JGH, Russo EMK, Novo NF (1980). Dosagem da testosterona, do sulfato de deidroepiandrosterona, da triiodotironina e da tiroxina pelo radioimunoensaio, da retenção da triiodotironina entre os silvícolas Paracanã. Rev Ass Med Bras 26:205.

Wehba J (1976). Avaliação da capacidade de absorção da lactose. Estudo em população de índios do Alto Xingu. Ph. D. Thesis, São Paulo: Escola Paulista de Medicina.

Weinstein ED, Neel JV, Salzano FM (1967). Further studies on the Xavante Indians. VI. The physical status of the Xavante of Simões Lopes. Am J Hum Genet 19:532.

Zegers BJM, Geerdink RD, Sander PC (1973). Serum immunoglobulin levels in Trio and Wajana Indians of Surinam. Vox Sang 24:457.

Diseases of Complex Etiology in Small Populations:
Ethnic Differences and Research Approaches, pages 325–344

Chapter 14

RISK TO DISEASE OF ANDEAN POPULATIONS INHABITING CONTRASTING ECOGEOGRAPHIC AREAS

F. Rothhammer[1], S. Castillo[2], W.J. Schull[3]

[1]Department of Cellular Biology and Genetics, [2]Department of Medicine, Faculty of Medicine, University of Chile, Santiago, Chile, [3]Center for Demographic and Population Genetics, University of Texas, Health Science Center, Houston, Texas

INTRODUCTION

Some twenty years ago, based largely on geographic logic and scanty archeological evidence, Wendell C. Bennett and Junius Bird (1964) provided a reconstruction of the principal migrational routes of the first South Americans. The nomadic hunters were supposed to have crossed the Isthmus of Panama and entered the Northern Andean Region by way of the Cauca and Magdalena Rivers. Some nomads were thought to have migrated eastward into Venezuela and others, after adjusting to the rigors of the Andes, southward into the mountains. More recent archeologic work has corroborated Bennett and Bird's reconstruction and suggested that that these events took place roughly 15,000 years ago (Fladmark, 1982).

On the western slope of the Andes mountains, between 17°30' and 20° latitude south, an abrupt altitudinal gradient exists that ranges from sea level to 6,000 m. This area, which comprises parts of northern Chile and western Bolivia, has been inhabited by _Homo sapiens_ since at least 7,500 B.C. (Rothhammer et al., 1982). It affords an exceptional opportunity to study the influence of a unique environment on risk to disease and the genetically established range of physiological responses to hypoxia (and concomitant factors) as seen in the Aymara speaking descendants of Andean Paleo-Indians.

The area of interest includes five geomorphological regions (Veloso and Kalin-Arroyo, 1982), namely, (1) the coastal mountain range which, extending along the Pacific Ocean, has at this latitude only 125 m of elevation, (2) the sierra rising to 3,800 m, (3) the western Andean range or Cordillera Central, (4) the high plateau or altiplano with an average elevation of 4,200 m, and finally (5) the eastern Andean range or Cordillera Oriental. These geomorphological regions differentiated from an ancient Miocene ryolithic plateau during the Pliocene-Pleistocene through tectonic activity. In the Quaternary, the high plateau relief was further modified through the appearance of new volcanoes. The high plateau is cold in winter, with temperatures below -12°C. During the summer the temperature may rise to 13°C. Relative humidity is low, especially in the winter. Precipitation is 450 mm annually.

Two rivers, the Lluta and San Jose, reach the Pacific Ocean in this area giving rise to fertile coastal valleys. From the climatic point of view, these valleys can be included in the tropical influence zone (Veloso and Kalin-Arroyo, 1982). The coastal range is strongly affected by the cold Pacific Ocean current, being dry and desertic with annual precipitation of 0.1 to 0.6 mm. Average temperatures are moderately high ranging between 18°C in the winter and 22°C in the summer months. The valleys exhibit high average humidity (74-79% monthly).

Some 3,000 Aymara-speaking Indians live presently in thirty or more villages with 60 to 400 inhabitants, scattered across the altitudinal gradient in Chile. Close to a million Aymaras live in the Departments of La Paz and Oruro on the Bolivian intermontane plateau.

Although several authors have worked in the Peruvian section of the altiplano among Quechua speaking Indians and called attention to various physiologic and pathologic features of this indigenous population, special interest has been directed towards describing cardiovascular characteristics including the negative correlation between overall blood pressure and altitude (Rotta, 1947; Hurtado et al., 1956; Penaloza et al., 1963; Buck et al., 1968; Zapata and Marticorena, 1968). Some investigators have claimed that hypertension and its cardiovascular and renal complications do not occur at high altitude (Baker, 1969; Hurtado, 1960) and others have maintained that high altitude protects against myocardial infarction.

EXAMINEES AND EXAMINATIONS

Most of the observations to be discussed in what follows were obtained as part of a multidisciplinary research effort involving professionals of Bolivia, Chile, Ecuador, Peru and the United States, termed the Multinational Andean Genetic and Health Program (Schull and Rothhammer, 1977). In the course of the program, between 1973 and 1975, some 2,500 Aymara-speaking Indians, inhabitants of 14 Chilean and Bolivian villages and hamlets distributed over the altitudinal gradient, were surveyed. Examinations and observations included physical, dental and oral cavity examinations; anthropometric measurements; resting electrocardiograms; pulmonary function, audiometric and psychomotor tests; medical, nutritional, reproductive and residential histories. A blood specimen was also obtained. Here we are concerned with the results of the physical examinations including a detailed appraisal of cardiovascular pathology. Other communications have been devoted to methodological, genetic, physiological, health, biochemical and growth and developmental aspects (Díaz et al., 1978; Palomino et al., 1978; Schull et al., 1979; Ferrell et al., 1978; Ferrell et al., 1980; Schull and Rothhammer, 1979; Goldsmith et al., 1977; Barton et al., 1976; Makela, et al., 1978 and Mueller et al., 1978).

The examinees ranged in age from under one year to over 90 and were about equally distributed between males and females. Selection of adult subjects was made on the basis of their willingness to participate. Village residents were invited by town leaders, schoolteachers and church officials to visit our medical field station. In addition, virtually all school children were examined. It should be noted that these examinations occurred for the most part in October and November, that is, in the southern hemispheric spring. Our data are, of course, cross-sectional and may confound seasonal as well as other transitory effects. All of the examinations were performed nevertheless in the springtime and summer and should, therefore, be reasonably comparable. Blood pressure measurements were taken with the subject in the sitting position using a mercury sphygmomanometer. The measurements were normally made on the right arm. Diagnostic impressions were coded according to the International Classification of Diseases (ICDA, 8th edition, 1968).

The inhabitants of the altitudinal gradient were subdivided in two groups on the basis of the linguistic origin of their maternal and paternal surnames. Individuals without either Aymara or Spanish names frequently used by the Aymara, were considered non-Aymara. All others, mestizo and putatively pure Aymara were considered Aymara. We excluded from the present study all individuals who were reported to have lived less than 90% of their lives in a given ecogeographic area.

Additional information was obtained during a genetic survey conducted by Chilean and German scientists in the Atacama desert oasis of Toconao located at 2,500 m, immediately east of the Atacama Salt Lake about 600 km south of the area just described. Some 260 Atacameno Indians from Toconao were examined in 1983. Observations were similar, with the exception that pulmonary function tests and electrocardiograms were omitted. The results of erythrocyte antigen and enzyme phenotyping, as well as the health status and the genetic response to drugs and environmental agents of this population have been reported elsewhere (Rothhammer et al., 1984; Goedde et al., 1984a; Goedde et al., 1984b; Castillo et al., 1984).

DISEASE AND DISABILITY

Some 150 ICDA codable pathologic conditions were encountered among the more than 2,700 individuals examined. Many involve only a few cases. Under these conditions any comparison among different ecogeographic areas or ethnic groups would be meaningless. We have consequently grouped diseases into broader categories and call the attention of the reader only to the most frequently encountered health problems.

Table 1. Distribution of diseases and disorders in Aymara members of the population of the Chilean altiplano, spending most of their lives in the area of residence, by sex.[1]

Disease category	Male		Female		Total	
	N	%	N	%	N	%
Infective, parasitic	15	4.6	10	3.2	25	3.9
Neoplasms	6	1.8	3	1.0	9	1.4
Endocrine, metabolic, nutritional	7	2.2	16	5.1	23	3.6
Blood	-	-	2	0.6	2	0.3
Mental disorders	-	-	-	-	-	-
Nervous system, sense organs	27	8.3	14	4.5	41	6.5
Circulatory system	31	9.6	30	9.6	61	9.6
Respiratory system	66	20.4	66	21.2	132	20.8
Digestive system	14	4.3	20	6.4	34	5.4
Genitourinary system	5	1.6	3	1.0	8	1.3
Pregnancy complications	-	-	-	-	-	-
Skin, subcutaneous tissue	36	11.2	49	15.7	85	13.4
Musculoskeletal, connective tissue	18	5.6	16	5.1	34	5.3
Congenital anomalies	14	4.3	15	4.8	29	4.6
Neonatal disease	-	-	-	-	-	-
Symptoms, ill-defined conditions	75	23.3	64	20.5	139	21.9
Accidents	9	2.8	4	1.3	13	2.0
Total[2]	323	100.0	312	100.0	635	100.0
People examined	227		250		477	

[1]Source: Díaz, et al., 1978, Tables 2a, 2b.
[2]Note that these are diagnoses and not persons; each individual is counted as many times as separate diagnosis occurred.

Table 2. Distribution of diseases and disorders in Aymara members of the population of the Bolivian altiplano, spending most of their lives in the area of residence, by sex.[1]

Disease category	Male		Female		Total	
	N	%	N	%	N	%
Infective, parasitic	23	11.0	24	13.3	47	11.9
Neoplasms	3	1.4	1	0.5	4	1.0
Endocrine, metabolic, nutritional	-	-	4	2.2	4	1.0
Blood	2	0.9	5	2.8	7	1.8
Mental disorders	-	-	-	-	-	-
Nervous system, sense organs	43	20.0	27	15.0	70	17.8
Circulatory system	21	9.8	22	12.2	43	10.9
Respiratory system	27	12.6	16	8.9	43	10.9
Digestive system	16	7.5	17	9.4	33	8.4
Genitourinary system	1	0.5	12	6.7	13	3.3
Pregnancy complications	-	-	2	1.1	2	0.5
Skin, subcutaneous tissue	20	9.2	25	13.9	45	11.4
Musculoskeletal connective tissue	16	7.5	10	5.5	26	6.6
Congenital anomalies	14	6.5	3	1.7	17	4.3
Neonatal disease	-	-	-	-	-	-
Symptoms, ill-defined conditions	24	11.2	12	6.8	36	9.2
Accidents	4	1.9	-	-	4	1.0
Total[2]	214	100.0	180	100.0	394	100.0
People examined		194		191		385

[1]Source: Murillo, et al., 1980, Table 3.
[2]Note that these are diagnoses and not persons; each individual is counted as many times as separate diagnoses occurred.

Inspection of Tables 1 and 2, which illustrate the distribution of disease and disability among the Chilean and Bolivian Aymara living in the altiplano above 3,800 m, reveals a higher prevalence of infectious, parasitic and sense organ diseases in Bolivian Aymara and a higher proportion of respiratory diseases in the Chilean Aymara. Chi-square analysis revealed that both distributions are statistically different ($X^2_{(16)}$=115.9, $p < 0.001$). This finding is not unexpected since the Bolivian and Chilean altiplano are different with respect to altitude, humidity,

Table 3. Distribution of diseases and disorders in Aymara members of the Chilean sierra, spending most of their lives in the area of residence, by sex.[1]

Disease category	Male N	Male %	Female N	Female %	Total N	Total %
Infective, parasitic	4	1.5	13	4.3	17	3.0
Neoplasms	1	0.4	2	0.7	3	0.5
Endocrine, metabolic, nutritional	10	3.8	5	1.6	15	2.6
Blood	-	-	-	-	-	-
Mental disorders	4	1.5	6	1.9	10	1.8
Nervous system, sense organs	21	8.0	25	8.2	46	8.2
Circulatory system	31	11.7	30	9.9	61	10.7
Respiratory system	42	15.9	56	18.4	98	17.2
Digestive system	6	2.3	6	1.9	12	2.1
Genitourinary system	-	-	4	1.3	4	0.7
Pregnancy complications	-	-	-	-	-	-
Skin, subcutaneous tissue	58	22.0	65	21.4	123	21.6
Musculoskeletal, connective tissue	13	4.9	10	3.5	23	4.0
Congenital anomalies	11	4.2	11	3.6	22	3.9
Neonatal disease	-	-	-	-	-	-
Symptoms, ill-defined conditions	53	20.0	67	22.0	120	21.2
Accidents	10	3.8	4	1.3	14	2.5
Total[2]	264	100.0	304	100.0	568	100.0
People examined	184		208		392	

[1]Source: Díaz et al., 1978, Tables 2a, 2b.

[2]Note that these are diagnoses and not persons; each individual is counted as many times as separate diagnoses occurred.

settlement patterns and availability of medical care.

Tables 3 and 4 which exhibit the prevalence for the various pathological conditions in the Chilean lower mountain region and the desert oasis of Toconao respectively, show similar trends to the Chilean sierra and altiplano villages, with the exception of

Table 4. Distribution of diseases and disorders in members of the population of the oasis of Toconao, by sex.

Disease category	Male		Female		Total	
	N	%	N	%	N	%
Infective, parasitic	8	17.0	4	4.7	12	9.1
Neoplasms	-	-	2	2.3	2	1.5
Endocrine, metabolic, nutritional	3	6.4	3	3.6	6	4.5
Blood	-	-	-	-	-	-
Mental disorders	3	6.4	5	5.9	8	6.1
Nervous system, sense organs	5	10.6	14	16.5	19	14.4
Circulatory system	5	10.6	4	4.7	9	6.8
Respiratory system	8	17.0	17	20.0	25	18.9
Digestive system	1	2.2	4	4.7	5	3.8
Genitourinary system	-	-	3	3.6	3	2.3
Pregnancy complications	-	-	-	-	-	-
Skin, subcutaneous tissue	3	6.4	8	9.4	11	8.3
Musculoskeletal connective tissue	3	6.4	7	8.2	10	7.5
Congenital anomalies	-	-	3	3.5	3	2.3
Neonatal disease	-	-	1	1.2	1	0.8
Symptoms, ill-defined conditions	8	17.0	7	8.2	15	11.4
Accidents	-	-	3	3.5	3	2.3
Total[1]	47	100.0	85	100.0	132	100.0
People examined	36		70		106	

[1]Note that these are diagnoses and not persons; each individual is counted as many times as separate diagnoses occurred.

Table 5. Distribution of diseases and disorders in Aymara members of the population of the Chilean coastal valleys of Azapa and Lluta spending most of their lives in the area of residence, by sex.[1]

Disease category	Male		Female		Total	
	N	%	N	%	N	%
Infective, parasitic	6	5.8	6	6.8	12	6.2
Neoplasms	1	0.9	2	2.3	3	1.6
Endocrine, metabolic nutritional	6	5.7	10	11.4	16	8.2
Blood	6	5.7	1	1.2	7	3.6
Mental disorders	-	-	1	1.2	1	0.5
Nervous system, sense organs	7	6.6	1	1.1	8	4.2
Circulatory system	20	18.9	11	12.5	31	16.0
Respiratory system	8	7.5	23	26.1	31	16.0
Digestive system	5	4.7	4	4.5	9	4.6
Genitourinary system	1	0.9	2	2.3	3	1.5
Pregnancy complications	-	-	-	-	-	-
Skin, subcutaneous tissue	11	10.4	11	12.5	22	11.3
Musculoskeletal connective tissue	5	4.7	4	4.5	9	4.6
Congenital anomalies	5	4.7	3	3.4	8	4.2
Neonatal disease	-	-	-	-	-	-
Symptoms, ill-defined conditions	24	22.6	9	10.2	33	17.0
Accidents	1	0.9	-	-	1	0.5
Total[2]	106	100.0	88	100.0	194	100.0
People examined	118		103		221	

[1]Source: Díaz, et al., 1978, Tables 2a, 2b.
[2]Note that these are diagnoses and not persons; each individual is counted as many times as separate diagnoses occurred.

dermatologic pathology, which seems to be more common in the sierra. The desert oasis of Toconao exhibits a higher prevalence of infectious pathology and diseases of the sense organs. In this respect, Toconao is more

Table 6. Distribution of diseases and disorders in the non-Aymara members of the population of the Chilean altiplano and sierra, spending most of their lives in the area of residence, by sex.[1]

Disease category	Male N	Male %	Female N	Female %	Total N	Total %
Infective, parasitic	-	-	-	-	-	-
Neoplasms	-	-	-	-	-	-
Endocrine, metabolic, nutritional	-	-	1	5.3	1	1.9
Blood	-	-	1	5.3	1	1.9
Mental disorders	1	3.0	-	-	1	1.9
Nervous system, sense organs	4	12.1	4	21.0	8	15.4
Circulatory system	6	18.2	1	5.3	7	13.6
Respiratory system	3	9.1	6	31.6	9	17.3
Digestive system	2	6.1	1	5.3	3	5.8
Genitourinary system	-	-	-	-	-	-
Pregnancy complications	-	-	-	-	-	-
Skin, subsutaneous tissue	2	6.1	2	10.5	4	7.7
Musculoskeletal connective tissue	4	12.1	1	5.2	5	9.6
Congenital anomalies	1	3.0	-	-	1	1.9
Neonatal disease	-	-	-	-	-	-
Symptoms, ill-defined conditions	10	30.3	1	5.3	11	21.1
Accidents	-	-	1	5.2	1	1.9
Total[2]	33	100.0	19	100.0	52	100.0
People examined	11		11		23	

[1]Source: Díaz et al., 1978, Table 2c.
[2]Note that these are diagnoses and not persons; each individual is counted as many times as separate diagnoses occurred.

similar to the Bolivian altiplano villages.

Next we turn to a discussion of the findings obtained among the Aymara living in the desert valleys

Table 7. Distribution of diseases and disorders in non-Aymara members of the population of the Chilean coastal valleys of Lluta and Azapa, spending most of their lives in the area of residence, by sex.[1]

Disease category	Male N	Male %	Female N	Female %	Total N	Total %
Infective, parasitic	1	0.9	1	0.9	2	0.9
Neoplasms	2	1.8	1	0.9	3	1.4
Endocrine, metabolic, nutritional	5	4.5	13	12.0	18	8.2
Blood	4	3.6	1	0.9	5	2.3
Mental disorders	2	1.8	3	2.7	5	2.3
Nervous system, sense organs	10	9.0	2	1.8	12	5.5
Circulatory system	24	21.6	30	27.5	54	24.5
Respiratory system	15	13.5	9	8.3	24	10.9
Digestive system	5	4.5	6	5.6	11	5.0
Genitourinary system	3	2.7	1	0.9	4	1.8
Pregnancy complications	-	-	-	-	-	-
Skin, subcutaneous tissue	10	9.0	19	17.4	29	13.2
Musculoskeletal, connective tissue	9	8.2	10	9.2	19	8.6
Congenital anomalies	1	0.9	2	1.8	3	1.4
Neonatal disease	-	-	-	-	-	-
Symptoms, ill-defined conditions	20	18.0	11	10.1	31	14.0
Accidents	-	-	-	-	-	-
Total[2]	111	100.0	109	100.0	220	100.0
People examined	77		92		169	

[1]Source: Díaz et al., 1978, Table 2c.
[2]Note that these are diagnoses and not persons; each individual is counted as many times as separate diagnoses occurred.

of Lluta and Azapa, close to sea level. Table 5 reveals that infectious diseases are slightly less common among the Aymara of the coast. However, the most relevant finding is that circulatory diseases are less frequent among the Aymara and Atacamenos living at higher altitudes than on the coast. The Atacameno village of Toconao shows the lowest prevalence of circulatory diseases. It should be noted, however, that in this village the assessment of cardiovascular health was made by a generalist not a cardiologist and electrocardiographic testing was not available.

In summary, in the middle and upper altitude Indian villages we find a slightly higher prevalence of respiratory diseases, with the exception of the Bolivian villages, and a lower prevalence of circulatory pathology. If we compute chi-square statistics between each of the five middle and high altitude Indian samples and the pooled observations we find $X^2_{(16)} = 328.1$, $p < 0.001$.

It seems of interest to find out if the tendencies observed among the Aymara are also present among the non-Aymara. In fact, Tables 6 and 7 show that the non-Aymara living on the coast exhibit a higher percentage of circulatory pathology and a lower prevalence of respiratory diseases. The difference is, however, not statistically significant ($X^2_{(16)} = 20.5$, $p > 0.20$). When comparing non-Aymara with Aymara living in the coastal valleys, it is noteworthy that the Aymara exhibit less circulatory and more respiratory pathology.

Focusing now on blood pressure, we find no important differences in acute hypertension between the Aymara of the altiplano, the sierra and the coast. Curiously, however, males are less affected by acute hypertension on the altiplano than on the coast; whereas females exhibit the opposite tendency (Table 8). The coastal Aymara show a higher prevalence of borderline hypertension, in contrast with the Aymara of the sierra and altiplano. Turning now to the non-Aymara, (Table 9), we observe less acute hypertension among the sierra and altiplano residents, and no difference in borderline hypertension.

The disorders discussed so far are either on the non-genetic extreme of the spectrum of diseases, as for example infections, or somewhere in the middle, e.g. cardiovascular problems. We presume that con-

Table 8. Distribution of diseases and disorders of the circulatory system in Aymara members spending most of their lives in the area of residence designated, by sex.[1]

Circulatory system disease	Coast				Sierra				Altiplano			
	Male		Female		Male		Female		Male		Female	
	N	%	N	%	N	%	N	%	N	%	N	%
Arterial hypertension ($\geq$160/95)	1	5.0	2	18.2	2	6.5	5	16.7	6	11.5	4	7.7
Borderline hypertension ($\geq$140/90)	7	35.0	3	27.3	5	16.1	6	20.0	12	23.1	15	28.8
Acute myocardial infarction	-	-	-	-	-	-	-	-	-	-	-	-
Other ischemic heart disease	-	-	-	-	-	-	1	3.3	3	5.8	1	1.9
All other heart disease	11	55.0	6	54.5	17	54.8	9	30.0	25	48.1	20	38.5
Cerebrovascular disease	-	-	-	-	1	3.2	-	-	-	-	-	-
All other circulatory disease	1	5.0	-	-	6	19.4	9	30.0	6	11.5	12	23.1
Total	20	100.0	11	100.0	31	100.0	30	100.0	52	100.0	52	100.0

[1]Source: Díaz et al., 1978, Table 2a, 2b and Murillo et al., 1980, Table 3.

Table 9. Distribution of diseases and disorders of the circulatory system in non-Aymara members spending most of their lives in the area of residence designated, by sex.[1]

Circulatory system disease	Coast Male N	Coast Male %	Coast Female N	Coast Female %	Coast Total N	Coast Total %	Sierra and Altiplano Male N	Sierra and Altiplano Male %	Sierra and Altiplano Female N	Sierra and Altiplano Female %	Sierra and Altiplano Total N	Sierra and Altiplano Total %
Arterial hypertension (≥160/95)	3	12.5	9	30.0	12	22.2	1	16.7	-	-	1	14.3
Borderline hypertension (140/90)	9	37.5	7	23.3	16	29.6	1	16.7	1	100.0	2	28.6
Acute myocardial infarction	-	-	-	-	-	-	-	-	-	-	-	-
Other ischemic heart disease	-	-	1	3.3	1	1.9	-	-	-	-	-	-
All other heart disease	9	37.5	7	23.0	15	27.8	-	-	-	-	-	-
Cerebrovascular disease	-	-	-	-	-	-	-	-	-	-	-	-
All other circulatory disease	3	12.5	6	23.3	10	18.5	4	66.6	-	-	4	57.1
Total	24	100.0	30	100.0	54	100.0	6	100.0	1	100.0	4	100.0

[1]Source: Díaz et al., 1978, Table c and Murillo et al., 1980, Table 3.

genital anomalies are closer to the genetic extreme. The anomalies exhibit similar prevalence in different altitudes among Aymara and non-Aymara subjects.

VALIDITY OF THE RESULTS AND CONCLUSIONS

First of all, it seems important to identify how representative our findings may be. As a consequence of the sampling procedures, we would expect to have examined most of the children in the fifteen villages represented in the study and probably a significant proportion of the adult population as well. This latter statement is particularly true for the Chilean villages where we have examined more than 70% of the ostensible censused population. One tends to assume that some individuals may have been physically unable to present themselves at our field stations and that therefore some pathological conditions may be underrepresented. However, since we remained more than three days in each village and the inhabitants knew of our presence there, in many instances they asked us to visit the acutely ill in their dwellings.

Three different but overlapping medical teams conducted the physical examinations in Chile and Bolivia. Given the subjectivity of the concept of morbidity, one tends to believe that some of the discrepancies observed are the consequence of different diagnostic criteria. We attempted to avoid this source of bias as much as possible by asking our physicians to follow a Reference Manual which was prepared <u>ex profeso</u> for the field studies.

It is noteworthy that the Aymara and Atacameno Indian populations of the villages located above 2,500 m exhibit a higher prevalence of infective, respiratory and sense organ diseases. We presume that these disorders are mostly due to the rigors of life inherent to high altitude ecogeographic habitats. On the other hand, low altitude Aymara speaking residents exhibit a higher prevalence of circulatory system disorders, especially borderline hypertension, than middle and high altitude Indian dwellers. Makela et al. (1978) have shown that systolic and diastolic blood pressure are significantly correlated with

Quetelet's Index (ratio weight/height^2) in our Aymara subjects across the Chilean altitudinal gradient, excluding those individuals diagnosed as hypertensive, i.e., systolic pressure greater than 160 mm Hg and / or diastolic pressure greater than 95 mm Hg. It is therefore conceivable that the differences we are observing are an indirect consequence of altitude and more directly related to relative weight or adiposity. The higher relative weight may, in turn, be explained by different occupational, living or nutritional habits.

When comparing the non-Aymara subjects residing above 3,000 m with those living on the coast, we observe a similar tendency. Altitude dwellers present a lower prevalence of circulatory system affections and higher rates of respiratory and infectious diseases, than coastal valley residents. A further comparison can be made between the Aymara and non-Aymara coastal valley inhabitants. Notably, the non-Aymara exhibit a higher prevalence of circulatory diseases, especially acute hypertension.

Concluding, Aymara speaking individuals tend to exhibit more respiratory diseases when living in the coastal valleys than non-Aymara individuals. Conversely, the Aymara tend to exhibit a lower prevalence of circulatory diseases at high and low altitude. This last finding may imply, provided that Aymara and non-Aymara have similar lifestyles and nutritional habits in the various regions, that ethnic factors play a role in the difference observed, particularly since it is known that genetic factors contribute to the variation in blood pressure among relatives (Cruz-Coke, 1981; Smith and Sing, 1977). In this context, it is of interest to compare the prevalence of circulatory diseases in the Aymara with that in a Caucasian rural community located at 1,000 m in the coastal mountain range of central Chile. Historic information reveals that Caleu has never been inhabited by Indians and was founded in 1550 by the Spanish attracted to the gold-bearing sands of a stream. Cruz-Coke (1962) examined without the aid of electrocardiograms the total population of the village, numbering 436 inhabitants, and found 14.1% had circulatory diseases. This author further subdivided the population of Caleu into natives and outsiders and detected prevalences of circulatory disorders of 10.1 and 23.8%, respectively. The prevalence among the Caleu natives is similar to the one exhibited by the Aymara at high altitude and the proportion of outsiders manifesting circulatory diseases is similar to the figures observed among non-Aymara living on the coastal valleys.

Even if we adjust these figures upward because the diagnoses were made without the aid of electrocardiograms, it turns out that the Caleu Caucasian natives still exhibit comparable proportions of circulatory diseases with the coastal Aymara and the Caleu outsiders, with the coastal non-Aymara. These findings are difficult to decipher, but they seem to indicate that the Aymara do no present unusually low figures of cardiovascular disease and that newcomers to an ecogeographic area present a higher risk of these diseases. This may be true for the Caleu outsiders and the Azapa valley non-Aymara.

We hesitate to resort to ethnic differences in susceptibility to explain our general findings. We suggest rather that the differences in circulatory system maladies observed among natives and outsiders, as well as Indian and non-Indian populations residing at different altitudes is due to distinct nutritional, occupational and living habits, as well as socio-economic factors which impinge on health care. This conclusion is in agreement with our previous results (Makela et al., 1978; Díaz et al., 1978; Murillo et al., 1980) and does not support the assertion that hypoxia protects directly against cardiovascular diseases.

ACKNOWLEDGEMENTS

This work was supported by NIH grant HL-15614, Proyecto 0339 from the Fondo Nacional de Ciencias, Conicyt-Chile B-518845F from the Direccion Desarollo de la Investigacion, University of Chile and a Deutsche Forschungsgemeinschaft-Conicyt Binational Research Program.

We are indebted to our examinees, to the members of our field teams and to numerous persons and institutions at the local levels in Chile and Bolivia. We are also grateful to Drs. Erika Taucher and Emöke J.E. Szathmary for a critical review of this article.

LITERATURE CITED

Baker P (1969). Human adaptation to high altitudes. Science 163:1149.

Barton S, Lenart V, Palomino H, Murillo F, Weidman W, Schull WJ (1976). High altitude, indigenous origin, and continuous cardiac monitoring. Aviat Space Environ Med 47:592.

Bennett WC, Bird J (1964). "Andean Culture History. Garden City." New York: The Natural History Press.

Buck A, Sadaki T, Anderson R (1968). "Health and Disease in Four Peruvian Villages: Contrasts in Epidemiology." Baltimore, Md: Johns Hopkins Press.

Castillo S, Rothhammer F, Goedde HW (1984) Algunos indices de salud de indios Atacameños. Rev Med Chile (in press).

Cruz-Coke R (1962). Medicina, enfermedad y miseria. Rev Med Chile 90:534.

Cruz-Coke R (1981). Etiology of essential hypertension. Hypertension 3(Suppl II):191.

Díaz B, Gallegos D, Murillo F, Covarrubias E, Covarrubias T, Rona R, Weidman W, Rothhammer F, Schull WJ (1978). The multinational Andean genetic and health program: II. Disease and disability among the Aymara. Bull Pan Amer Hlth Organ 12:219.

Ferrell RE, Bertin T, Barton SA, Young R, Murillo F, Schull WJ (1978). The Aymara of western Bolivia. IV. Gene frequencies for 8 blood groups and 20 serum protein and erythrocyte enzyme systems. Am J Hum Genet 30:539.

Ferrell RE, Bertin T, Barton SA, Rothhammer F, Schull WJ (1980). A multinational Andean genetic and health program. IX. Gene frequencies and rare variants of 20 serum protein and erythrocyte enzyme systems in the Aymara of Chile. Am J Hum Genet 32:92.

Fladmark KR (1982). Le peuplement de l'Amerique. La Recherche 137:1110.

Goedde HW, Rothhammer F, Benkmann HG, Bogdanski P (1984a). Genetic response to drugs and environmental

agents in Atacameño Indians. Hum Genet (in press).
Goedde HW, Rothhammer F, Benkmann HG, Bogdanski P (1984b). Erythrocyte enzymes and serum proteins of Atacameño Indians. Ann Hum Biol (submitted).
Goldsmith RI, Rothhammer F, Schull WJ (1977). Mydriasis and heredity. Clin Genet 12:128.
Hurtado A, Velasquez Y, Reynafarje C, Lozano R, Chavez R, Salazar H, Reynafarje B, Sanchez C, Munoz J (1956). Mechanisms of Natural Acclimatization. San Antonio, Tx: School of Aviation Medicine, U.S. Air Force, Randolph Air Force Base, Report 56-1.
Hurtado A (1960). Some clinical aspects of life at high altitudes. Ann Int Med 53:247.
International Classification of Diseases, (1968). Adapted for Use in the United States, 8th Revision, Public Health Service Publ No 1693. Washington, DC: Superintendent of Documents, US Government Printing Office.
Makela M, Barton SA, Schull WJ, Rothhammer F (1978). The multinational Andean genetic and health program. IV. Altitude and the blood pressure of the of the Aymara. J Chron Dis 31:587.
Mueller WH, Schull VN, Schull WJ, Soto P, Rothhammer F (1978). A multinational Andean genetic and health program: V. Growth and development in an hypoxic environment. Ann Hum Biol 5:329.
Murillo F, Barton SA, Palomino H, Lenart V, Schull WJ (1980). The Aymara of western Bolivia: Health and disease. Bull Pan Amer Hlth Organ 14:52.
Palomino H, Barton SA, Murillo F, Schull WJ (1978). The Aymara of western Bolivia: II. Maxillofacial and dental arch variation. Am J Phys Anthrop 49:157.
Penaloza D, Sime F, Bancher N, Gamboa R, Cruz J, Marticorena E (1963). Pulmonary hypertension in healthy men born and living at high altitudes. Am J Cardiol 11:150.
Rothhammer F, Cocilovo, JA, Quevedo S, Llop E (1982). Microevolution in prehistoric Andean populations: I. Chronologic craniometric variation. Am J Phys Anthrop 58:391.
Rothhammer F, Goedde HW, Llop E, Acuña M, Carvajal P (1984). Erythrocyte and HLA antigens of Atacameño Indians. Am J Phys Anthrop 65:243.
Rotta A (1947). Physiologic condition of the heart in the natives of high altitude. Am Heart J 33:669.

Schull WJ, Rothhammer F (1977). A multinational Andean genetic and health program: A study of adaptation to the hypoxia of altitude. In Weiner JS (ed): "Physiological Variation and its Genetic Basis," Society for the Study of Human Biology, Vol 17, London: Taylor and Francis, p 139.

Schull WJ, Ferrell RE, Rothhammer F (1979). Genes, enzymes and hypoxia. In Brussard P (ed): "Ecological Genetics, Proceedings in the Life Sciences," New York: Springer-Verlag, p 73.

Schull WJ, Rothhammer F (1979). Analytical methods for genetic and adaptational studies. In Laughlin WS, Harper A (eds): "The First Americans: Origins, Affinities and Adaptations," New York: G. Fischer, p 241.

Smith DG, Sing CF (1977). Genetic environmental interactions in the variation of blood pressure in Tecumseh, Michigan. J Chron Dis 30:781.

Veloso A, Kalin-Arroyo M (1982). Caracteristicas del medio fisico. In Veloso A, Bustos-Obregon E (eds): "El Ambiente Natural y las Poblaciones Humanas de los Andes del Norte Grande de Chile," Vol 1, Santiago, Chile: Universidad de Chile, p 5.

Zapata B, Marticorena E (1968). Presion arterial sistemica en el individuo senil de altura. Arch Inst Biol Andina 2:220.

Diseases of Complex Etiology in Small Populations:
Ethnic Differences and Research Approaches, pages 345–365

Chapter 15

PHYSICAL ENVIRONMENTAL, SOCIOCULTURAL AND ETHNIC CORRELATES OF HUMAN BIOLOGY IN SOME POPULATIONS OF WEST BENGAL, INDIA AND NEIGHBORING REGIONS: MORTALITY DIFFERENTIALS

A. Basu, R. Gupta, P. Bharati,
B. Mukhopadhyay, and S.K. Roy

Human Adaptability Program, Biological Sciences Division, Indian Statistical Institute, Calcutta, India

INTRODUCTION

A multidisciplinary study program on the nature and extent of adaptation of human populations to various environmental stresses was initiated under the general title of Human Adaptability Program in the Indian Statistical Institute in early 1976. The short-term objective of the program was to identify and measure (1) the impacts of three sets of factors, namely physical environmental, sociocultural and ethnic/genetic, on health; and (2) the impacts of human health and activity patterns on environment. These arose from recommendations of the IBP/HA panel (Weiner, 1969) and UNESCO/MAB program (UNESCO, 1973). The long-term objective was to determine the limits to human adaptation. The latter were defined as follows: (1) lower limit - the quantum of stress(es), single or multiple (and if multiple, of their interaction effects), beyond which survival at the population level was no longer possible; and (2) upper limit - the quantum of withdrawal/absence of stress(es) and/or presence of favorable stimulus(i) beyond which the chances of survival and well-being did not improve.

"Well-being" was defined as a state of harmonious relationship with physical, biological and sociocultural environments, and the "feeling of satisfaction" derived from this. "Health" was defined narrowly in terms of physical well-being and lack of disease and infirmity, although we are aware of WHO's

(1971) broader definition that includes complete physical, mental and social well-being. Health was assessed with such parameters as mortality, adult body dimensions, child growth, hematological status, intestinal parasitic prevalences, and disease patterns. The measures of ill health used in this presentation are simply infant and adolescent mortalities, on the assumption that death denotes complete lack of well-being – physical, mental, and social.

The Human Adaptability program started with a study of the impact of altitude on the health-related parameters mentioned above following the standard method, suggested by the IBP/HA panel (Weiner, 1969) and modified by Baker and Dutt (1972). A native high altitude population with its migrant counterparts in lower altitudes, in this case the Sherpas of Upper Khumbu, Nepal (above 3000m), and their lower altitude migrant counterparts in the Kalimpong subdivision (1500-2000m), Darjeeling district, West Bengal, India were compared. By "altitude" we meant a set of physical environmental stresses, for example, hypoxia, cold, and terrain.

Differences were found between the high and low altitude Sherpas in fertility, adult body dimensions, child growth measurements, and hematological traits. However, the nature of some of these differences were unlike those seen in other studies, and differences were not found in other traits. It was felt that there was a logical fallacy in ascribing the differences that were found to altitude-related physical environmental stresses, because it could not be ruled out that such differences arose from the impacts of concomitant sociocultural stresses. It was noted that there were two major differences between human and experimental animal population studies, from which the initial impetus for high altitude human biological studies was drawn: (1) while in animal studies all conditions except the one that was to be studied could be made similar between the high and low altitude subgroups, such standardization could hardly be achieved in human studies; and (2) the vast domain of the sociocultural environment which virtually did not exist in animal studies might act in addition to, or even override the effect of, physical environmental stresses in human studies.

Altitudinal differences between subpopulations of the same population in mortality have been found in both animal and human populations. Generally, high altitude subgroups have higher mortality (Dutt, 1980; Grahn and Kratchman, 1963; Harrison et al., 1969; Mazess, 1965). However, there are exceptions, suggesting that the high altitude physical environmental stress effects (e.g., hypoxic effects) on pre- or post-natal mortality are neither inevitable nor universal (Baker, 1978; Baker and Dutt, 1972; Way, 1976).

In view of this, the purposes of this presentation are (1) to consider some data from Himalayan populations to detect altitudinal variations, if any, in mortality in this region; (2) to investigate whether altitudinal variations, if any, in mortality are necessarily due to high altitude physical environmental stresses, or to concomitant sociocultural ones (that is, can the latter be ruled out?); (3) if the latter cannot be ruled out, to assess the possible effects of sociocultural factors independent of altitude; and (4) thereby, to address ourselves to the basic question: "is altitude a specialized environment at all in the human case?".

MATERIALS AND METHODS

Research Design

Populations were studied in the sub-Himalayan and deltaic zones. In the sub-Himalayan zone, infant and adolescent mortality rates were compared between the high and low altitude Sherpas of Upper Khumbu, Nepal and Kalimpong subdivision, northern West Bengal, respectively to detect the effects of altitude-related physical environmental factors. Comparisons were also made between Buddhist and Christian subgroups of the Lepchas and among occupational subgroups of the Sherpas, and between Sherpas and Lepchas inhabiting similar altitudes of Kalimpong subdivisions and practicing similar occupations, to detect the effects

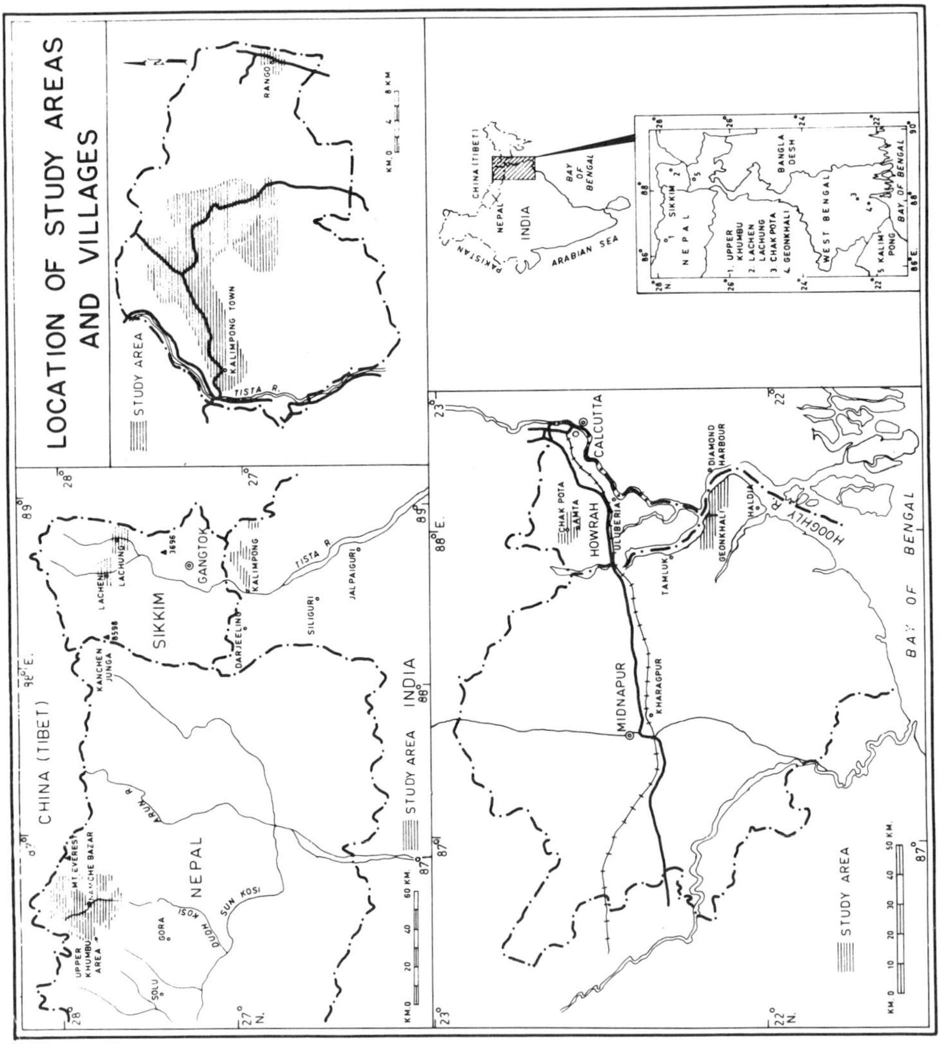
LOCATION OF STUDY AREAS AND VILLAGES
CHINA (TIBET)
NEPAL
SIKKIM
INDIA
STUDY AREA
UPPER KHUMBU AREA
MT EVEREST
NAMCHE BAZAR
GORA
SOLU
DUDH KOSI
SUN KOSI
ARUN R.
KANCHEN JUNGA
LACHEN
LACHUNG
GANGTOK
KALIMPONG
DARJEELING
SILIGURI
JALPAIGURI
TISTA R.
KALIMPONG TOWN
RANGO
CALCUTTA
HOWRAH
CHAK POTA
AMTA
ULUBERIA
DIAMOND HARBOUR
GEONKHALI
HALDIA
TAMLUK
KHARAGPUR
MIDNAPUR
HOOGHLY R.
BAY OF BENGAL
ARABIAN SEA
PAKISTAN
BANGLA DESH
WEST BENGAL
1. UPPER KHUMBU
2. LACHEN LACHUNG
3. CHAK POTA
4. GEONKHALI
5. KALIMPONG

Figure 1. Map.

of sociocultural and ethnic factors, respectively. In the same zone, comparison was also made between two mountain populations of northern Sikkim, both belonging to the same ethnic group, Bhutia, and inhabiting similar altitudes, but exposed periodically to different physical environmental and/or sociocultural factors because of their differential transhumance practices. In the deltaic zone, comparisons were made among Christian, Hindu and Muslim populations of neighboring villages of the Geonkhali area, Tamluk subdivision, southern West Bengal and subgroups of one Hindu caste group to detect the effects of cultural factors related to religion. The economic subgroups of the the population of a single village of the Uluberia subdivision, southern West Bengal were also compared to detect the effects of micro-economic conditions. Locations of the study areas are shown in Figure 1.

Population Description

The Sherpas of Upper Khumbu are an offshoot of the larger Tibetan population which migrated from eastern Tibet to their present habitat (above 3000m) around 1533 AD (Haimendorf, 1964; Oppitz, 1974). These Sherpas still speak a Tibetan dialect and follow the Tibetan sect of Buddhism. In the past, they practiced potato and yam cultivation/yak breeding and trade with Tibet, but with closure of the border with Tibet and development of tourism and mountaineering they have changed to a cash economy, working as tourist guides and high altitude porters (Haimendorf, 1964). They eat a cereal-dominated diet, live in poorly ventilated houses, suffer from high intestinal parasitic infestations and iodine deficiency (Hirai et al., 1975; Lang and Lang, 1971; Sacherer, 1974). Their cash earnings are variable and generally restricted to tourist seasons and much of them are spent on expensive consumer goods (Sacherer, 1974), so that they end up with an overall low standard of living. The Sherpas of Kalimpong migrated from Upper Khumbu to their present habitat (1500-2000m) about 200 years ago (Gupta, 1980). They have variable occupations with one cluster of settlements practicing agriculture, another plantation labor and yet another wood cutting-cum-selling and other forest-based activities. They eat variable high meat-milk-vegetables to high cereal diets, live in houses having variable hygienic standards, suffer from high intestinal parasitic infestations (Bhattacharya, 1980; Bhattacharya et al., 1981) and generally have variable standards of living.

The Lepchas are generally believed to be indigenous to the medium altitudes of Sikkim-Darjeeling Himalaya. They generally practice agriculture, often inhabit (in the Kalimpong region) villages adjacent to those inhabited by the Sherpas, eat more cereal-dominated diets that the Sherpas do, and mostly live in rather unhygienic houses and suffer from high intestinal parasitic infestations as in the case of Sherpas (Bhattacharya et al., 1981). Unlike in the case of Sherpas, a large proportion of the Lepchas profess Christianity. The Sherpas of Rango Medicinal Plantation, Government of West Bengal live at the same altitude as the Lepchas. These Sherpas work as wage laborers in the plantation, live in its unhygienic colonies at about 1500m, eat cereal-dominated diets and suffer from heavy intestinal parasitic infestations (Bhattacharya et al., 1981).

The two highest altitude villages in northern Sikkim (Lachen, 2600m; Lachung, 2300m) are both inhabited by Bhutia. These people belong to the Tibetan sect of Buddhism and eat mainly cereal-dominated diets. One group, the Lachen-pa, migrates seasonally to still higher altitudes, spending four to five months a year at this altitude for potato cultivation. The other group, the Lachung-pa, migrates to much lower altitudes and spends about the same length of time there for maize cultivation. Both groups are therefore recurrently exposed to different physical environmental and/or sociocultural factors.

The Mirpurians (Christian) claim to have descended from twelve Portuguese gunners, who settled down in the Geonkhali area of southern West Bengal and founded their village in the mid/late 1700s. The wives of these gunners were local to this area. The Mirpurians are mainly, but not exclusively, agriculturists. Their dietary status varies considerably with the average household's protein-calorie intake being lower than the recommended allowances made by the Indian Council of Medical Research (Basu et al., 1980). Housing conditions also vary considerably, intestinal parasitic infestations are high (Bhattacharya, 1980; Bhattacharya et al., 1981) and the standard of living is generally low. The Namasudras (Hindu) are a numerically dominant caste of West Bengal, the majority of which are landless agricultural laborers (Risley, 1891). The Namasudras of Balaramchak, like anywhere else, seemingly have a poor standard of living. The Mahishya (Hindu) is a traditionally agricultural and numerically dominant caste of deltaic West Bengal (O'Malley and Chakravarti, 1909). The Mahishyas of Gopalchak and Bamanchak primarily practice their traditional occupation, but a relatively greater number of individuals in Bamanchak have other occupations, for example teaching, other services, and business. These individuals have urban contact, seemingly are economically better off and have a higher standard of living. The Muslims of this region are, impressionistically, quite similar to their Hindu neighbors, particularly the Namasudras, in economic condition and standard of living.

The Mahishyas of Chakpota are primarily agriculturists, but as in Bamanchak many of them have other occupations. Most have high intestinal parasitic infestations (Bhattacharya et al., 1984) and their dietary status, economic conditions and standard of living are variable.

Data Collected

The number of households surveyed is given in Table 1. The following demographic data were collected using questionnaires. Age, sex, marital status, and birthplace of all household members were obtained from household heads. Individual reproductive performance, namely, the number of live births, dead children and reproductive wastages were obtained from married women. No statistical sampling procedure could be followed in the field. Difficulties were encountered in the assessment of age as there was no birth registration, or other types of written records available. Age was therefore estimated with the help of traditional calendars in populations in which these existed, or by reference to important local events, in others. The Chakpota Mahishya population was also classified into three economic subgroups using as cut-off points the conventional "poverty line" of Rs.50.00 (US $5.00 approximately) and the locally defined "sufficiency line" of Rs.100.00 (US $10.00 approximately) representing monthly per capita income. All information was cross checked from several sources and on subsequent visits.

Table 1. Number of households surveyed by population/religion.

Area/village/ subgroup	Population/ religion	No. of households
Upper Khumbu	Sherpa	110
Kalimpong	Sherpa	250
Agri. lab.	Sherpa	50
Plantation lab.	Sherpa	59
Forest lab.	Sherpa	141
Kalimpong	Buddhist Lepcha	53
Kalimpong	Christian Lepcha	105
Rango	Sherpa	53
Lachung	Bhutia	96
Lachen	Bhutia	37
Mirpur	Mixed Portuguese-Bengali (Christian)	56
Gopalchak	Mahishya	115
Bamanchak	Mahishya	150
Balaramchak	Namasudra	89
Balaramchak	Muslim	72
Balaramchak Tantipara	Muslim	26
Barchand Patra	Namasudra	119
Chakpota	Mahishya	255
Low econ. subgroup	Mahishya	80
Med. econ. subgroup	Mahishya	108
High econ. subgroup	Mahishya	67

The data on infant mortality rate (IMR) and adolescent mortality rate (AMR) are presented in this paper.

RESULTS AND DISCUSSION

The data presented in Table 2 show that contrary to expectation generated by animal experiments, as well as some Andean human population studies, there is no significant differences in IMR between high and low altitude Sherpas of Upper Khumbu and Kalimpong, respectively. This suggests that altitude-related physical environmental effects on mortality are not detectable in this case. On the other hand, among the groups inhabiting similar altitudes, the pooled Kalimpong Sherpa sample does differ significantly from the remote Rango Sherpa sample in IMR as does the Buddhist Lepcha sample (Kalimpong urban area) from the Christian Lepcha sample from the same area. These findings suggest detectable effects of urban nearness/contact in the case of the Sherpas, and educational, economic, and other factors associated with religion in the case of the Lepchas. The differences between Sherpas and Buddhist Lepchas of the same Kalimpong habitat suggests that ethnic factors which may be sociocultural and/or genetic in nature may also have important effects.

The Lachen and Lachung populations in north Sikkim provide an interesting demonstration of how physical environmental and sociocultural factors may get intertwined. For instance, the Lachen-pas' periodic visits for potato cultivation to a high altitude area at about 4000m are culturally determined but they in their turn lead to recurrent exposure of the people to high altitude physical environmental stresses. On the other hand, the Lachung-pas' periodic visits for maize cultivation to a lower altitude area at about 1500m, that is also culturally determined, lead to their recurrent exposures to a much milder physical environment. The point to note here is that even if the mortality differences between Lachen and Lachung are determined by the different physical environmental stresses associated with their temporary habitats at 4000 and 1500m, respectively, exposures to these differential physical environmental stresses are themselves determined by the sociocultural factor of differential transhumance pattern. Accordingly, the idea of distinguishing between physical environmental, and sociocultural stress effects, which remain inextricably intertwined in this situation, becomes meaningless. Distinguishing among the effects of different sociocultural factors is also a problem. For example, IMR does not differ significantly among the agricultural laborer, plantation laborer and forest economy-practicing subgroups of the low altitude Kalimpong Sherpas (Table 3). This suggests that sociocultural factors that may differ among these subgroups do not have any detectable effects on mortality in this case.

Table 2. Infant and adolescent mortalities by population/religion:Mountain zone.

Area	Population/ religion	No. of live births	IMR (%)	AMR (%)
Upper Khumbu	Sherpa	33	7.2	13.2
Kalimpong	Sherpa	1186	6.6	17.1
Kalimpong	Buddhist Lepcha	240	11.7	22.9
Kalimpong	Christian Lepcha	517	3.5	10.1
Rango	Sherpa	253	13.8	24.5
Lachung	Bhutia	354	7.6	14.7
Lachen	Bhutia	94	22.3	39.4

Binomial test for equality of proportions (Test statistic, $T_1 + T_2$):

Comparison	IMR	AMR
Up.Kh.Sh. vs. KPG Sh.	0.006±0.016	0.039±0.023
KPG SH. vs. Rango Sh.	0.073±0.019*	0.074±0.030*
KPG Ch.Lep. vs. KPG Bu.Lep.	0.231±0.035*	0.129±0.027*
Lachung Bh. vs. Lachen Bh.	0.147±0.036*	0.247±0.046*

*Significant at the 5% level.

Thus, while there are no detectable effects of

high altitude physical environmental factors on IMR, effects of sociocultural and/or ethnic factors are demonstrated in these mountain-dwelling populations residing between 1500m and 2600m, one of them being exposed to the high altitude environment at 4000m for a large part of the year. Therefore, the possibility of sociocultural factors operating even in high altitude populations cannot be ruled out. Claimed "altitudinal" differences in mortality in reality may be attributed to "concomitant sociocultural" differences.

Table 3. Infant and adolescent mortalities by occupational groups:Sherpa.

Occupational group	No. of live births	IMR (%)	AMR (%)
Agriculture practicing	181	6.1	14.9
Plantation labor	279	6.8	17.9
Forest labor	726	6.6	17.4

Binomial test for equality of proportions (Test statistic, $T_1 + T_2$):

Comparison	IMR	AMR
KPG Ag.Sh. vs. KPG Pl.Sh.	0.007±0.024	0.030±0.035
KPG Pl.Sh. vs. KPG Fo.Sh.	0.002±0.018	0.006±0.027
KPG Ag.Sh. vs. KPG Fo.Sh.	0.005±0.019	0.024±0.031

Note:The test results were non-significant.

Sociocultural and ethnic effects on mortality independent of altitude are shown in Table 4. The significant Mirpur Christian vs pooled Hindu, and Mirpur Christian vs pooled Muslim, differences in the Geonkhali area further confirm the effects of ethnic and/or sociocultural factors. Furthermore the significant Low vs Medium, and Low vs High, differences between the economic subgroups of the population of Chakpota village (Table 5), suggest that economic differences within the same micro-region/village/population exposed to very similar physical environmental as well as, in the latter case, traditional caste-related-sociocultural characteristics, but differing in micro-sociocultural including micro-economic characteristics, may also have considerable effects.

Table 4. Infant and adolescent mortalities by population/religion:Deltaic zone.

Village	Population/ religion	No.of live births	IMR (%)	AMR (%)
Mirpur	Mixed Port.-Beng.(Christian)	325	6.2	12.9
Gopalchak	Mahishya	579	12.9	21.8
Bamanchak	Mahishya	913	13.3	21.9
Balaramchak	Namasudra	485	13.4	23.5
Balaramchak	Muslim	462	12.9	19.0
Balaramchak Tantipara	Muslim	200	15.0	30.5
Barchand Patra	Namasudra	775	14.2	23.4

Binomial test for equality of proportions (Test statistic, $T_1 + T_2$):

Comparison	IMR	AMR
Mir.Ch. vs. Pooled Hin.	0.073±0.020*	0.096±0.024*
Mir.Ch. vs. Pooled Mus.	0.074±0.021*	0.096±0.027*
Pooled Hin. vs. Pooled Mus.	0.001±0.015	0.001±0.018

*Significant at the 5% level.

Differences in AMR are generally analagous in nature to those in IMR. Adolescent mortality rates are greater in magnitude than infant mortality rates, presumably because duration of exposure to the stresses (whatever the nature of the stresses) is longer and consequently their cumulative effects more severe by adolescence.

Overall then, while the effects of altitude-related physical environmental factors on mortality are not demonstrated from our data, the effects of sociocultural factors even of small magnitudes, are clearly demonstrated in our data from two contrasting ecological zones, except in the case of Kalimpong Sherpa occupational subgroups. Further, the ethnic differences that are shown may also be due to sociocultural factors. However, the present data do not permit elimination of possible genetic effects on mortality, so that interpretation of the causes of the observed ethnic differences should best be reserved at this stage.

Table 5. Infant and adolescent mortalities by economic subgroup: Chakpota.

Economic subgroup	No. of live births	IMR (%)	AMR (%)
Low economic	462	14.7	23.2
Medium economic	811	10.5	16.0
High economic	439	8.4	14.4

Binomial test for equality of proportions (Test statistic, $T_1 + T_2$):

Comparison	IMR	AMR
Low vs. medium	0.042±0.020*	0.071±0.022*
Low vs. high	0.063±0.020*	0.088±0.027*
Medium vs. high	0.020±0.017	0.017±0.022

*Significant at the 5% level.

Lack of universality of altitude effects on human biological traits is also borne out by other types of data on the Sherpas. For instance, adult body dimensions are larger among the high altitude Sherpas than among the low altitude ones (Gupta and Basu, 1981), while in most animal experiments as well as some Andean human studies adult body dimensions are smaller in the high altitudes. The high and low altitude Sherpa physical growth curves are very similar for many measurements (for example, height, weight). For other traits, while curves are lower and the adolescent growth spurt is lacking in the high altitude sample, differences between the high and low altitude curves are smaller than in other studies (Frisancho, 1978). Lastly, for yet other traits the altitudinal differences in growth curves do not seem to follow any definite pattern. In hematological parameters, the high altitude Sherpas do have higher values, as in the case of other studies, but the differences in magnitude between high and low altitude Sherpas is much smaller than in others. Occupational subgroups of the Kalimpong Sherpas do not differ significantly thereby ruling out socioeconomic effects, but the Lepcha-Sherpa differences (male: Sherpa > Lepcha; female:Sherpa < Lepcha) may indicate interesting socioculturally determined ethnic effects. Among the Lepchas, for example, social norms demand that females get the largest share of the available food. No such norms exist among the Sherpas (Basu et al., 1984b). Such sex differential dietary intake norms may be reflected in the sex differential patterns of Sherpa-Lepcha difference in hematological parameters (Gupta et al., 1983).

Absence of universality of altitude effects is also demonstrated by other studies. For instance, Goldstein et al. (1983) have shown that in some high altitude Himalayan populations fertility is as high as in many low altitude populations instead of being lower. They have questioned the very concept of fertility reduction due to the effects of altitude-related physical environmental traits. Basu and Gupta (1984) generally subscribe to this view, although not as emphatically, despite Goldstein et al.'s (1983) scathing, if largely unfounded, criticism of Gupta's (1980) earlier study. Conspicuous lack of evidence of altitude effects on fertility in Himalayan populations has also been indicated by Basu et al. (1984a). Harrison et al. (1969) have shown that fertility is higher and mortality lower in higher altitudes in the Simien mountains, unlike the physiological expectation. Mueller et al. (1981) who studied children in three altitude zones in the Andes observed that "Presumably the differences in illness incidence and mortality rates due to different causes relates to sociocultural factors, geographical isolation, access to medical care, nutrition, and other undetermined factors related to living at high altitudes rather than to (altitude related) physiological changes per se" (p. 69).

That altitude may not have any uniform or universal effect on mortality is also apparent from macrolevel data. For instance, a glance through the data provided in 'World Population 1977' and the accompanying map (US Department of Commerce, 1978) reveals that the high mortality (20 or more deaths per 1000 population) countries of the world are scattered over diverse physical environmental zones, rather than being concentrated in the high altitude areas. Further, data provided in 'World Development Report 1982' (World Bank, 1982) show positive relationships between life expectancy (another measure of mortality), on the one hand, and GNP (Figure 2) and adult literacy (Figure 3), on the other. Effects of various sociocultural and biological, exogenous and endogenous, factors (e.g., socioeconomic condition, household and family size, maternal age, birth order, breastfeeding pattern, medical innovation, maternal nutrition, genetic/congenital malformation/disorder, trauma of different kinds, organic and infectious diseases) have also been studied in some details at both macro- (Ashworth, 1982) and microlevels (Brennan, 1983).

It thus appears from the limited data presented above that high altitude (as generally defined in terms of the physical environmental stresses of hypoxia, cold, and terrain) may not constitute a specialized environment with universal and uniform effects as far as human biological traits are concerned. It is far more likely, as has been suggested by Baker (1978), Cruz-Coke (1978), Basu et al. (1984a) and Goldstein et al. (1983) that varied concomitant sociocultural and other factors operating differentially in different high altitude populations/ regions have varied effects on different human biological traits in high as much as low altitude environments. The ethnic factor may introduce an additional causative variable.

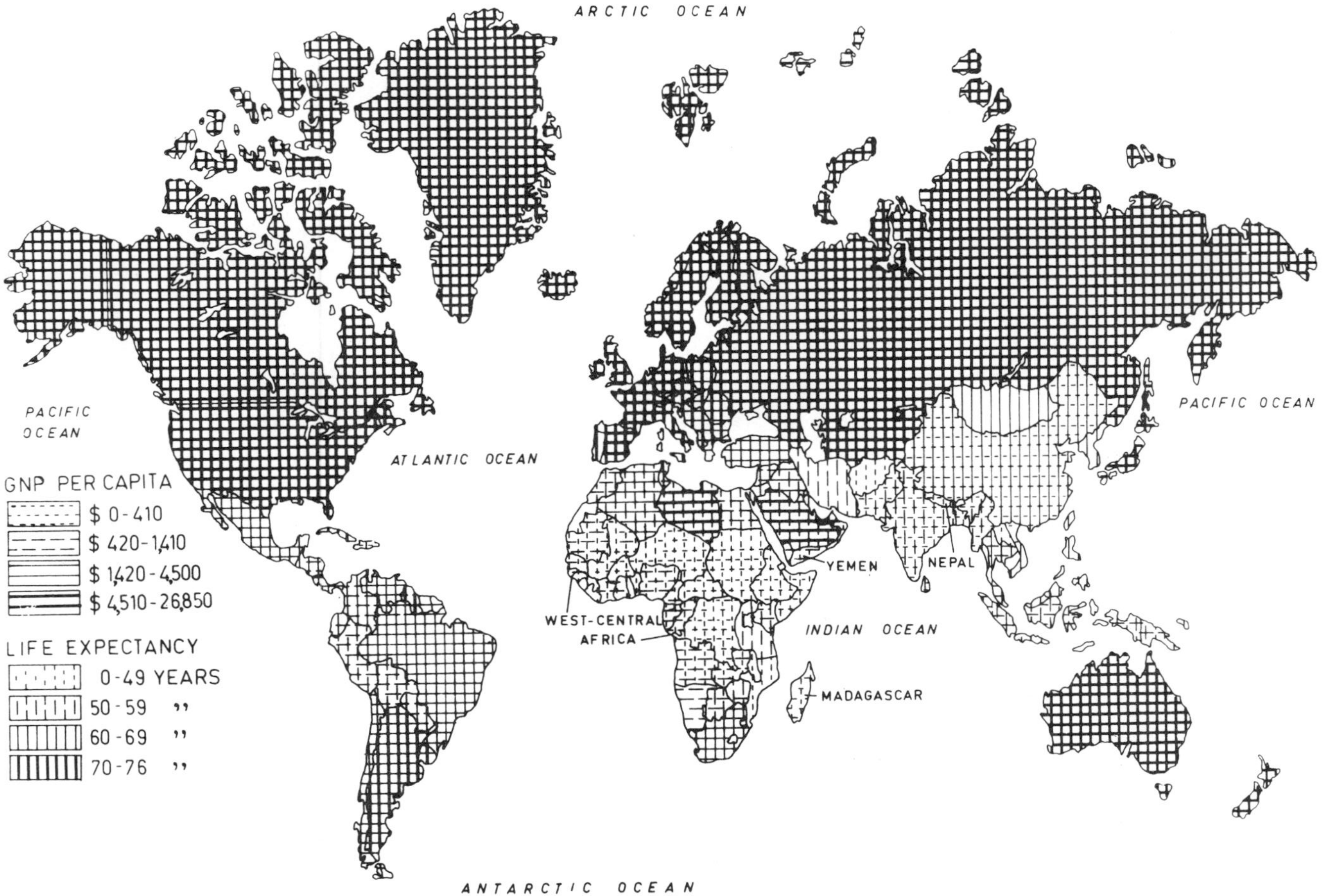

Figure 2. Relationship between life expectancy and gross national product.

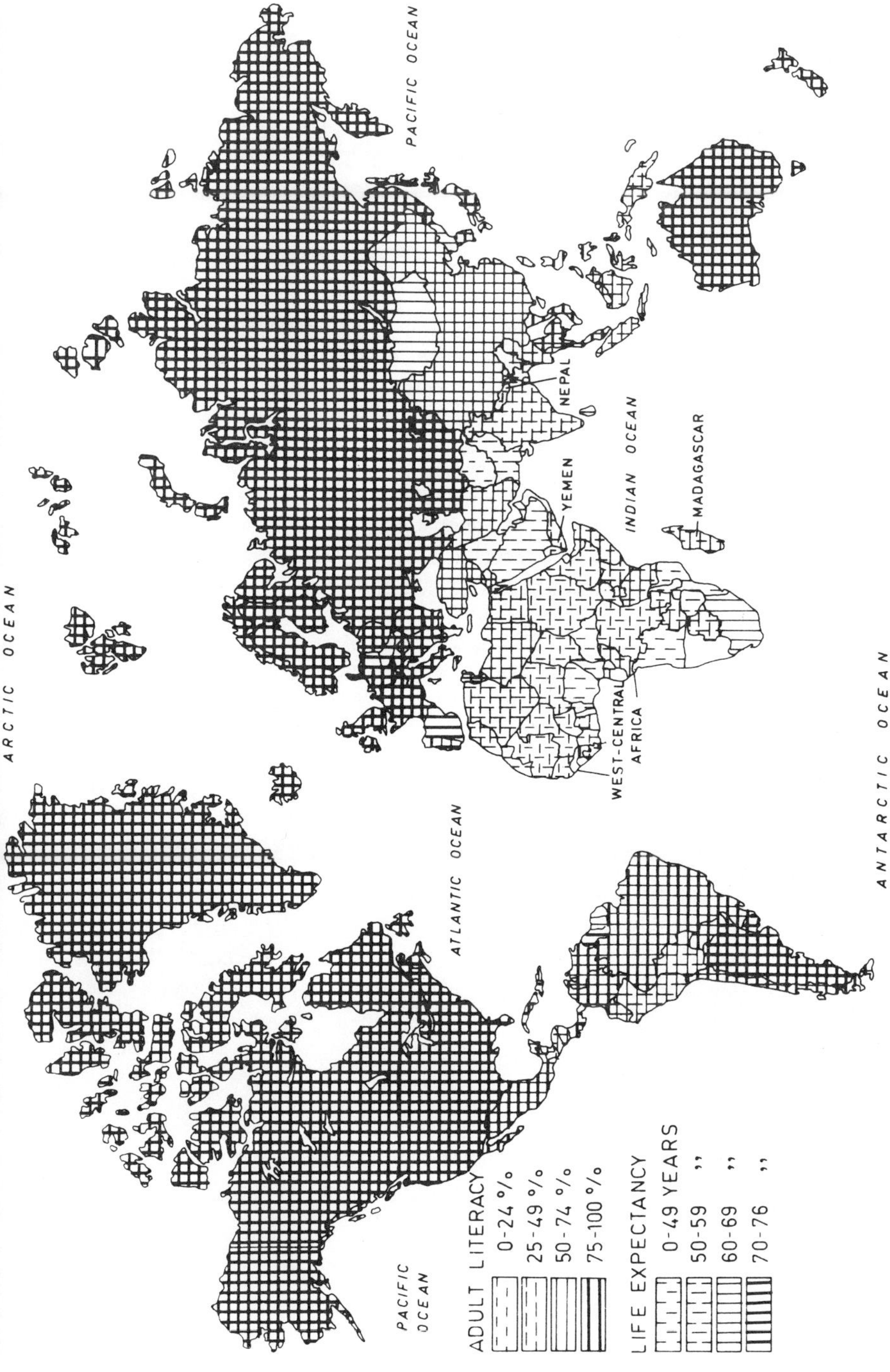

Figure 3. Relationship between life expectancy and adult literacy.

It is therefore to the detection and measurement of relative effects of individual physical environmental, sociocultural and ethnic/genetic factors, and of factor-complexes, on individual human biological traits, as well as trait-complexes which may together be treated as a composite index of community health, that we plan to address ourselves to, especially with reference to Indian populations, in the future.

ACKNOWLEDGEMENTS

We are indebted to the people of our study areas for their help and cooperation to our studies; to His Majesty's Government of Nepal, the Tribhuvan University, Kirtipur, the National Park and Wildlife Conservation Office, Kathmandu and the Indian Embassy, Kathmandu for providing permission and help to carry out field work in Upper Khumbu; to the subdivisional authorities, Kalimpong, Scheduled Castes and Tribes Welfare Department, Directorate of Cinchona and other Medicinal Plants, Government of West Bengal for organizational help in Kalimpong; to the district authorities, Midnapore district for organizational help, and the authorities of the Geonkhali High School for providing accommodations, in Geonkhali; to the Archdeacon of Calcutta and parish priest of the Roman Catholic Church in Mirpur for permission to work there; to the district authorities, Howrah district, and Sanskriti a cultural organization in Chakpota, for organizational help in Chakpota; to Dr. P.P. Majumder for statistical help to Mr. B. Dey for technical help; to Mr. P.C. Kumar for preparing the diagrams; to Mr. P. Adhikary for preparing the manuscript; and to the authorities of the Indian Statistical Institute, UNESCO and XI ICAES Secretariat for financial and logistic support to the work.

LITERATURE CITED

Ashworth A (1982). International differences in infant mortality and the impact of malnutrition: A review. Human Nutrition: Clinical Nutrition 36C:7.

Baker PT (ed) (1978). "The Biology of High-altitude

Peoples." Cambridge: Cambridge University Press.
Baker PT, Dutt JS (1972). Demographic variables as measures of biological adaptation: A case study of high altitude populations. In Harrison GA, Boyce AJ (eds): "The Structure of Human Populations," Oxford: Clarendon Press, p 352.
Basu A, Gupta R, Bhattacharya KK (1980). A demographic study of Mirpur: A village in coastal Midnapore district, West Bengal J Biosoc Sci 12:227.
Basu A, Gupta R (1984). Comments on "High altitude hypoxia, culture and human fecundity/fertility: A comparative study". Am Anthropologist (in press).
Basu A, Gupta R, Mukhopadhyay, B (1984a). Anthropological demography of populations of the eastern Himalayas. In Lukacas JR (ed): "People of South Asia," New York: Plenum Press, p 343.
Basu A, Roy SK, Mukhopadhyay B, Bharati P, Gupta R, Majumder PP (1984b). Each according to his need? Intrahousehold food distribution in some contrasting populations/subpopulations of West Bengal, India. Paper presented at the Symposium on "The Sharing of Food--From Phylogeny to History", 3-5 December, 1984, Bad Homburg, West Germany.
Bhattacharya SK (1980). Intestinal parasitic infestations in two populations inhabiting contrasting habitats. In Singh IP, Tiwari SC (eds): "Man and His Environment," New Delhi: Concept Publishing Company, p 177.
Bhattacharya SK, Mukhopadhyay B, Bharati P, Gupta, R, Dey B, Basu, A (1981). Intestinal parasitic infestations in populations inhabiting similar and contrasting ecological zones. Hum Ecol 9:485.
Bhattacharya SK, Bharati P, Mukhopadhyay B, Moitra N (1984). Intestinal parasitic prevalences in relation to economic status in a village population of Howrah district, West Bengal. Indian J Pub Hlth (in press).
Brennan ED (ed) (1983). Mortality patterns in anthropological populations (A collection of papers). Hum Biol 55:1.
Cruz-Coke R (1978). A genetic description of high altitude populations. In Baker PT (ed): "The Biology of High-altitude Peoples," Cambridge: Cambridge University Press, p 47.
Dutts JS (1980). Altitude and fertility: The confounding effect of childhood mortality - a Bolivian

example. Soc Biol 27:101.
Frisancho AR (1978). Human growth and development among high altitude populations. In Baker PT (ed): "The Biology of High-altitude Peoples," Cambridge: Cambridge University Press, p 117.
Goldstein MC, Tsarong P, Beall CM (1983). High altitude hypoxia, culture and human fecundity/fertility: A comparative study. Am Anthropologist 85:28.
Grahn D, Kratchman J (1963). Variation in neonatal death rate and birth weight in the United States and possible relations to environmental radiation, geology and altitude. Am J Hum Gen 15:329.
Gupta R (1980). Altitude and demography among the Sherpas. J Biosoc Sci 12:103.
Gupta R, Basu A (1981). Variations in body dimensions in relation to altitude among the Sherpas of eastern Himalaya. Annals Hum Bio 8:145.
Gupta R, Das SK, Bhattacharya SK (1983). Altitude and haematology among the Sherpas and Lepchas of the eastern Himalaya. ISI Tech. Report No. Anthrop 1/83.
Haimendorf C Von F (1964). "The Sherpas of Nepal." Calcutta: Oxford Book Company.
Harrison GA, Kuchemann CF, Moore MAS, Boyce AJ, Baju T, Mourant AE, Godber MJ, Glasgow BG, Kopec AC, Tills D, Clegg EJ (1969). The effects of altitudinal variations in Ethiopian populations. Phil Trans of the Roy Soc London B 256:147.
Hirai K, Okuda T, Fukuwatari M (1965). Observations of living of the Sherpa tribe in Nepal and their dietary survey. Reports on the Science of Living 23: 27.
Lang SDR, Lang A (1971). The Kunde hospital and a demographic survey of the Upper Khumbu, Nepal. New Zealand Med J 74:1.
Mazess RB (1965). Neonatal mortality and altitude in Peru. Am J Phy Anth 23:209.
Mueller WH, Schull WJ, Rothhammer F (1981). Studies of the Aymara of highland, intermontane, and coastal Chile. In Bastien JW, Donahue JM (eds): "Health in the Andes," Pt.2:Andean Environment: Altitude, Nutrition, and Coca. Washington, DC: American Anthropological Association, p 69.
O'Malley LSS, Chakravarti M (1909). "Bengal District Gazetteer, Howrah". Calcutta: Bengal Secretariat Book Depot.

Oppitaz M (1974). Myths and facts:Reconsidering some data concerning the clan history of the Sherpas. In Von F Haimendorf C (ed): "Contribution to the Anthropology of Nepal," Warminster: Aris and Phillips Ltd., p 232.

Risley HH (1891). "The Tribes and Castes of Bengal." Vol.I, Calcutta: Bengal Secretariat Press.

Sacherer JM (1974). Sherpas of Rolwaling valley: Human adaptation to a harsh mountain environment. Objects et Mondes 14:317.

UNESCO (1973). Programme on man and the biosphere (MAB). Working group on project 6:Impact of human activities on mountain and tundra ecosystems. Final Report. Paris: UNESCO.

US Department of Commerce (1978). World Population 1977. Recent Demographic Estimates for the Countries of the World. Washington, DC: Bureau of the Census.

Way AB (1976). Morbidity and postneonatal mortality. In Baker PT, Little MA (eds): "Man in the Andes. A Multidisciplinary Study of High-altitude Quechua," Strodsburg: Dowden, Hutchinson and Ross, Inc., p 147.

Weiner JS (1969). "A Guide to the Human Adaptability Proposals." IBP Handbook No. 1. Oxford: Blackwell Scientific Publ.

World Bank (1982). World Development Report 1982. New York: Oxford University Press.

WHO (1971). Family planning in health services. World Health Organization Technical Report Series No. 476.

Diseases of Complex Etiology in Small Populations:
Ethnic Differences and Research Approaches, pages 367–397

Chapter 16

AN ANTHROPOLOGICAL PERSPECTIVE ON THE EPIDEMIOLOGY OF HEMOGLOBIN DEFECTS AND GLUCOSE-6-PHOSPHATE DEHYDROGENASE DEFICIENCIES IN THE NORTHERN HALF OF THE AFRICAN CONTINENT

Ph. Lefèvre-Witier

Centre National de la Recherche Scientifique, Centre d'Hémotypologie, Toulouse, France

INTRODUCTION

The northern part of Africa is a distinct region in its geoclimatic characteristics and its populations. In this immense area, arid or subarid climate constitutes a major biological constraint that requires some similar adaptations from all inhabitants. Most of the population is extremely dispersed. Settlements are separated by large distances and linked together by very poor means of communication.

Although aridity is a common factor in the region, its influence is variable. Accordingly when we speak about people and diseases of northern Africa, we have to distinguish different climatic zones (Figure 1): (1) The Mediterranean coastal areas (e.g. Tell in Maghrib) that have a somewhat cold winter, and rainfall in the spring and fall; (2) The northern Sahara, a severe desert with oases that have permanent water supplies; (3) The Sudano-Atlantic Sahara that is less severe due to mist and to the presence of large rivers, the Senegal and the Niger; (4) The Central Sahara mountains (Tassili, Ahaggar, Air, Tibesti, Voltaic and Ethiopian plateaus) where altitude modifies the heat and aridity; (5) The Sahel that can be divided into two subareas: the northern one is a steppe where only extensive cattle-herding exists; the southern one permits poor seasonal agriculture; and

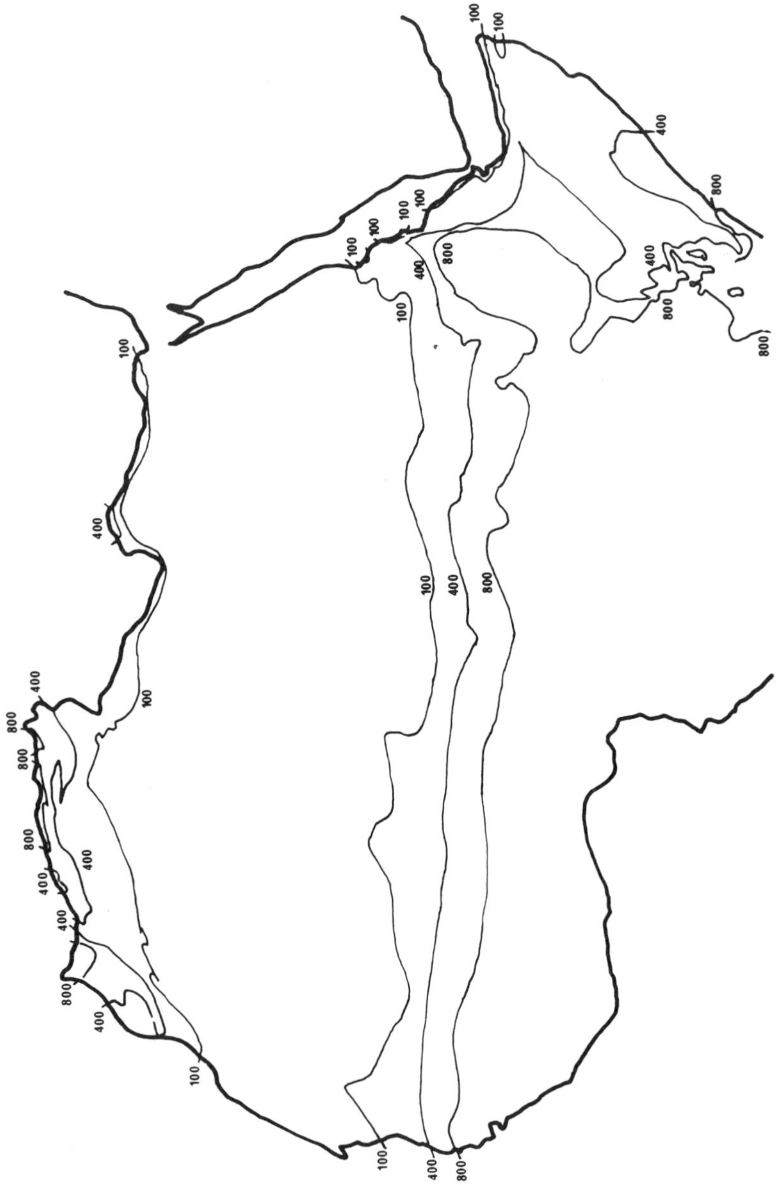

Figure 1. Rainfall limits in the northern part of Africa (100 mm Sahara desert, 100-800 mm Sahel and Steppe, 800 mm humid forest).

(6) The Sudanese savanna that appears south of the 500 mm. rainfall limit and stretches to the humid tropical forest. The primary forest occupies most of the central part of the half continent but its extension is limited in the western and eastern extremities.

In most of the northern arid areas two morphotypes exist. One is more Caucasoid, for example, the Arabo-Berbers of the Maghrib, Machrek and Egypt, the Moors of the Atlantic Sahara, and the Tuaregs of the Central Sahara; one is more Negroid, for example, the Tubu of the Tibesti, the Harratin of the Saharan oases, and the Fulani of the Sahel. Nevertheless, dolichocephaly, slenderness, and resistance to heat and thirst are common features that can be seen in all these groups. Indeed these peoples differ more culturally in their ways of life, nomadic or sedentary, than they differ genetically in their gene pools.

The sedentary populations of the southern Sahel and tropical forest are black-African. Despite the different morphotypes encountered, almost all the populations seem autochthonous to this part of Africa. The only well-known macro-migration that occurred during the last three thousand years is that of the Arabs, especially the Hilallian during the eleventh and the thirteenth centuries A.D. However, this Arabic migration was probably limited in demographic terms (De Planhol, 1968).

In its desire to build simplified epidemiological models, colonial anthropology often tried to link ways of life, pathology and morphotypes. In the Sahara this resulted in an opposition established between the "white man, camel rider" and the "black man, palm tree cultivator" (Sergent, 1960). This model hid the fact that pastoralism and agriculture were practiced equally by the two "types" of populations. According to Monod (1969), "to know a country of that size, one should not refer to the simplified or caricatural schemes of textbooks, but rather one should humbly accept the reason of reality and advance slowly step by step."

This statement should guide all those wishing to

make correlations between pathology and populations in the northern part of Africa. Evidently the observed forms of pathology reveal certain contrasts: On the one hand, diabetes mellitus, hypertension, gallstones, stomach ulcers, and tuberculosis are very widespread north of the 32nd parallel; on the other hand, some major tropical parasitoses, for example, malaria, river eye blindness, filariasis are progressively found south of the 16th parallel. However, in the Mediterranean countries of Africa there are also some serious parasitoses due to amoebas, taenia, echinococcus, schistosomiasis, and malaria. Thus it seems that it would be possible to determine geographical specificities and to map out easily the pathological risks, not necessarily by following ethnic classifications, but by surveying regional areas. The failure to use such an approach is due in many cases to the lack of basic data on the prevalence and the incidence of the diseases listed above. In many other cases the approach is not attempted because the diseases appeared very recently. Moreover, in places where some surveys have been conducted, where some sanitary structures have been installed, financial and/or human means have not enabled the research to be continued or the data to be analysed. Many of the surveys are also often obsolete because they were done during colonial times. Data acquired by young African nations are sometimes limited to restricted geographical areas or to current epidemics. Nevertheless, the desire for knowledge and prevention, is encouraged by the WHO, and by recent African ministries of health. In Algeria especially, special research was initiated in order to have a better understanding of the sanitary map of the country. Although African medical congresses and foreign teams of medical researchers have tried to compare their results, an important synthesis has yet to be produced. These problems are shared with many other developing countries, especially the least advanced countries, several of which are located in the northern part of Africa.

In this paper, therefore, we have chosen to describe a model of pathology in which the original data come from numerous systematic surveys on blood groups and other genetic markers. This model concerns

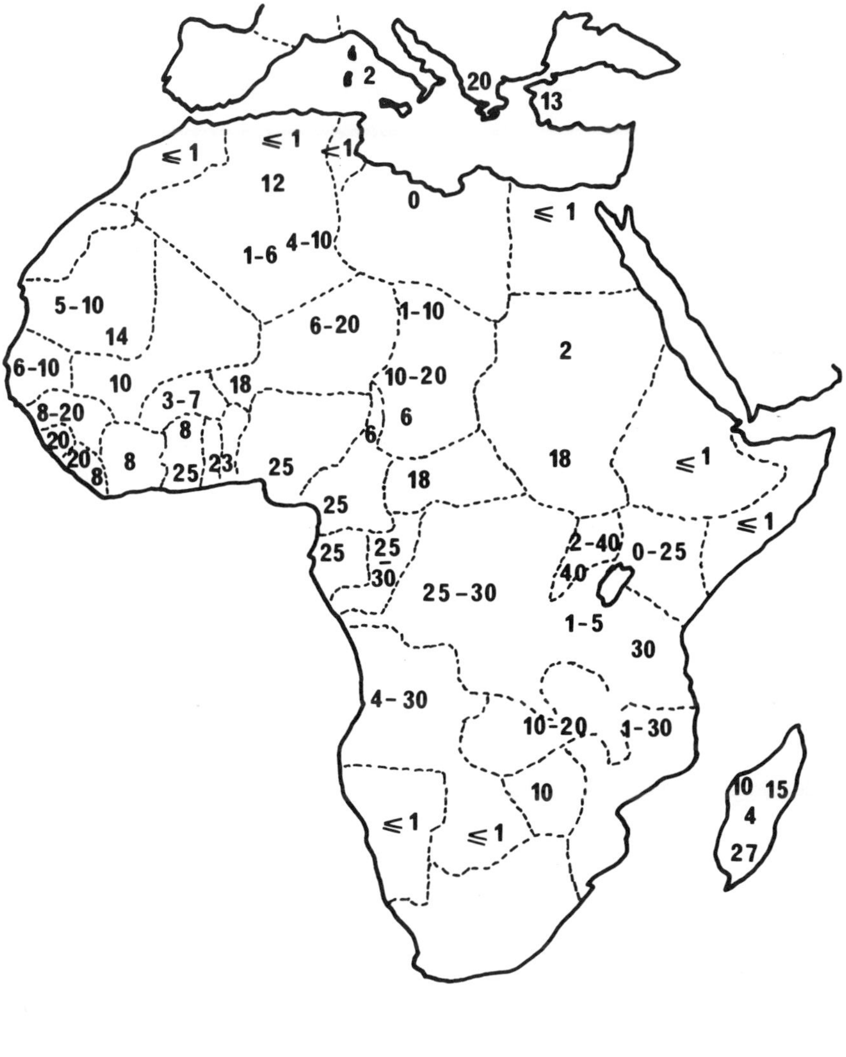

Figure 2. Sickle cell trait frequency in Africa.

the study of the following red cell genetic defects: abnormal hemoglobins S and C, beta-thalassemia and glucose-6-phosphate dehydrogenase deficiencies. The distribution and physio-pathological consequences of these disorders are closely related to the location and the history of the populations, to their demographic and mating structures and finally to their food production modes and life styles.

DISTRIBUTION OF GENETIC DEFECTS AND VARIANTS IN NORTH AFRICA

The Distribution of Hb S and Hb C

The distributions of the hemoglobin beta mutations S and C (and a few others: O, J, D ...) and beta thalassemia are better known than those of glucose-6-phosphate dehydrogenase (G6PD). For the latter the inventory of variants began in the seventies with only the deficiencies being noted before that date.

The distribution of the sickle cell trait in Africa has been mapped out in the broad lines (Charmot and Lefèvre-Witier, 1977). A look at the map of the sickle disease belt (Figure 2) reveals a clear-cut distribution by latitude (zonal bands). The maximum frequency zone (Hb S=25% to 30%) straddles the Equator extending 10 degrees north and south and thus it practically does not belong to the northern part of Africa as defined above. The medium frequency zone (Hb S=10% to 20%) stretches from Senegal to the northeastern province of Kenya. This zone includes all the countries that have wooded savannas and corresponds to the southern part of the Sahel. A third zone is formed by the steppe of the Sahel and by the Sahara in which frequencies are constantly lower than 10%. Finally, all of the coastal zones from the Atlantic and Mediterranean Sea to the Red Sea and the Indian Ocean show frequencies of Hb S lower than 1%.

The Hb C mutation affects the 6th amino acid position from the N terminated end of the beta chain as does the mutation for Hb S. The distribution of Hb C is limited to the western part of northern Africa as

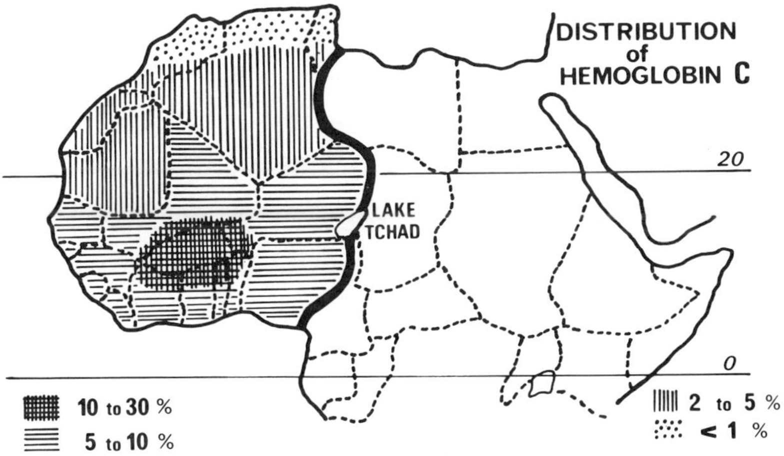

Figure 3. Hb C distribution in north-west Africa and its eastern limit.

proved by studies in populations of the Algero-Lybian border in Tassili n'Ajjer (Cabannes et al., 1967). This distribution remains valid today (Figure 3). However, more recent surveys in Algeria by Benabadji and collaborators have shown that this Hb C abnormal hemoglobin was two to three times less frequent in this country than Hb S, contrary to earlier reports (Adjrad, 1981; Trabuchet, 1977). It should be noted that in most of the western Sahel countries, and especially in Upper Volta and Niger, the Hb C frequencies are often equal to or greater than the Hb S frequencies (see Figure 4 and Cabannes, 1964).

The Distribution of β-Thalassemia

In Africa beta thalassemia results from many different mutations affecting the beta chain gene. The classification used here is as bioclinical as genetical. One can distinguish: beta O thalassemia, beta + thalassemia, delta-beta thalassemia or F thalassemia. The 20% occurrence of the beta thalassemia trait found in most of the other Mediterranean countries and in

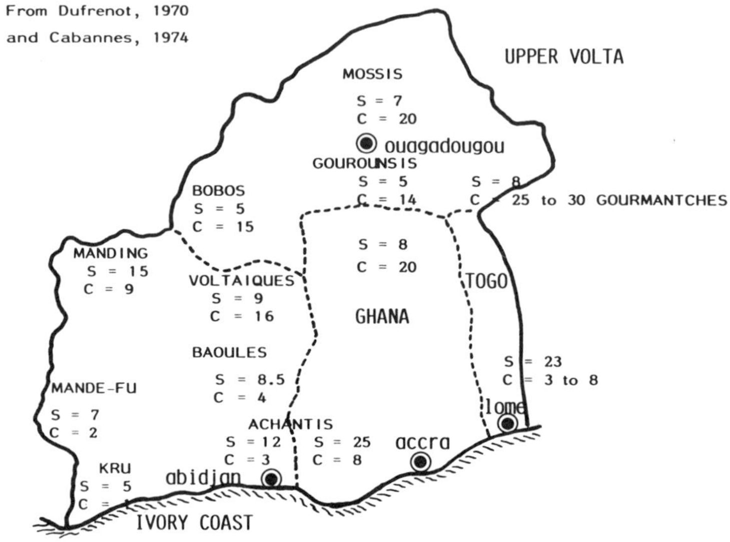

Figure 4. Distribution of Hb S and Hb C traits in some populations of the Guinea gulf.

Egypt contrasts sharply with the 10% maximum found in the populations of the Maghrib, the Machrek and northern Sahara. Even though northern Algeria shows only 2.12% frequency of the trait (Trabuchet et al., 1977), higher frequencies occur in some populations of the Sahara, for example, in the Tuareg of the Ahaggar (3%) and Tassili plateau (7.2%) (Benabadji, 1984; Cabannes, 1967) (Figure 5). The 7.2% frequency was computed in 1967 on samples examined with a less accurate methodology. This population of north-eastern Tuareg should be tested again. In the Sahel the frequency of beta thalassemia is no more than 1% with as many cases of delta-beta thalassemia seen as in Liberia (Willcox, 1975). However, it should be mentioned that systematic surveys are very infrequent in most of these countries as are evaluations of the relative distribution of the different beta thalassemia traits. Algeria alone has conducted accurate studies which in particular enable exploration of the DNA polymorphism of the β-like globin gene (Mears et al., 1981), to estimate the distribution of delta-beta thalassemia (0.05% in the Tell and 0.68% in the

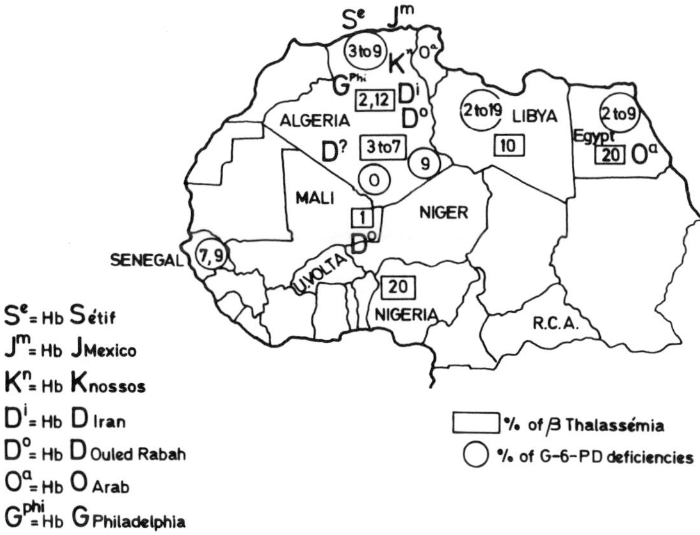

Figure 5. Distribution of some other hemoglobin mutations and of G6PD deficiencies in the nothern half of the African continent.

Ahaggar Sahara) (Adjrad, 1981) and to determine the frequency of the F-Sardinia gamma chain mutation (10% in the normal newborns and 30% of the newborns with homozygotic beta-thalassemia) (Morle et al., 1984).

Other Hemoglobin Mutations

The hemoglobin mutations that we have considered above are the most common as well as the most pathological. However, several others exist, such as the mutations concerning the 22nd and 121st amino acid of the beta chain. Mutations of the 22nd amino acid produce hemoglobin D-Iran (Beta 22, B1, Glu → Gln) and hemoglobin G-Coushatta (Beta 22, B1, Glu → Aln). Both of them have been found in Algeria, especially D-Iran in El Oued in the northern Sahara by Elion et al. (1973). Mutations of the 121st amino acid produce hemoglobin D-Punjab (Beta 121, B1, Glu → Gln) and the hemoglobin O-Arab (Beta 121, B1, Glu → Lys). Hb O-Arab was identified in several locations of northern

Africa, including Egypt and Tunisia (Figure 5). D-Punjab has not yet appeared in Africa. Another D hemoglobin, D-Ouled-Rabah (Beta 19, B1, Asn → Lys), has been identified in one person born in Aures (Algeria) and also among the Tuareg Iwellemeden, of the Nigerian and Malian Sahara (Lehmann et al., 1977). In the course of recent research in Ahaggar three new D hemoglobins were detected: one in the Saoura valley and two in Tamanrasset (Algeria) (Benabadji and Lefèvre-Witier, 1984). The exact mutations in these hemoglobins have not yet been determined. Very recently a case of hemoglobin Knossos (beta chain, 27th amino acid mutation) was discovered in an Algerian family of the Aures mountain (Rouabhi et al., 1983). Different alpha chain mutations have also been found in surveys: Hb J-Mexico, Setif, and G-Philadelphia (Figure 5) and also alpha-thalassemia in Algeria (Trabuchet, 1977).

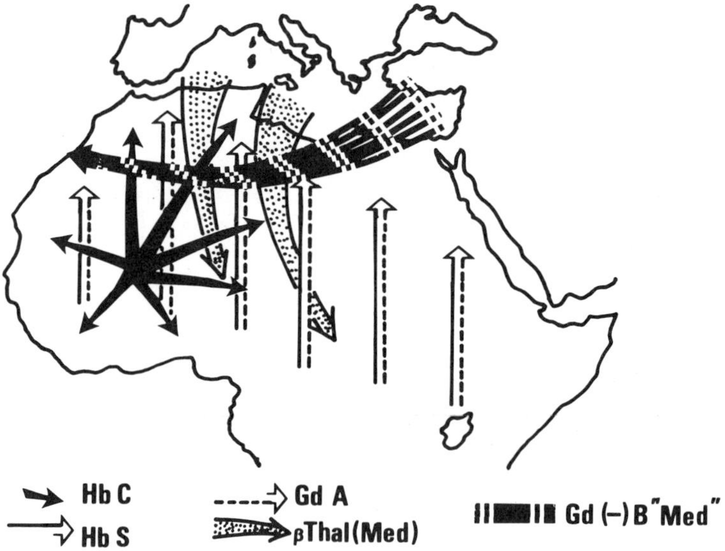

Figure 6. Clines of some hemoglobin and G6PD mutations in the nothern part of Africa.

The Distribution of G6PD Deficiencies

The glucose-6-phosphate dehydrogenase mutations show an original distribution in the Mediterranean area and in northern Africa. First of all, the mutations are numerous and every survey conducted in the past ten years has revealed new types of G6PD: normal, fast or slow. More than thirty types, half of which are deficient, have been found from Egypt to the Ivory Coast. The distribution of G6PD deficiencies has two major characteristics: (1) A decreasing North-East/ South-West cline can be observed (Figure 6). Indeed, the frequency of the deficiency is 2% to 19% in Egypt and Libya (McCurdy et al., 1974; Kamel et al., 1975), 3% to 9.3% in Algeria (Kabylia, Northeastern Sahara, Djanet) (Benabadji, 1977), less than 3% in Western Algeria, Ahaggar and Mali (Tuareg Iwellemeden) and less than 1% in Morocco. In contrast, all the indigenous subsaharan populations of Africa show a constant 10% to 20% frequency of deficiency. (2) The type of deficiency varies widely according to the population studied. In Egypt, the "Mediterranean" Gd B- is common but other types exist. In 37 G6PD deficient families, 17 abnormal variants were found by McCurdy et al. (1974). Some of these appear as local types found in Saharan oases: Gd(-) El Karga, Gd(-) Siwa, Gd(-) El Fayum (Table 1). In contrast in the Algerian Tell and plateaus, the "Mediterranean" B-type has not been found. In that country some other fast, slow or normal mutations are responsible for the deficiency. Gd(-) Kabyle, Gd(-) El Oued, and Gd(-) Laghouat are some examples of those found most frequently. In the central Sahara, Gd(-) Kabyle is responsible together with some other types such as Gd(-) Madrona (Vergnes et al., 1979) Gd(-) Ahnef, Gd(-) El Mihane, and Gd(-) Ibadan Austin, identified in the Djanet oasis (Table 1) (Benabadji, 1977).

In Sahelian and subsaharan Africa, the most common deficient type is the Gd(-) A fast variant. Its frequency is twice less but varies parallel to the normally active A+ variant; the cline for which is characteristic of the northern part of Africa. Gd A+ frequency in the Mediterranean coastal regions is 1.8%. In the Algerian Tell it is 3.4%, in

Table 1. Enzyme Deficient Molecular Variants of Glucose-6-Phosphate Dehydrogenase in the Northern Part of Africa.

G6PD Variants		Geographical Regions*									
		1	2	3	4	5	6	7	8	9	10
Normal:	B-	+			+	+	+				
	Blida	+									
	El Oued		+								
	Colombus						+				
	Chicago					+					
	El Kharga						+				
	El Fayoum						+				
Slow:	Alger	+									
	Thenia	+									
	Titteri	+									
	Igli		+								
	Ibadan Austin		+	+			+			+	+
	Ramatgan					+	+				
	Athen-like					+					
	Tell-Hashomer					+					
	Madrona		+				+		+		
	West-Bengal						+				
	Siwa						+				
Fast:	A-	+	+	+	+		+				
	Kabyle	+	+	+		+	+				
	Debrousse-Constantine	+				+	+				
	Laghouat		+	+							
	Ohio						+				
	Tahta						+				
	Djanet		+	+							
	Ahnef			+							
	El Mihane			+							
	Dakar							+			
	Mali							+			

*Geographical Regions are: (1) Algeria North, (2) Algerian Sahara, (3) Djanet Algerian Sahara, (4) Ideles Algerian Sahara, (5) Egypt Delta, (6) Egypt Sahara, (7) Senegal, (8) Mali, (9) Nigeria, and (10) Republic of Central Africa.

Tripolitania and in Cyrenaica, 6% (Kamel, 1974) and increases up to 15.6% in Ideles, a village of Ahaggar (Lefèvre-Witier, 1977), as in some other parts of the central Sahara and Sahel. Still higher frequencies include 16.3% in Libyan Fezzan (Kamel et al., 1975), 16% in the Egyptian oasis of El Dakhla (McCurdy, 1974), 18% in the Malinke of Senegal (Vergnes et al., 1974), and 26% in the Bororo Fulani of Niger (Treilhou, 1963). This high frequency is the apex of the cline and remains stable in Black African populations (Figure 6).

The G6PD Tacoma-like variant described by Vergnes et al. (1975) in the Malinké and Bedik of the Senegal is closely similar to Gd(-) Ibadan Austin and Gd(-) Madrona but its enzyme activity looks normal. G6PD Dakar and Mali described by Kahn et al. (1971) shows a very moderate enzyme deficiency.

Disease Severity Associated with Hemoglobinopathies and G6PD Deficiency

Homozygous sickle cell anemia can be lethal everywhere but its clinical manifestations are variable among individuals and populations. This has been demonstrated in Italy (Siniscalco et al., 1962), in the United States, and in India (Saha and Banerjee, 1973), in the Arabian peninsula (Perrine et al., 1978) and in Black Africa (Allison, 1954; Garlick, 1960; Lambotte, 1974). In these populations, the fitness value of the trait or genotypes depends on many factors of the biotope and perhaps also on other genetical factors (Wajcman and Labie, 1981). The problems caused by this clinical variability are now elaborated by systematic surveys on the natural history of sickle cell anemia, especially in the United States and in Jamaica (Powards, 1975; Serjeant, 1972).

Hemoglobin C is normally stable and functional. Only a small number of homozygous individuals might encounter some clinical risks. Anemia appears more regularly when Hb C mutation is associated with other abnormal hemoglobin defects such as Hb S or beta thalassemia in heterozygous individuals because Hb C compensates less for the more severe genetic defect than does Hb A. Some other severe anemias due to Hb O-Arab and D-Punjab, especially when associated with Hb S, have been described in the Near East and in India (Ozsolu, 1970). However, hemoglobin D-Iran and D-Ouled-Rabah and alpha chain variants found in northern Africa do not show any pathological symptoms.

The beta chain production deficiencies are responsible for a wide variety of well described diseases (Weatherhall and Clegg, 1972; Spritz and Forget, 1983). Such a variety requires a simplified distinction between lethal diseases like Cooley's anemia and the unclassifiable intermediary forms. These forms pool together homo- or heterozygous "bioclinical" genotypes for beta +, beta O and delta beta genes and probably many others that are sometimes linked with alpha-thalassemia. It is worth noting that while the beta thalassemia trait is sometimes almost clinically inapparent, it can sometimes induce anemia and hypodevelopment in any child and adolescent suffering from a nutritional deficiency. In Algeria the beta thalassemia syndromes have been thoroughly studied by Benabadji, Labie and Colonna (Belhani et al., 1977). In that country they create serious problems, especially when associated with hemoglobin S and C. These double heterozygous forms present a rank order of severity. In microdrepanocytosis or S-beta thalassemia, the symptoms differ from one patient to another, but hemolytic anemia can be severe, especially in S-beta O thalassemia. S-delta-beta thalassemia is rare. C-beta thalassemia is tolerated less in Algeria than in Black Africa or in black people of the United States.

The G6PD deficiencies present a similar variability in the northern part of Africa. The activity levels of the different molecular variants and deficiencies that they provoke are as varied as the sensitivity of the male carriers of the trait and the nutritional factors responsible for the hemolytic crisis. For example, the clinical symptoms of the deficiency due to the Gd(-) B "Mediterranean" are much more severe than those due to the Gd(-) Algerian or Saharan variants or to Gd(-) A of subsaharan Africa.

This paper emphasizes the variety of hemoglobin

genes, and their genotype and phenotype frequencies because the northern half of the African continent is the only part of the world where the major beta chain variants, such as Hb S, Hb C, and beta thalassemia, co-exists. Moreover it is in North Africa where they can be associated with alpha chain defects and with G6PD enzyme deficiencies, even in the same individuals.

Other Genetic Polymorphisms

The rich polymorphism observed for hemoglobin is also characteristic of many other systems of genetic markers. In northern Africa, mutations specific to Caucasoid, Negroid and sometimes Saharan populations exist together. Their gene frequencies are intermediate to the characteristic frequencies seen in Europe, Black Africa and the Near East. Over time the different Saharo-Sahelian populations have had recurrent contacts with the three large neighboring population groups mentioned above. Thus differentiation and hybridization produced not only a great number of molecular variants or haplotypes but also subtle clines stretching from north to south or sometimes from east to west of this half-continent (Ruffié and Lefèvre-Witier, 1972). Examples of such clines are provided by the $\underline{R}^{o}$ and $\underline{r}$ haplotypes of the Rhesus system and of the c^3 antigens of the Gm system (Figure 7).

Little data exist for the HLA system in this part of Africa. However, a survey of the Tuareg Iwellemeden of Mali (Kel Kummer) and Niger (Kel Nan) revealed a rich HLA polymorphism (Colombani et al., 1972). A similar polymorphism has been observed in north Africa in the Gm system, more than 24 antigens and 12 haplotypes have been identified to date (Blanc and Lefèvre-Witier, 1981). The rich polymorphisms that are typical of several systems could offer many fitness values to natural selection. The clines of most of the genetic markers allow genetic definitions, comparisons of populations, and analyses of their probable migrations.

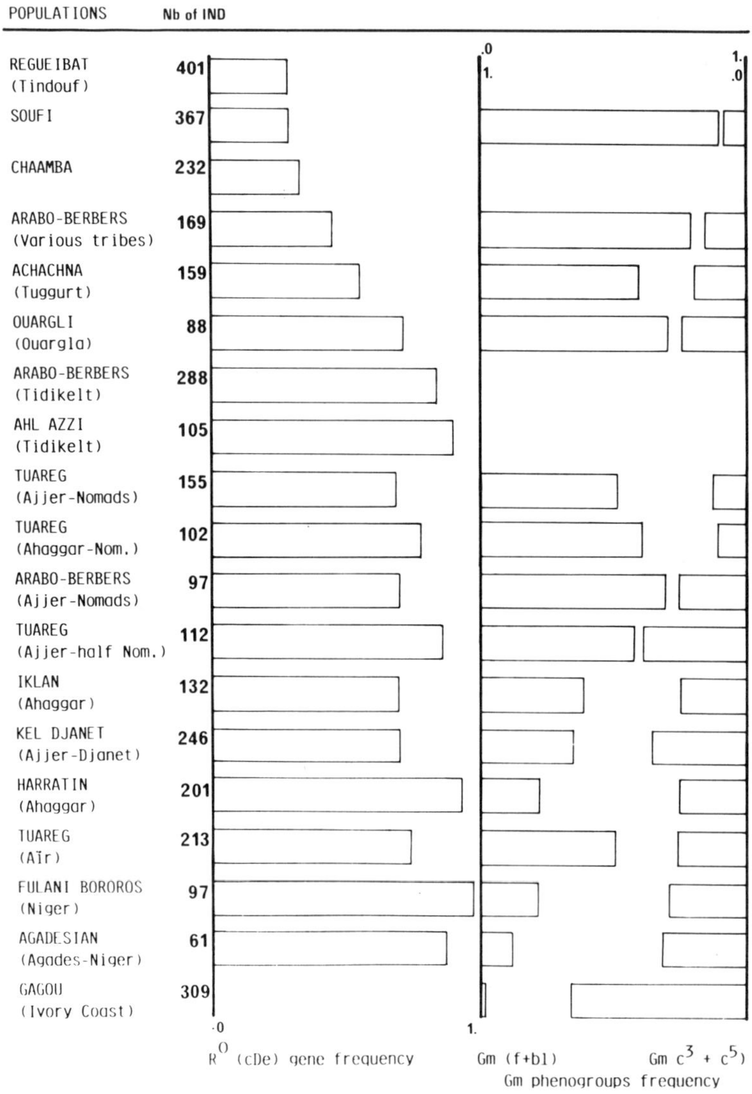

Figure 7. Clines of the $\underline{R}^0$ gene of Rhesus blood group and of two Gm phenogroups from the Mediterrean sea to Central West Africa.

INFLUENCE OF POPULATION STRUCTURE AND ECOLOGY ON GENETIC DISEASE

The pathological risk induced by the beta variants of hemoglobin and G6PD deficiencies depends on the past and present evolution of the population's genetic structure in its own biotopes. This dynamic will now be examined in the context of three different factors: bioclimate, migration and socio-economic influences.

Bioclimatic Factors

Different types of bacteria, viruses and parasites correspond to the macro- and micro-climates that have already been described. Many authors have studied how these infectious micro-organisms could give an advantage, through selection, to certain heterozygous genotypes and maintain polymorphism. The relationships between the plasmodium of malaria and the beta chain defects of hemoglobin seem among the most evident of the phenomenon of balanced polymorphism.

Three specific points should be mentioned concerning the northern part of the African continent: 1) In many places homozygous sickle cell anemia kills children and its fitness value can be estimated as zero (Livingston, 1976). However, this does not occur for some of the homozygous beta thalassemias. 2) The heterozygotes Hb AC and Hb A/beta thalassemia can have a slight advantage with respect to malaria. 3) the fitness value of the S mutation in the heterozygotes appears clearly only in the zone where *Plasmodium falciparum* is hyper-endemic, that is, in the humid tropical forest. The evolution of hyperendemic malaria is the key to the formation of the African sickle cell anemia belt (Figure 8). There is strong evidence linking hyper-endemic malaria with deforestation and multiplication of the *Anopheles* mosquitos due to the Bantu culture of 2000 years B.C. The HB S mutation has developed parallel to the beginning of agriculture in this culture, thus providing a good example of the association between a complex biological phenomenon (balanced polymorphism) and a

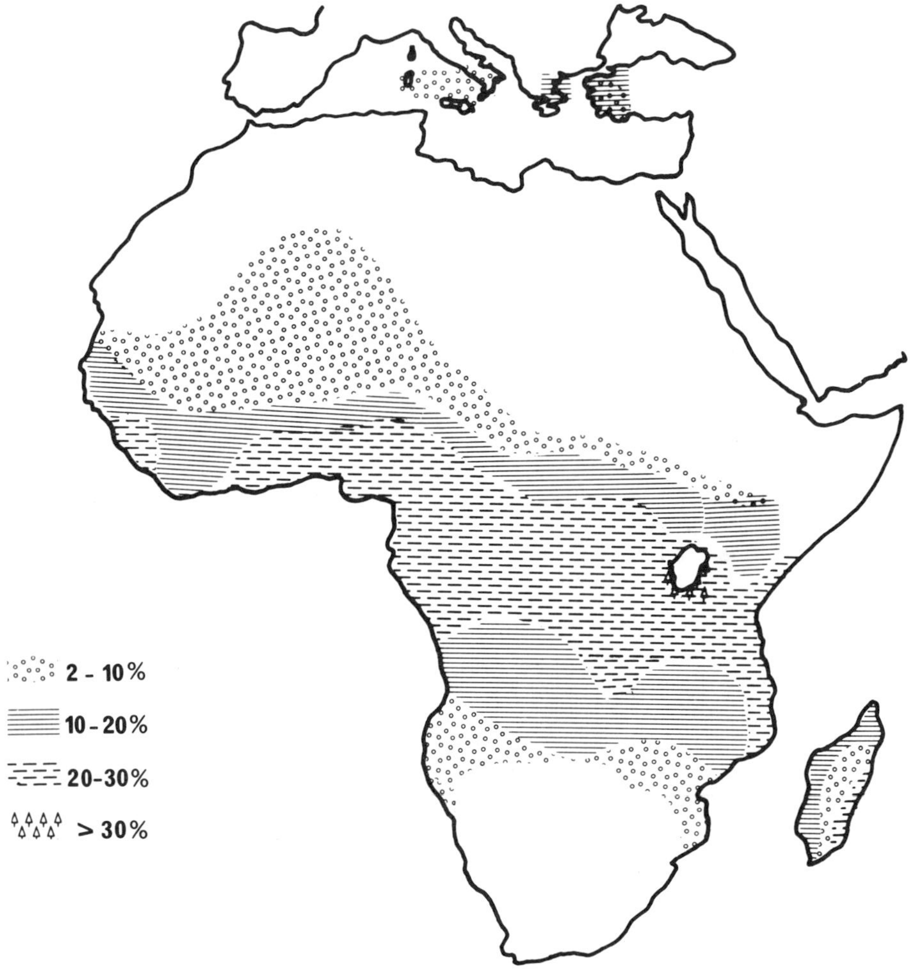

Figure 8. Sickle cell anemia belt (Lambotte, 1974).

specific technological development that may have been accompanied by population migration. Indeed, the same link can be observed in the western Sudanese area, on the coast of the Gulf of Guinea. In this region the linguistic map of the two language families (Sudanese and Bantu) (Oliver and Fage, 1970) corresponds exactly to the highest Hb S frequency zones.

By numerous computer simulations, Livingstone (1976) was able to establish a correlation between the actual clines of genotype frequencies at equilibrium of the three major hemoglobin beta chain mutations and the time span required for their formation. He estimated a depth of 160 generations (2000 B.C. to 1077 A.D.). In the paper by Livingstone (1976), one generation equals 25 years. Livingstone's data were collected in some coastal countries of the Gulf of Guinea where malaria is hyper-endemic.

In order to have a better understanding of the clines observed in the wooded-savanna and the steppe and of the time required to reach equilibria by the Hb S mutation in the populations of these areas it would be worthwhile to repeat the same simulations. Indeed the selective power of Plasmodium falciparum seems different in those regions where the dry season strongly modifies the epidemiology of malaria. The following changes are noticeable in the arid savanna and steppe: 1) In the savanna, malignant malaria often becomes holo-endemic with seasonal transmission from host to man. 2) During the dry season, other diseases sometimes play a role as important as malaria in selection. 3) The time required to build a strong anti-malarial immunity is much longer in the savanna for both Hb AS and Hb AA individuals than in the forest because they have less contact with the parasite. Hence, the epidemics of malaria are particularly dangerous in the savanna. 4) The protection provided in the hyper-endemic areas to Hb AS women in terms of miscarriage and stillborn decreases in the holo-endemic areas. 5) A discrete renal pathology can often be observed in Hb AS heterozygotes. The red cell sickling process results in a reduction of the kidney's ability to concentrate electrolytes, and this is aggravated by any dehydration. Thus in this case the adaptability of the Hb AS heterozygotes could be lower north of the 800 mm. rainfall limit, the limit of the tropical forest.

These observations suggest a decrease in the selective advantage of the Hb AS phenotype towards malignant malaria in the savanna and the steppe. However, the selective advantages of the other beta chain variant genotypes are maintained. Because there is no specific selective advantage for the S hemoglobin mutation in holo-endemic steppe area it was probably unable to increase in frequency, in the populations where beta thalassemia or other abnormal hemoglobins are found. This could have been the case for the Nilotic people of the Sudan (Nuer, Dinka, Shilluk) (Livingstone, 1976) and for the Libyco-Berber Tuareg studied in the Algerian Sahara (Lefèvre-Witier, 1982).

Malaria seems to be the major factor in determining the genotypic and phenotypic frequencies of the red cell defects considered in this paper. However, the main underlying mechanism which regulates genetic structures is not malaria but, aridity. The latter transforms the ecology of the plasmodium and of the host intermediaries, it modulates the immune response, and it accelerates sickle cell formation.

Migration Effects

Many plausible explanations for gene flow are provided by various theories of migration. They have often been used to explain the distribution of the hemoglobin beta chain mutations and the G6PD variants. In order to analyze these theories, we have to consider climatic evolution during the African neolithic. Approximately 5000 years ago increasing aridity in the tropics significantly disturbed the demographic patterns of northern Africa, not only in the forest areas but also in the Sahara and the Sahel. The inhabitants of these regions either adapted to the dessication or fled elsewhere. Fishing disappeared in the latter areas and gathering and hunting became more and more hazardous. In the Maghrib and the Machrek, the Capsian neolithic populations expanded from the Atlas mountains to the coastal areas. In the Sahara, some populations settled at the foot of sand dunes and the mountains where water was still available. In the Sahelian savannas, a limited agriculture consisting of barley and millet farming appeared. The Bovidian herdsmen (8,000 B.C.) had to adjust to reduced grazing grounds from the Libyan plateaus and the Fezzan to the Tassili n' Ajjer and to move to areas corresponding to the present Chad, Niger and Senegal. Their descendants are probably part of the Fulani (Hampate ba and Dieterlen, 1966) of the southern Tuareg, the Dazza of the Tibesti and, in the East, the Nilotic peoples of the Bahr El Ghazal, the Omo River, and Mt. Kilimanjaro.

For a long time it was considered necessary to explain the distribution of hemoglobin S mutation in both Africa and India by a dispersion out of a "Veddoid" center located in the Near East (Lehmann, 1954). The introduction and the diffusion of S hemoglobin in Africa was correlated with the transcontinental migration of Bovidian herdsmen. This migratory theory was rapidly challenged by the polycentric theory which postulated the appearance of the S mutation in different locations.

The most recent research (Kan and Dozy, 1980; Mears et al., 1981; Pagnier et al., 1984) seems to confirm this theory. Indeed, the treatment of DNA in chromosome 11 by restriction enzymes reveals a polymorphism linked to the beta chain gene. The resulting haplotypes correspond to the beta A normal gene or beta S or beta C abnormal genes. Those linkages show an interesting distribution in the northern part of the African continent. For example, if we consider only the restriction site named Hpa I, the beta S and beta C genes are linked to a 13 kilobase DNA fragment by the lack of the Hpa I site, or to a 7.6 kilobase DNA fragment when the site exists. The beta S or C and the 7.6 kilobase Hpa I linkage is the most common among black populations of Atlantic west Africa, the central Bantu forest and east Africa. However, the beta S or C linkage to the 13 kilobase fragment appears in an area stretching from Togo, Benin and Upper Volta to Maghrib. This mutation could have diffused when the Sahara was more humid. It could have been maintained by malaria selection in the relatively large neolithic populations and augmented more recently by the historical micro migrations across the desert.

Socio-cultural and Economic Factors

Tribal structures still exist in the northern part of Africa, not only among the nomadic herdsmen and in the villages, but also in the towns where marriage frequently occurs between kin, including parallel or cross, cousins. The resulting consanguinity, either remote or close, has been fully studied in many small isolated African populations where over a few generations the gene frequencies can vary due to a strong "founding effect". Under such conditions drift appears more efficient than selection itself, as Livingstone (1976) stated for the beta chain mutations.

Several small isolated populations that we studied in northern Africa can serve to illustrate drift effects resulting from demography and inbreeding. In each of these populations we have completely analyzed the family trees and mating patterns. The observations below are drawn from Ideles, a sedentary community of 500 individuals in the Algerian Ahaggar (Lefèvre-Witier, 1982).

Firstly, the Hb S and Hb C genes are carried almost entirely by the Negroid components of Ideles (Harratin and Iklan) whereas the beta thalassemia trait is carried equally by Negroid and Caucasoid (Merabtine and Tuareg) family groups (Table 2). Secondly, the G6PD deficient genes Gd(-) A and Gd(-) B found in both population groups have an overall frequency in Ideles of only 1%. The variant Gd(+) A found equally in both groups shows an overall frequency of 12%.

The marriage between Iklan and Harratin have been frequent over generations. Thus it is easy to follow the hereditary transmission of beta chain mutations and the appearance of abnormal hemoglobin associations. At Ideles we found only one Hb SC double heterozygote. One can postulate that in such a harsh environment, the abnormal hemoglobin associations and the homozygous genotypes were systematically lethal in utero and in infancy. A similar genealogical study has been in progress since 1977 among Isseqqamaren Tuareg in the Ahaggar and Tassili to verify the transmission of beta thalassemia and delta-beta thalassemia.

Table 2. Distribution of hemoglobin beta chain mutations and G6PD variants in Ideles (Ahaggar, Algeria).

	Nb	HbS (%)	HbC (%)	Beta-Thal (%)	Gd(+)A	Gd(-)A	Gd(-)B
Merabtine and Tuareg	194	1.0	1.0	8.24	8 men	0	1 man
Harratin and Iklan	187	5.9	11.7	6.4	6 men	1 woman	1 man

The research on small isolated populations in the northern part of Africa has shown that gene flow is maintained and that geographical distance does not represent a barrier. As we have already seen above, environmental conditions can play an important role in the diffusion of hemoglobin beta chain mutations and G6PD deficiencies and simulate ethnic barriers as proved by the two following examples. 1) The frequencies of Hb S trait are different between two Bantu populations, settled on both banks of the Zambesi River. The explanation of these differences could lie in the fact that the high Hb S frequency population of the left bank lives in the forest and the low Hb S frequency population of the right bank lives in the savanna. 2) The differences of Hb S trait frequencies between the Nilotic Lwo and Nuer can also be explained by their respective settlements in the humid forest (Uganda) and the wooded-savanna (Sudan). However, true social barriers to the hemoglobin S transmission exist between the Tuareg and their Iklan (excaptives) as between the Tedda of Tibesti and their black Kamadja shepherds (Cabannes, 1961). Also, the same barriers exist for hemoglobin C between Tuareg and Tedda who marry infrequently.

Food problems are fundamental in the clinical pathology of the mutations mentioned throughout this paper. The hemolytic crisis of the G6PD deficiency seems to appear spontaneously sometimes. However, in most cases it is provoked by consumption of food or chemicals which aggravate the metabolic defect of the red cells, thus causing their destruction. The fava bean is the most common agent followed by the synthetic anti-malarial drugs (Nivaquine, Primaquine, etc...) and even by acetyl-salicylic acid. The fava bean is found everywhere in the Mediterranean area and thus in the Maghrib countries, Libya and Egypt. Favism is very common in Egypt due to Gd(-) B "Mediterranean" but is infrequent in Morocco, Algeria and Tunisia. In these Maghrib countries hemolytic anemia is caused by other strongly deficient variants. There is such variable individual or familial sensitivity to the pollen or to the fava bean itself that a special genetic control has been postulated (Stamatoyannopoulos, et al., 1966).

The prevalence of favism justifies systematic surveys in Egypt but not in the Maghrib. Prevention of access to fava beans is almost unconceivable in countries where this food is so popular and inexpensive. Moreover, recent studies (Goldenser, 1983) tend to support the notion that fava beans provide protection against malaria similar to that of G6PD deficiency. A similar dilemma exists for G6PD deficiency and anti-malarial drugs. Thus, some hemolytic accidents do appear during mass anti-malarial prevention campaigns. Fortunately most of these campaigns are carried out in subsaharan Africa where Gd(-) A is alone responsible for minor hemolytic accidents. Fortunately, acetyl-salicylic acid, a common drug in Africa, is very rarely responsible for hemolytic accidents.

The pathology of beta thalassemia and of the associations between abnormal hemoglobins, especially Hb S and Hb C, and beta thalassemia appear to be more severe in economically deprived families and/or areas in Africa as well as in Asia. The genetic anemias caused by the hemoglobin abnormalities are aggravated by folic acid, iron, and protein deficiencies due to hyponutrition and malabsorption, especially in instances of intestinal parasitosis. A recent systematic survey in the Algerian Sahara (Ahaggar) (Benabadji, 1984) has proven both the importance of intestinal parasitosis and the frequency of chronic nutritional anemia among women and children (20% show a weight of hemoglobin inferior to 11 grams per liter).

Finally, socio-administrative structures play a role in evaluating pathological risks in northern Africa. Indeed, any traditional population, and especially the pastoral ones, benefit from only limited sanitary control. The rural dispensaries have difficulties in detecting the red cell genetic defects and even if they are suspected in one individual or family, there are no laboratories to confirm their presence. Homozygous and heterozygous children with severe anemia die in infancy but these deaths are not officially listed because civil records are not yet well established in many of the communities. Even if the genetic disease is diagnosed, treatment by transfusion and hospitalization would be difficult in most cases. Thus, it is easy to understand that systematic detection, as well as counselling before marriage with blood tests would be inconceivable in most areas, especially rural ones. By contrast, in the big towns where pre- and post-natal care is more organized and where some hospital laboratories exist, the detection and treatment of abnormal hemoglobin diseases and G6PD deficiencies are more and more successfully undertaken. However, pre-natal diagnoses in utero by fetal blood sampling (to examine the production of hemoglobin genes) or by amniotic liquid sampling (to examine the DNA of cells by enzymes specific to the mutations) still present serious cultural, technological and financial problems.

CONCLUSION

Aridity, selection due to malaria and considerable genetic variation make the northern part of the African continent an exceptional place for the study of hemoglobin beta chain mutations and of the glucose-6-phosphate dehydrogenase variants. Their pathological risks and natural histories constitute an excellent model of complex epidemiology and human ecology. Currently this model is not evolving into a more simplified one. In the different countries considered in this paper, its new pattern depends on two main distinct causes: the improvement of health care facilities and migration to urban areas. These two factors accelerate the detection of red cell genetic defects. The urban increase of population density also favors genetic exchange and consequently the association between hemoglobin or G6PD abnormalities.

Social change in rural societies, often parallel to emigration, contributes to the decrease of traditional consanguinity. Conversely, the resulting micromigrations create new communities accompanied by strong genetic "founding effects". These new populational patterns modify the distribution of the frequencies and of the pathological risks.

The malaria eradication program, whose progress is constant although sometimes limited, does not really reduce the incidence of the above considered genetic anemias because the pool of the heterozygotes is very important, especially in the forest eco-system.

As specialized hospital services are more and more involved in detecting and treating these genetic diseases, their economic cost regularly increases. However, antenatal detection, genetic counseling and medical care improve greatly the conditions of life of the groups at risk.

In the northern part of Africa, as well as in the rest of the world, the greatest hope for patients lies perhaps in the repair of the DNA mutation or the replacement of the gene function by genetic engineering, despite the limited success of such recent repair attempts.

LITERATURE CITED

Adjrad L, Azizi K, Arbane M, Benabadji M (1981). Les hémoglobinopathies en Algérie. Paper read at the Congrès Médical Maghrebin.

Allison A C (1954). Protection afforded by sickle-cell trait against subtertian malarial infection. Brit Med J 1:290.

Belhani M, Dahmane M, Richard F, Trabuchet G, Benabadji M, Colonna P, Labie D (1977). Aspects cliniques et biologiques des betathalassémies: à propos de 176 observations. Sem Hop Paris 53:891.

Benabadji M, Benlatrache C, Merad F, Suaudeau C, Benmoussa M, Kornprobst G, Cladel G (1977). Glucose-6-phosphate dehydrogenase deficiency in Algeria. Sem Hop Paris 16:899.

Benabadji M, Lefèvre-Witier Ph (1984). Hémoglobinoses et anémies en Ahaggar. Nouvelle Revue Française d' Hématologie (submitted).

Blanc M, Lefèvre-Witier Ph (1981). Marqueurs des immunoglobulines (Gm) chez les Touaregs du Sahara, en particulier chez les Touaregs ISSEQQAMARENES du Hoggar. Paper read at the 15ème Colloque des Anthropologistes de Langue Française, Bruxelles.

Cabannes R, Ruffié J (1961). Les types hémoglobiniques dans les populations des massifs montagneux du Sahara central (Hoggar et Tibesti). L'Anthropologie 65:467.

Cabannes R (1964). Les types hémoglobiniques des populations de la partie occidentale du continent africain. A Monographie du Centre d'Hémotypologie. Paris: Hermann, p 148.

Cabannes R, Accurso A, Nicolas C, Arne D (1974). Répartition des hémoglobines abnormales dans les populations Akan de Côte d'Ivoire. Ann Univ Abidjan 8:158.

Cabannes R, Lefèvre-Witier Ph, Sendrail A (1967). Etude des hémoglobines dans les populations du Tassili n'Ajjer (Sahara central). Bull et Mém Soc Anthrop Paris 1:434.

Capot-Rey R (1953). Le Sahara Français. Paris: Presses Universitaires de France.

Charmot G, Lefèvre-Witier Ph (1978). Géographie de la drépanocytose. Les causes de sa répartition dans l'Afrique au sud du Sahara. Méd Trop 38:167.

Colombani J, Dego L, Petrignani C, Chaventré A, Lefèvre-Witier Ph, Jacquard A (1973). HLA gene structure of Kel Kummer Tuareg. In Dausset J, Colombani J (eds): "Histocompatibility Testing," Copenhagen: Munksgaard, p 153.
De Planhol X (1968). Les fondements géographiques de l'histoire de l'Islam. Paris: Flammarion.
Dufrenot MM, Legait JP (1970). Contribution à l'étude de la répartition des genes S et C hémoglobiniques en Haute-Volta, au Mali et au Niger. Bull Soc Path Ex 63:606.
Elion J, Belkhodja O, Wajcman H, Labie D (1973). Two variants of hemoglobin D in the Algerian population: Hemoglobin D Ouled Rabah (beta 19 (BI) asn → lys) and hemoglobin D Iran (beta 22 (B4) glu → gln). Biochim Biophys Acta 310:360.
Garlick JP (1960). Sickling and malaria in South-west Nigeria. Trans Roy Soc Med Trop Hyg 54:146.
Golenser J, Miller, J, Spira DT, Navok T, Chevion M (1983). Inhibitory effect of a fava bean component on the in vitro development of Plasmodium falciparum in normal and glucose-6-phosphate dehydrogenase deficient erythrocyte. Blood 3:507.
Hampate ba A, Dieterlen G (1966). Les fresques d'époque bovidienne du Tassili n'Ajjer et les traditions des Peul: Hypothèse d'interprétation. J de la Société des Africanistes 36:151.
Kahn A, Boivin P, Hakim J, Lagneau J (1971). Hétérogénéité des glucose-6-phosphate deshydrogénases érythrocytaires déficitaires dans la race noire. Etude cinétique et description de deux nouvelles variantes Gd(-) Dakar et Gd(-) Mali. Nouvelle Revue Française d'Hématologie 11:741.
Kamel K, Umar M, Ibrahim W, Mansour A, Gaballah F, Selim O, Azim A, Hamza S, Sabry F, Mofy N, El Naggar A, Hoerman K (1975). Anthropological studies among Libyans. Erythrocytic genetic factors, serum haptoglobin phenotypes and anthropometry. Am J Anthrop 43:103.
Kan YW, Dozy AM (1980). Evolution of the hemoglobin S and C genes in world populations. Science 209:388.
Lambotte C (1974). La sicklémie de l'enfant en Afrique Noire. Ann Soc Belge Méd Trop 54:177.
Lefèvre-Witier, Ph (1974). Un isolat du Sud Sahara: les Kel Kummer. VI-Structures génétiques des systèmes sanguins érythrocytaires et sériques.

Population 3:518.
Lefèvre-Witier Ph (1982). Ecology and biological structure of pastoral Isseqqamaren Tuareg. Crawford MH, Mielke J (eds): "Current Developments in Anthropological Genetics," Vol 2, New York: Plenum, p 93.
Lefèvre-Witier Ph (1982). Ideles (Ahaggar-Algérie): structures et dynamique génétiques d'une comunauté rurale du Sahara central. Thèse de Doctorat d'Etat en Biologie Humaine. Toulouse: Université Paul Sabatier.
Lefèvre-Witier Ph, Vergnes H (1977). Enzyme polymorphisms of Ideles populations (Ahaggar, Algeria) and the Iwellemeden Kel Kummer Tuareg (Menaka, Mali). Hum Hered 27:454.
Lehmann H (1954). Distribution of the sickle cell gene. A new light on the origin of the East Africans. Eugen Rev 46:101.
Livingstone FB (1976). Hemoglobin history in West Africa. Human Biology 48:487.
Mauran-Sendrail A, Lefèvre-Witier Ph, Lehmann H, Casey R (1977). Haemoglobin D-Ouled Rabah beta 19, BI, asy → lys, in a Tuareg tribe of the southern Sahara. J Méd Genetics 14:245.
Mauran-Sendrail A, Lefèvre-Witier Ph, Rosa J, Garrigues G (1977). Hb D-Ouled Rabah (beta 19, asn → lys), in the Iwellemeden Kel Nan: a Tuareg tribe in Niger. IRCS Med Sc Hem 5:374.
McCurdy PR, Kamel K, Selim O (1974). Heterogeneity of red cell glucose-6-phosphate (G6PD) dehydrogenase deficiency in Egypt. J Lab Clin Med 5:673.
Mears JG, Beljord C, Benabadji M, Alaoui-Belghiti Y, Baddou MA, Labie D, Nagel RL (1981). The sickle gene polymorphism in North Africa. Blood 58:599.
Mears JG, Lackman HM, Cabannes R, Amegnizin KPE, Labie D, Nagel RL (1981). Sickle gene: its origin and diffusion from West Africa. J Clin Invest 68:606.
Monod, Th (1969). Sahara d'hier et d'aujourd'hui. Revue Atlas No. 34:14.
Morle L, Arbane M, Morle F, Rouyer-Fessard P, Feingold J, Bouhass R, Benabadji M, Aguercif M, Beuzard Y (1984). Genetic control of the proportion of gamma chain of human hemoglobin. Brit J Haem (submitted).
Oliver R, Fage JD (1970). "A Short History of Africa." 3rd Ed. Harmondsworth, England: Penguin Books.
Ozsolu S (1970). Homozygotes hemoglobin D-Pundjab.

Acta Haemat 43:353.
Pagnier J, Mears JG, Dunda-Bekhodja O, Rego KE, Beljord C, Nagel RL, Labie D (1984). Evidence for the multicentric origin of the Hb S gene in Africa. Proc Nat Acad Sci USA 81:1771.
Perrine RP, Pembrey ME, John P, Perrine S, Shoup FD (1978). Natural history of sickle cell anemia in Saudi Arabs. A study of 270 subjects. Annals Int Med 88:1.
Rouabhi F, Chardin F, Boissel JP, Beghoul F, Labie D, Benabadji M (1983). Silent β-thalassemia associated with Hb Knossos Beta (27(B9) Ala → Ser) in Algeria. Hemoglobin 7:555.
Ruffié J, Lefèvre-Witier Ph (1972). Ergebnisse serologischer forschungen in der Sahara. In "Die Sahara und ihre randgebiete," Vol 2, Humangeographie München: Weltforum Verlag, p 255.
Saha N, Banerjee B (1973). Hemoglobinopathies in the Indian subcontinent: a review of literature. Acta Genet Med Gemello (Roma) 22:117.
Sergent E, Parrot L (1960). Contribution de l'Institut Pasteur d'Algerie à la Connaissance humaine du Sahara (1900-1960). Alger: Institut Pasteur d'Algérie.
Serjeant GR, Serjeant BE (1972). A comparison of erythrocyte characteristics in sickle cell syndromes in Jamaica. Br J Haemat 23:205.
Siniscalco M, Bernini L, Latte B, Motulsky AG (1961). Favism and thalassemia in Sardinia and their relationship to malaria. Nature 190:1179.
Spritz RA, Forget BG (1983). The thalassemias: molecular mechanisms of human genetic disease. Am J Hum Genet 35:333.
Stamatoyannopoulos G, Fraser GR, Motulsky G, Fessas P, Akrivakis A, Papayannopoulos TH (1966). On the familial predisposition to favism. Am J Hum Genet 18:253.
Thompson BW (1965). "The Climate of Africa." Oxford: Oxford University Press.
Trabuchet G, Belhani M, Richard F, Hamladji RM, Benabadji M, Colonna P (1977). Premières observations d'alpha-thalassémie en Algérie. Sem Hop Paris 53:885.
Trabuchet G, Dahmane M, Benabadji M (1977). Hémoglobines anormales en Algérie. Sem Hop Paris 53:879.

Treilhou JP (1969). Nomades et sédentaires d'Agadès (République du Niger). Etude hémotypologique. Thèse Médecine Toulouse Purpan: Université Paul Sabatier.
Vergnes H, Gherardi M, Bouloux C (1975). Erythrocyte glucose-6-phosphate dehydrogenase in the Niokolonko (Malinke of the Niokolo) of eastern Senegal. Identification of a slow variant with normal activity (Tacoma-like). Hum Hered 25:80.
Vergnes H, Gherardi M, Lefèvre-Witier Ph, Jaeger G, Benabadji M (1979). Genetic variants of human glucose-6-phosphate dehydrogenase in a Saharian and Pygmy family. Human Hered 29:50.
Wajcman H, Labie D (1981). Aspects actuels de la biologie de la drépanocytose. Ann Méd Interne 132:568.
Weatherhall DJ, Clegg JB (1972). "The Thalassemia Syndromes." Oxford: Blackwell.
Willcox MC (1975). Thalassemia in northern Liberia. A survey in the Mount Nimba area. J Med Genet 12:55.

EPILOGUE AND SUMMARY

Diseases of Complex Etiology in Small Populations:
Ethnic Differences and Research Approaches, pages 401–411

EPILOGUE AND SUMMARY

F. Vogel

Institute f. Anthropologie und Humangenetik, University of Heidelberg, Federal Republic of Germany

DEFINITIONS AND CONCEPTS

In the foregoing contributions, aspects of genetic epidemiology have been discussed. Using these contributions as examples, some generalizations will now be tried. According to Ward's (Ch 8.) definition,

"Genetic epidemiology aims to identify the distribution of genetic risk in terms of the underlying etiology of disease, by analyzing the distribution of diseases, and associated risk factors, in groups of related individuals."

In order to delineate genetic epidemiology from other types of genetic analysis, I would like to specify this definition somewhat more precisely by altering the last sentence as follows: "... in well-defined populations compared with groups of related individuals".

The first epidemiological studies were performed almost 150 years ago on infectious diseases. Analyzing local distributions of cases in epidemics of cholera or typhoid often allowed to identify and eliminate the source (see Roberts, Ch. 1). More recently, epidemiological approaches have been used to identify external "risk factors" for common disorders of middle and advanced age, such as cardiovascular disease or cancer. In this way, the significance of high blood cholesterol and hypertension for coronary heart disease, or of cigarette smoking for lung cancer were established (see Doll and Peto, 1981). This "risk factor" philosophy, however, oversimplified the real situation by neglecting individual differences: Not all cigarette smokers develop lung cancer. Is this just a matter of good luck or are there genetic differences in disease susceptibility?

Since Williams (1956) published his treatise on "biochemical individuality", evidence has accumulated for an enormous amount of genetic variability at the biochemical level within human populations. Only considering all sources of interindividual variability analyzed so far at the gene product level, not even two living human beings (excepting monozygotic twins) will probably be identical genetically. While some of this variation may simply be caused by random mutations in combination with genetic drift (Kimura, 1983), much of it has been shown to be of some functional significance and may have influenced natural selection. The associations between ABO blood groups (Vogel and Helmbold, 1972), or HLA-types (Dausset and Svejgaard, 1977), and many common diseases, or individual differences in metabolism, main effect and side effects of drugs (see Vogel and Motulsky, 1979) are specific examples.

The first studies in genetic epidemiology were concerned with incidence, prevalence, genetic subtypes, mutation and selection of monogenic diseases, such as achondroplasia, hemophilia, or Duchenne muscular dystrophy. Series of surveys during the 1940's and 1950's, in Kemp's Copenhagen institute, Becher's (1939-1952) study on the Duchenne disease in Südbaden, the numerous surveys in the state of Michigan (Neel, Schull and their coworkers), and in Northern Ireland (Stevenson) mark the first important period in genetic epidemiology (for a review see Vogel and Rathenberg, 1975). Methods for aspects of such studies (for example, ways of ascertainment; calculation of relative fertility and selective advantages and disadvantages; analysis of genetic heterogeneity; mutation rate estimates) were developed and many basic facts could be established.

This development came to an end, when fascinating

approaches were introduced into human genetics: Cytogenetics, single cell genetics, biochemistry and molecular biology opened up new paths for analysis of genetic mechanisms in health and disease. No wonder that most human geneticists retreated from the field into the laboratory. For a time, almost no epidemiological studies were started. However, it soon became clear that this could not last long. The genetic problems posed by the fast development of our societies are too urgent. How will our modern civilization change the biological composition and fitness of future generations? In which ways will it influence important parameters such as mutation rates, natural selection, or susceptibility of certain genotypes to "civilization" diseases? For answering such questions, epidemiological evidence is needed. Therefore, it is not surprising that in recent years, interest in epidemiological problems has increased again (see for example, Morton, 1982).

Compared with the early studies, there is an interesting shift in emphasis from monogenic diseases to more complex ones whose etiology is described conventionally but not very satisfactorily as "multifactorial". This shift is accompanied by two trends: On the one hand, single causative factors such as genetic polymorphisms and their interaction with specific environmental agents are analyzed. Such an analysis is often cumbersome; it can only proceed stepwise and requires a thorough knowledge of pathophysiology of the biological systems involved. Therefore, a shortcut seems to offer itself: Could application of complex statistical models be helpful for a much faster and even more thorough analysis? For some authors, the term "genetic epidemiology" is more or less equivalent with development and application of such models (see, for example, Morton and Chung 1978). contrary to this, however, others have stressed the absurdity of the hope to contribute essentially to the genetic analysis of a disease (or group of diseases) without knowing anything about its physiological basis (Murphy, 1981). Sound research designs and statistical methods are essential for epidemiological analysis. Ward, in this volume, is right in stating that "elementary epidemiological principles are often sacrificed" in genetic epidemiology. But statistics cannot be the leading methodology. Statistical methods are at their best when used for answering clearly stated biological questions.

SPECIAL METHODOLOGICAL PROBLEMS DISCUSSED IN THIS VOLUME

Study of the contributions in this volume opens our eyes for many methodological problems involved in epidemiological studies. Let us start with some ostensibly very simple things: Primitive populations, for example, are of special interest since the influence of environmental factors on a certain genetic constitution can often be studied much more easily than in populations living under more "advanced" conditions. Moreover, new disease patterns, a consequence of changing living conditions, may help for a better understanding of gene-environment interactions even in populations of industrial countries. Anomalies of glucose metabolism and diabetes are good examples (see the contributions by Kirk et al., Ch. 6; and by Szathmary, Ch. 9). Often, however, genetic analysis in primitive populations meets with special difficulties; in some Amerindians, for example, it is difficult simply to establish pedigrees (Szathmary, Ch. 9). Moreover, longitudinal studies (as performed in classical epidemiological work on risk factors such as the Framingham study) would often be required (Ward, Ch. 7) whereas only cross-sectional surveys are feasible technically. Important environmental parameters, such as malnutrition (Haas and Greska, Ch. 11) need a more precise definition. Even problems that, at first glance, seem to have been solved in the first period of genetic epidemiology during the 1940's and 50's, such as estimation of relative fitness of various genotypes, need a fresh look (Adams and Smouse, Ch. 12). We cannot hope first to develop a perfect arsenal of methods and, then, to apply these methods to our epidemiological problems. Rather, refinement of methods goes hand in hand with their actual application. There are few if any prescriptions in the literature on a "standard methodology" for such studies. Almost each situation requires a research design of its own. Before such a design is developed, it is always a good idea to read as many research reports of experienced investigators as possible.

What is true for the seemingly simple cases mentioned above, applies still more for the complex problems posed by "multifactorial diseases", where quantitative genetic models are necessary for analysis (Smalley et al., Ch. 4), or where the multipoint linkage approach using genetic markers or DNA polymorphisms opens up, at least in principle, a new way to analysis of genetic heterogeneity (Lathrop and Lalouel, Ch. 5). To evaluate critically the scientific merits of an epidemiological study, we should check it, beginning with the basic steps (ascertainment of diseased and healthy subjects; reliability of pedigree information; collection of the basic data; criteria for medical diagnosis) to the final statistical analysis. As a rule, negligence in careful data collection is much more common and leads to devastating results more often than inadequate statistics.

MONOGENIC AND CHROMOSOMAL DISEASES

As mentioned, the first phase of genetic epidemiology was concerned mainly with monogenic diseases; when methods of chromosome analysis had been introduced during the late 1950's and 1960's, "population cytogenetics" of chromosomal aberrations added another important aspect (Court Brown, 1967). The advantage of working with these diseases is the (at least in principle) clear-cut definition of basic data. Looking at incidences in various populations, we can be reasonably sure that identical phenomena are compared. Whatever inferences are drawn, for example, on genetic risks due to mutagenic agents such as ionizing radiation, we are on relatively safe ground (see the UNSCEAR Report, 1982; Vogel 1985). A thorough analysis of specific cases of natural selection has also been possible for some monogenic disorders (for details, see Vogel and Motulsky, 1979). Here, the reader of the present volume will find especially interesting new data and considerations on our classical example of balancing selection, the sickle cell malaria case (Lefèvre-Witier, Ch. 16).

For example, do all sickle cell mutations go back to only one, or to several sources? Why is the clinical course of the same disease so different in various populations? What are the special conditions of malaria selection in the arid steppes of the Sahel?

Another, probably monogenic and possibly autosomal recessive disease is the type of hypoacusia on the island of St. Barthélemy that is being investigated by Mayer et al. (Ch. 10). This is a "classical" isolate study; the genealogies have been traced back to the founder generation. The study promises more precise characterization of a possibly new type of inherited hypoacusia and deafness. It demonstrates the usefulness of isolate studies in medical genetics.

MULTIFACTORIAL DISEASES

Most contributions, however, are concerned with the so-called "multifactorial diseases". Here, problems are much more complex at all levels and a combination of various strategies is required to elucidate the genetic basis, and to analyze the all-pervading heterogeneity (see, for example, Sing et al., Ch. 3). Analysis may proceed "from top to bottom", i.e. it may start from a complex phenotype and try to analyze its components. Or it may proceed "from bottom up", by first identifying one or several basic components and then, finding out how these components interact to produce a phenotype. Examples from the first approach are the studies of Rothhammer et al (Ch. 14) and Basu et al. (Ch. 15) on the effects of living in high altitudes on risks, for example, for circulatory diseases or mortality. New methods, such as calculation of "model-free" risk figures (Chakraborty, Ch. 2), belong into this category. Here, it is always good to remember that heritability estimates, so commonly used in quantitative genetics, only apply to the specific population for which they have been estimated (Roberts, Ch. 1). The same holds true for empiric risk figures for "multifactorial" diseases and birth defects: The predominating genetic components of the same or a very similar phenotype might be quite different in different populations.

This has been demonstrated, for example, by Roberts (Ch. 1) using both analytical approaches "from bottom up" and "from top to bottom". Earlier studies had shown an association of a special HLA-type, B7, with multiple sclerosis. In Roberts' Newcastle data, this association did not exist. Genetic analysis among populations of the Shetland and Orkney Islands showing the highest prevalence of multiple sclerosis gave evidence for a polygenic basis in combination with a strong environmental component; heritabilities were, however, quite different. Moreover, the relative significance of a specific genetic factor such as HLA-B7 within such a multifactorial system varies from one population to the next.

Another example for an analysis "from bottom to top" is diabetes. Various approaches in the last decade from "classical" twin studies (Tattersall and Pyke, 1972) to analysis of genetic variation in the insulin molecule, and insulin receptors (see Vogel, 1982; Rüdiger and Dryer, 1983) have done much to solve the riddles posed by the group of diabetic phenotypes that had made diabetes before the "nightmare of medical geneticists" (Neel et al., 1965). The present volume contributes interesting aspects to this analysis. The Kirk group, for example, presents evidence that the well known association of type I diabetes with HLA-D3 and D4 (see Dausset and Svejgaard, 1977) is not the only contribution of a genetic polymorphism to disease liability (Kirk et al., Ch. 6). Among Polynesians, the Gc*1 allele of the vitamin D-binding protein is increased significantly in diabetics, and there is a consistent increase of the 6PGD*A allele in various populations. The studies of the Kirk group on diabetes are a good example, how "top to bottom" and "from bottom up" strategies may be combined in genetic analysis.

Type 2 diabetes and obesity are common in many Amerindian populations. There is now an increasing number of studies in which this problem is examined from various angles (see Szathmary, Ch. 9). One important "bottom up" approach is the study of blood glucose levels in normal populations. Here, the hypothesis of a bimodal distribution that would point to a major gene difference was refuted for the Dogrib

Indians of Northwestern Canada. But even if a bimodal distribution could be demonstrated for a continuously distributed physiological parameter such as blood glucose in diabetics and normals, this would not necessarily point to a major gene effect: "Pathological" variants of physiological parameters often show a tendency for self-enhancement: A high blood glucose level may put the B-cell system of the pancreas under stress; this may lead to a decrease of insulin production, and to a further increase of blood glucose etc. Such vicious circles are common in "multifactorial" diseases. Weiss (Ch. 8) presents evidence that such "phenotype amplifications" may cause, for example, the high prevalence of gallbladder cancer in New World peoples, where it is 3 to 6 times as common as in the rest of the U.S. population. This is largely a post-war phenomenon. It is known that cholesterol gallstones are a common precursor of gallstone cancer. Gallstones, however, are very common among Amerindians; they appear to be part of the New World "syndrome" which also includes obesity and type 2 diabetes. This syndrome is apparently the reaction of special genotypes to the "unnatural" living conditions of the recent past: More food, especially more calorie-rich carbohydrates and fat; less motoric activity, for example.

Similar self-amplifying mechanisms are very probably common in other "multifactorial diseases, for example in hypertension and its complications. High blood pressure damages the walls of arteries; this damage, by reducing elasticity, leads to still higher blood pressure, etc. Such pathogenetic mechanisms will be elucidated only when the research workers are acquainted equally well with principles of genetic analysis and with pathophysiology of the disease they want to analyze.

FUTURE PROSPECTS

The foregoing considerations are a small (and, admittedly, subjective) selection of those stimulated by reading the contributions in this volume. Scientifically, genetic epidemiology is a fascinating field that offers many tricky problems for the analytically minded scientist. Moreover, it is important practically for many reasons, only a few of which will be mentioned in the following:

(1) Prediction of the amount of genetic damage due to mutagenic agents;

(2) component analysis of genetic and environmental factors influencing susceptibility to etiologically complex disease;

(3) influence of cultural and economical changes on such disease liabilities in relation to the genetic background;

(4) calculating appropriate genetic risk figures for genetic counseling;

(5) planning of population screening programs for prevention of genetic damage;

and many others. However, an appropriate development of genetic epidemiology meets with a number of difficulties. Some of them come from the society at large, but others have their roots within the scientific community of human geneticists themselves. Difficulties from the society at large are caused by an increasing sensitivity of most populations against being used as "guinea pigs" for research programs. This leads, for example, to more and more prohibitive rules for protection of individual data. If this development continues, it may become disastrous for many studies in genetic epidemiology. It is possible that anonymous data may be of limited use in some problems, for example, in cancer genetics. They are certainly useless in genetic epidemiology where precision usually depends on diagnosis and physiological parameters in a complete set of family members that must be checked and rechecked by personal examination. In the past, some scientists may not have used personal data with due restraint; to gain confidence in the society at large, we should strictly keep to these rules. But we should also try to convince the societies in which we are living that epidemiological research is performed for the common benefit, and that overemphasizing individual rights and sensitivities may cause severe harm for all of us. However, some difficulties for the development of genetic epidemiology are intrinsic; they are rooted within our scientific community. Scientific development in human genetics has been dominated in recent years by almost incredible advances in the analysis of the human genome. Entirely new paths have been opened by introduction of methods from molecular biology. It is only understandable that the great majority of young, creative and ambitious scientists feel attracted by the bright prospect of relatively fast and conspicuous success in this field. Epidemiological research on diseases, on the other hand, is usually time-consuming; success even of brilliantly designed and carefully performed work is usually much less glamorous. Such problems often attract scientists who like and are gifted for solving mathematical problems, and playing with sophisticated mathematical models. However, these scientists have a tendency to overrate the analytical power of their methods, underestimating at the same time the problems involved in simple data collection and diagnosis, and in pathophysiology of the diseases to be analyzed. The skills of these mathematically minded scientists are urgently needed; but they should be prevented from going wild. They should be checked by critical "practitioners", who have a sound medical and pathophysiological background, and know from experience the down-to-earth problems of data collection and assessment. At present, there are much too few such practitioners, especially in the younger generation of scientists, and those who get interested in epidemiology are in danger of being overawed by their counterparts, the mathematicians. They should realize that formal sophistication is often combined with an incredible naivety in setting up the basic assumptions, and that it is their task to control this.

It is a big advantage of this volume that these possible shortcomings have largely been avoided. Therefore, it may document an important step toward a sound genetic epidemiology.

LITERATURE CITED

Court Brown WM (1967). "Human Population Cytogenetics." Amsterdam: North Holland.
Daussett J, Svejgaard A (eds) (1977). "HLA and Disease." Copenhagen: Munksgaard.
Doll R, Peto R (1981). The causes of cancer:

Quantitative estimates of avoidable risks of cancer in the United States today. J Nat'l Cancer Inst 66:1192.
Kimura M (1983). "The Natural Theory of Molecular Evolution." Cambridge: Cambridge University Press.
Morton NE (1982). "Outline of Genetic Epidemiology." New York: Academic Press.
Morton NE, Chung CS (eds) (1978). "Genetic Epidemiology." New York: Academic Press.
Murphy EA (1981). Only authorized persons admitted: The quantitative genetics of health and disease. Johns Hopkins Med J 148:114.
Neel JV, Fajans SS, Conn JW, Davidenson RT (1965). Diabetes mellitus. In: Neel JV, Shaw MW, Schull WJ (eds): "Genetics and the Epidemiology of Chronic Disease." Washington, D.C.: Gov't Printing Office, p 105.
Rüdiger HW, Dreyer M (1983). Pathogenetic mechanisms of hereditary diabetes mellitus. Hum Genet 63:100.
Tatersall RB, Pyke DA (1972). Diabetes in identical twins. Lancet ii:1120.
United Nations Sources and Biological Effects of Ionizing Radiation (1982). United Nations Scientific Committee on the Effects of Atomic Radiation, 1982 Report to the General Assembly, with annexes. New York: United Nations Publications No. E82.IX.8.
Vogel F (1982). Die bedeutung der humangenetik für eine theorie der Krankheit. Verh Dtsch Ges Path 66:1.
Vogel F (1985). Gesichertes und hypothetisches im bereich der strahlengenetik. In Leppin W, Meißner J, Börner W, Messerschmidt (eds): "Die Hypothesen im Strahlenschutz," Stuttgart: Thieme, p 144.
Vogel F, Helmbold W (1972). Blutgruppen - Populationsgenetik und statistik. In Becker PE (ed): "Humangentik - ein Kurzes Handbuch," Vol I/4, Stuttgart: Thieme, p 129.
Vogel F, Motulsky AG (1979). "Human Genetics - Problems and Approaches." Heidelberg: Springer.
Vogel F, Rathenberg R (1975). Spontaneous mutation in man. Adv Hum Genet 5:223.
Williams RJ (1956). "Biochemical individuality." New York: John Wiley & Sons.

Index